IAP MEC Textbook of
Medical Education Technology

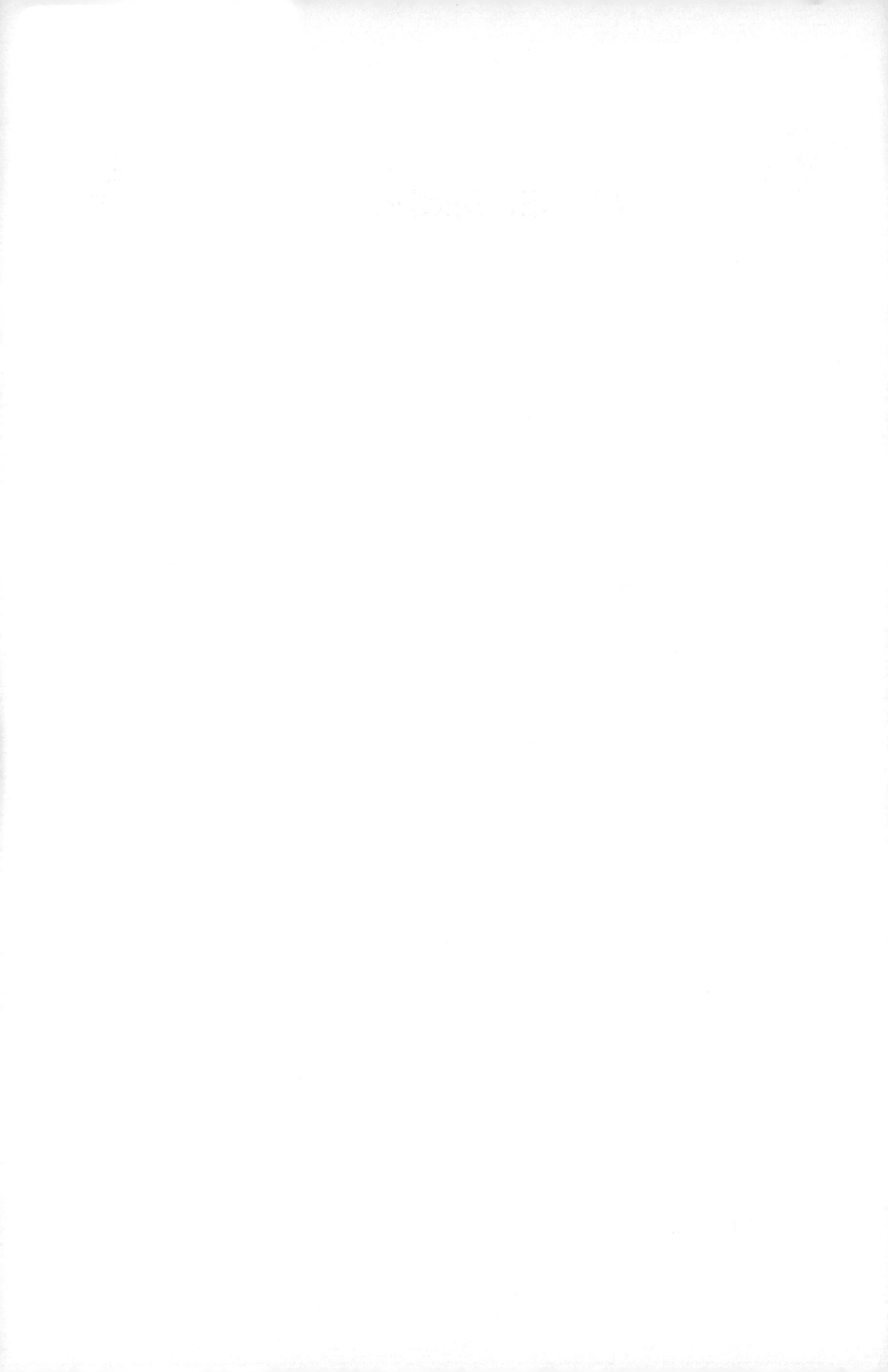

INDIAN ACADEMY OF PEDIATRICS ©

IAP MEC

MEDICAL EDUCATION CHAPTER

IAP MEC Textbook of
Medical Education Technology

Editor-in-Chief

Harish K Pemde

MD FIAP
Director Professor
Department of Pediatrics
Lady Hardinge Medical College
New Delhi, India

Editors

Pawankalyan Pinnamaneni

MD FACI FIAP Fellow in Pediatric Pulmonary and Sleep Medicine (AUS)
Professor Department of Pediatrics
Dr Pinnamaneni Siddhartha Institute of Medical Sciences and Research Foundation
China Avutapally, Andhra Pradesh, India

Vishnu Mohan PT

MBBS MD Fellowship in Neonatology PGDHM PGDMLS
Senior Consultant
Department of Neonatology
Aster Malabar Institute of Medical Sciences
Calicut, West Bengal, India

Ajay Gaur

MD PhD ACME FIAP FRCPCH (UK)
Professor and Head
Department of Pediatrics
GR Medical College
Gwalior, Madhya Pradesh, India

Forewords

Vasant M Khalatkar
Neelam Mohan
GV Basavaraja
Yogesh N Parikh
C Nirmala

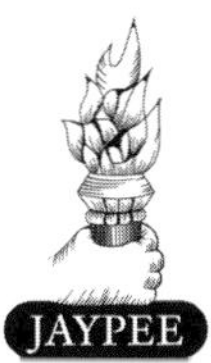

JAYPEE BROTHERS MEDICAL PUBLISHERS

The Health Sciences Publisher

New Delhi | London

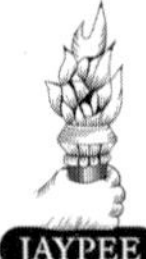

JAYPEE **Jaypee Brothers Medical Publishers (P) Ltd**

Headquarters
EMCA House, 23/23-B
Ansari Road, Daryaganj
New Delhi 110 002, India
Landline: +91-11-23272143, +91-11-23272703
+91-11-23282021, +91-11-23245672
e-mail: jaypee@jaypeebrothers.com

Corporate Office
4838/24, Ansari Road, Daryaganj
New Delhi 110 002, India
Phone: +91-11-43574357
Fax: +91-11-43574314
e-mail: jaypee@jaypeebrothers.com

Overseas Office
JP Medical Ltd.
83, Victoria Street, London
SW1H 0HW (UK)
Phone: +44-20 3170 8910
e-mail: info@jpmedpub.com

EU GPSR Authorised Representative
Logos Europe, 9 rue Nicolas Poussin
17000, La Rochelle, France
Phone: +33 (0) 6 67 93 73 78
e-mail: contact@logoseurope.eu

Website: www.jaypeebrothers.com
Website: www.jaypeedigital.com

Inquiries for bulk sales may be solicited at: jaypee@jaypeebrothers.com

IAP MEC Textbook of Medical Education Technology

First Edition: **2026**

ISBN: 978-93-7545-718-3

Printed at: Samrat Offset Pvt. Ltd.

IAP MEC Executive Board

Contributors

Aarushee Jhunjhunwala
Medical Student
Datta Meghe Medical College
Nagpur, Maharashtra, India

Abhishek Ramesh Jain MD (Pediatrics)
Assistant Professor
Department of Pediatrics
Government Medical College
Chhatrapati Sambhaji Nagar, Maharashtra, India

Ajay Gaur MD PhD ACME FIAP FRCPCH (UK)
Professor and Head
Department of Pediatrics
GR Medical College
Gwalior, Madhya Pradesh, India

Akash Bang
MD DNB MNAMS PGDMLS IDPCCM
Professor
Department of Pediatrics
All India Institute of Medical Sciences
Nagpur, Maharashtra, India

Anant Khot MD ACME
Additional Professor
Department of Pharmacology
All India Institute of Medical Sciences
Nagpur, Maharashtra, India

Aniket Sarwade MD
Assistant Professor
Department of Pediatrics
Government Medical College and Hospital
Chhatrapati Sambhaji Nagar, Maharashtra, India

Anil Gurtoo MD (Medicine)
Head
Department of Medicine
Sitaram Bharatia Institute
New Delhi, India
Formerly Vice Principal, and Coordinator Medical Education Unit, Lady Hardinge Medical College
New Delhi

Anurag Tomar MBBS MD (Pediatrics)
Professor, Pediatrics; Director, NIMS University Pediatrics
National Institute of Medical Science and Research, NIMS University
Jaipur, Rajasthan, India

Archana Dhok MBBS MD M-Phil (HPE)
Professor and Head
Department of Biochemistry
Jawaharlal Nehru Medical College, DMIHER (DU)
Wardha, Maharashtra, India

Archana Malik MD (Pulmonary Medicine)
Associate Professor and Head
Department of Pulmonary Medicine
All India Institute of Medical Sciences
Deoghar, Jharkhand, India

Arunita Tushar Jagzape
MD (Physiology) PhD (Physiology) MPhil in Health Professions Education, GSMC–FAIMER
Professor
Department of Physiology
All India Institute of Medical Sciences
Raipur, Chhattisgarh, India

Aswathy Rajan MD (Pediatrics)
Associate Professor
Department of Pediatrics
AJ Institute of Medical Sciences and Research
Mangaluru, Karnataka, India

Chandra Mohan Kumar
MD (Pediatrics) MAMS FIAP
Professor and Head
Department of Pediatrics
All India Institute of Medical Sciences
Patna, Bihar, India

Deepti Thandaveshwara
MBBS MD Fellowship in Neonatology
Assistant Professor
Department of Pediatrics
JSS Medical College, JSS Academy of Higher Education and Research
Mysore, Karnataka, India

Ghanshyam Das MD (Pediatrics)
Professor
Department of Pediatrics
Gajra Raja Medical College
Gwalior, Madhya Pradesh, India

Ghanshyam N Ahir MD (Community Medicine)
Associate Professor and In-charge Head
Department of Community Medicine (PSM)
Government Medical College
Bhavnagar, Gujarat, India

Girish Chandra Baniya
MBBS MD (Psychiatry) FIPS ACME
Associate Professor and Head
Department of Psychiatry
Government Medical College
Barmer, Rajasthan, India

Harish K Pemde MD FIAP
Director Professor
Department of Pediatrics
Lady Hardinge Medical College
New Delhi, India

Joseph John MD (Ped) DNB (Ped)
Professor
Department of Pediatrics
All India Institute of Medical Sciences
Bhubaneswar, Odisha, India

Kush D Jhunjhunwala MD
Professor of Pediatrics
Datta Meghe Medical College
Nagpur, Maharashtra, India

Latha Ravichandran
MBBS DCH DNB (Pediatric Medicine) FAIMER Fellow, International Fellowship in Medical Education (USA)
Master's in Health Professions Education
Dean – Education and Professor
Sri Ramachandra Institute of Higher Education and Research
Chennai, Tamil Nadu, India

Madhulika Monga MD (Physiology)
Direct and Professor
Department of Physiology
Lady Hardinge Medical College
New Delhi, India
Co-coordinator, Medical Education Unit, Lady Hardinge Medical College, New Delhi

Meenal Batta MD
Department of Physiology and Pediatrics
Guru Gobind Singh Medical College
Faridkot, Punjab, India

Nilofer Mujawar MD (Pediatrics) PGDN
Department of Pediatrics
NKP Salve Institute of Medical Sciences
Nagpur, Maharashtra, India

Pawankalyan Pinnamaneni
MD FACI FIAP Fellow in Pediatric Pulmonary and Sleep Medicine (AUS)
Professor
Department of Pediatrics
Dr Pinnamaneni Siddhartha Institute of Medical Sciences and Research Foundation
China Avutapally, Andhra Pradesh, India

Prabha B Khaire (More) MD (Pediatrics)
Professor and Head
Department of Pediatrics
Government Medical College
Chhatrapati Sambhaji Nagar, Maharashtra, India
Member, BOS medicine and allied MUHS Nashik

Prashanth SN MBBS MD DNB (Pediatrics)
Professor and Head
Department of Pediatrics
JSS Medical College, JSS Academy of
Higher Education and Research
Mysuru, Karnataka, India

Praveen Singh
MBBS PhD FAIMER Fellow
Professor of Anatomy and Medical Education
Convenor, NMC-Nodal Centre for MET
Department of Anatomy and Medical Education
Convenor, NMC-Nodal Centre for MET
Pramukhswami Medical College
Karamsad, Gujarat, India

Priyanka Gupta
MD ACME PSG-FRI FAIMER Fellow
Professor
Department of Pediatrics
ESIC Medical College and Hospital
Faridabad, Haryana, India

Puja Dulloo
MBBS MD (Physiology) MHPE (Keele University, UK)
FAIMER Fellow PGDHHM ACME
Professor and Head
Department of Physiology
Parul Institute of Medical Sciences and Research
Vadodara, Gujarat, India

Ravi Ambey MD (Pediatrics)
Professor
Department of Pediatrics
Gajra Raja Medical College
Gwalior, Madhya Pradesh, India

Richa Ambey DCH
Medical Officer
Department of Pediatrics
Gajra Raja Medical College
Gwalior, Madhya Pradesh, India

Richie Dalai MD (Pediatrics) DM (Neonatology)
Assistant Professor
Department of Neonatology
All India Institute of Medical Sciences
Patna, Bihar, India

Roosy Aulakh MD (Pediatrics) MBA (HHSM)
Professor
Department of Pediatrics
Government Medical College and Hospital
Chandigarh, India

Sagar V MD
Senior Resident
Shri Atal Bihari Vajpayee Medical College
and Research Institution
Bengaluru, Karnataka, India

Sahil Saini MD (Pediatrics)
Senior Resident
Department of Pediatrics
Gajra Raja Medical College
Gwalior, Madhya Pradesh, India

Sandeep Shrivastava MBBS MS DNB ACME PhD
Director Professor
Department of Orthopedics
Jawaharlal Nehru Medical College, DMIHER (DU)
Wardha, Maharashtra, India

Sanghamitra Ray MBBS MD (Pediatrics) MNAMS
Assistant Professor Pediatrics
Department of Pediatrics
Vardhman Mahavir Medical College and
Safdarjung Hospital
New Delhi, India

Sanjiv Lewin MD DNB MBA (HHSM)
Professor and Pediatrician
Family Medicine, Pediatrics, Clinical Ethics
and Medical Education
St. John's Medical College and Hospital
Bengaluru, Karnataka, India

Santosh T Soans MD DCH FIAP FRCPCH (UK)
Professor and Head
Department of Pediatrics
AJ Institute of Medical Sciences and Research
Mangaluru, Karnataka, India

Sara Dhanawade MD (Pediatrics)
Professor of Pediatrics and Medical Superintendent
Department of Pediatrics
Bharati Vidyapeeth (Deemed to be University)
Medical College & Hospital
Sangli, Maharashtra, India

Saroj Kumar Tripathy MD (Pediatrics)
Associate Professor
Department of Pediatrics
All India Institute of Medical Sciences
Deoghar, Jharkhand, India

Sarthak Das MD (Pediatrics)
Professor and Head
Department of Pediatrics
All India Institute of Medical Sciences
Deoghar, Jharkhand, India

Satvik Bansal
MBBS (Gold Medalist) MD Fellowship (Neonatology)-University of Oxford UK Fellowship (Neonatology)-Indian Academy of Pediatrics
Associate Professor
GR Medical College
Gwalior, Madhya Pradesh, India

Sharmila Banerjee Mukherjee
MD (Pediatrics)
Director Professor (Pediatrics)
Lady Hardinge Medical College
New Delhi, India

Shashi Kant Dhir MD
Department of Physiology and Pediatrics
Guru Gobind Singh Medical College
Faridkot, Punjab, India

Shilpa KL MD
Associate Professor
Bangalore Medical College and Research Institute
Bengaluru, Karnataka, India

Shipra Jain MBBS MD ACME
Professor
Department of Pharmacology
Mahatma Gandhi Medical College and Hospital
Jaipur, Rajasthan, India

Shivaprakash Sosale C MD
Associate Professor
Bangalore Medical College and
Research Institute
Bengaluru, Karnataka, India

Somashekhar Nimbalkar MD (Pediatrics)
Professor of Neonatology
Department of Neonatology
Pramukhswami Medical College
Anand, Gujarat, India

Sonali Suresh Purhe MD (Pediatrics)
Assistant Professor
Department of Pediatrics
Government Medical College
Chhatrapati Sambhaji Nagar, Maharashtra, India

Suman Singh
MBBS MD (Microbiology) PhD (Microbiology) Advance Course in Medical Education
Professor
Department of Microbiology
Pramukhswami Medical College
Anand, Gujarat, India

Swarna Rekha Bhat MD (Pediatrics)
Former Professor
Department of Pediatrics and Neonatology
St John's Medical College
Bengaluru, Karnataka, India

Tushar Bharat Jagzape
MD (Pediatrics) MPhil in Health Professions Education, GSMC–FAIMER Diploma in Allergy and Asthma (CMC)
Professor
Department of Pediatrics
All India Institute of Medical Sciences
Raipur, Chhattisgarh, India

Vikram Bhaskar
MD (Pediatrics) FACEE (Peds Emergency)
Associate Professor
Department of Pediatrics
University College of Medical Sciences
New Delhi, India

Vinod H Ratageri MD DCEH
Professor and Head
Department of Pediatrics
Karnataka Medical College and
Research Institute
Hubli, Karnataka, India

Vishnu Mohan PT MBBS MD Fellowship in
Neonatology PGDHM PGDMLS
Senior Consultant
Department of Neonatology
Aster Malabar Institute of Medical Sciences
Calicut, West Bengal, India

Foreword

It is a privilege to write the Foreword for the *IAP MEC Textbook of Medical Education Technology,* a resource designed for all medical teachers and aspiring teachers, while retaining special relevance for pediatricians associated with the Indian Academy of Pediatrics. In a rapidly changing academic and clinical environment, medical colleges and training programs need teachers who are not only clinically competent but also educationally skilled, reflective, and future-ready.

The organization of this textbook reflects that vision. The initial section lays the foundations by addressing the landscape of medical education in the country, curriculum and syllabus design, competency-based medical education, the role of Medical Education Units, group dynamics, and systems approach, which are applicable across disciplines and institutions. The subsequent Teaching and Learning section covers core teaching skills and methods for undergraduate and postgraduate learners, large and small group teaching, aligning competencies with teaching–learning methods, understanding learner needs, microplanning of sessions, self-directed learning, and progression across learning domains.

A robust set of chapters on assessment provides practical guidance on principles and methods of assessment of knowledge and clinical skills, question paper setting, assessment of professionalism and ethics, workplace-based and community-based assessment, assessment for and of learning, selection processes, and internal assessment. These topics are central to any modern competency-based curriculum and will support departments in designing fair, transparent, and educationally sound examinations and workplace assessments.

The final section brings together several contemporary and emerging themes that are particularly important for those involved in IAP training activities and other faculty development programs: online teaching–learning and assessment, faculty development, mentor–mentee and doctor–student programs, educational feedback, reflection writing, educational networks, scholarship and publications, simulation-based education, and teaching of evidence-based medicine. Inclusion of a dedicated chapter on the use of artificial intelligence in medical education is especially timely, given the rapidly expanding role of AI in personalized learning, assessment, simulation, and academic productivity.

This book will be useful not only to pediatricians but also to medical teachers in all specialties, participants of IAP and national faculty development programs, and colleagues who undertake training, workshops, and teaching assignments under the banner of the Academy. The editors and authors are to be commended for producing a concise, practical, and context-relevant resource that will strengthen the educational capabilities of faculty and support better learning experiences for our students.

We warmly congratulate the editorial team and recommend this textbook to all who are committed to improving the quality of medical teaching and training in India.

Vasant M Khalatkar
President (2025)

Neelam Mohan
President (2026)

BV Basavraja
President (2024)

Yogesh N Parikh
Honorary Secretary General (2024–25)
Indian Academy of Pediatrics

C Nirmala
Chairperson
IAP Medical Education Chapter (2025)

Preface

IAP MEC Textbook of Medical Education Technology has been conceived as a practical and India-centric resource for all medical teachers and aspiring teachers—across all clinical and preclinical disciplines—while drawing on the rich experience of pediatric educators and the ongoing educational initiatives of the Indian Academy of Pediatrics. The book is intended for faculty members, residents with an interest in teaching, and colleagues who participate in or conduct training programs, workshops, and other educational assignments under IAP and similar platforms.

The first section introduces the broader context of medical education in the country, including curriculum and syllabus, competency-based medical education, the role of the Medical Education Unit, group dynamics, and systems approach. These chapters aim to give readers a conceptual framework that can be applied in any discipline, enabling them to understand why educational reforms are needed and how institutional structures can support them.

The "Teaching and Learning" section focuses on day-to-day educational practice: teaching–learning methods for undergraduate and postgraduate students, core teaching skills, large and small group teaching, matching competencies with methods, assessing learner needs, microplanning of sessions, promoting self-directed learning, and facilitating progression across cognitive, psychomotor, and affective domains. Each chapter seeks to bridge theory and practice, offering strategies that can be implemented in typical Indian medical college settings with real-world constraints.

The "Assessment" section consolidates essential knowledge and skills for designing and implementing meaningful assessments, including principles of assessment, tools for assessing knowledge and clinical skills, question paper setting, assessment of professionalism and ethics, workplace-based and community-based assessments, assessment for and of learning, selection processes, and internal assessment. The goal is to help teachers to move beyond routine examinations to a more holistic and competency-oriented view of assessment that supports learning.

The final section addresses thematic areas that are increasingly central to educational practice and faculty development: online teaching–learning and assessment, faculty development programs, doctor–student and mentor–mentee relationships, educational feedback, reflection writing, educational networks and growth, scholarship and publications, simulation-based education, and evidence-based medicine and its teaching. A dedicated chapter on artificial intelligence (AI) in medical education explores opportunities and cautions in using AI for personalized learning, simulation, assessment, and educational administration, recognizing that AI will increasingly shape how teachers and learners work.

This textbook is designed to support those who attend or conduct IAP training activities, such as conferences, workshops, and faculty development programs, by providing a common conceptual language and a set of practical tools that can be adapted to local needs. The editors are deeply grateful to the Indian Academy of Pediatrics, all contributors and reviewers, and the many learners and colleagues whose questions and feedback inspired these chapters. Any limitations remain the responsibility of the editors, and constructive suggestions for future editions will be received with appreciation.

On behalf of all editorial board members,

Harish K Pemde
Pawankalyan Pinnamaneni
Vishnu Mohan PT
Ajay Gaur
Editors of IAP MEC Textbook of Medical Education Technology

Acknowledgments

Grateful acknowledgment is first due to the Indian Academy of Pediatrics (IAP) and the IAP Medical Education Chapter for their vision, encouragement, and unwavering support in conceiving and nurturing this textbook on medical education technology. Special thanks are also extended to the Executive Boards of IAP and of the IAP Chapter on Medical Education for the years 2024 and 2025 for their continued trust, guidance, and endorsement of this initiative.

Heartfelt gratitude is extended to the distinguished members of the Editorial Board and contributors whose expertise and commitment have significantly enriched this textbook. Their thoughtful inputs, critical appraisal, and encouragement have been invaluable throughout the conceptualization and development of this work.

Special thanks are due to Prof Dr GV Basavaraja, Dr Vasant Khalatkar, Dr Neelam Mohan, Prof Dr Yogesh Parikh, Dr Atanu Bhadra, Dr Santosh Soans, Dr Sanjay Lalwani, Dr Somashekhar Nimbalkar, Dr C Nirmala, Dr M Singaravelu, Dr Pawankalyan Pinnamaneni, Dr Vishnu Mohan PT, Dr Ajay Gaur, Dr Anurag Tomar, Dr Tushar Bharat Jagzape, Dr Roosy Aulakh, Dr Guduru Vijay Kumar, Dr Sanjiv Lewin, Dr Latha Ravichandran, and Dr Vinod H Ratageri for their constructive feedback and academic support. Their collective experience in medical education has helped to refine the content to meet the needs of learners and teachers alike.

Grateful acknowledgment is also made to Dr Pravin Singh, Dr Puja Dullo, Dr Ghanshyam Ahir, Dr Shipra Jain, and Dr Sandeep Shrivastava for their valuable guidance, collaboration, and support during various stages of this project. Their dedication and professional camaraderie have played a crucial role in bringing this textbook to fruition.

Finally, sincere thanks are due to Shri Jitendar P Vij (Group Chairman), Mr Ankit Vij (Managing Director), Mr MS Mani (Group President), Ms Pooja Bhandari [Director–Production (Books and Journals)], Mr Sabyasachi Hazra (Director—PG and PNR Content), Mr Akhilesh Saxena (Development Editor), and the team of M/s Jaypee Brothers Medical Publishers (P) Ltd, New Delhi, for their professionalism, meticulous editorial and production support, and for transforming this manuscript into a high-quality academic resource for medical educators and learners. Their behind-the-scenes efforts are deeply appreciated.

Harish K Pemde
Editor-in-Chief
IAP MEC Textbook of Medical Education Technology

Contents

SECTION 1: Introduction

SECTION 2: Teaching and Learning

SECTION

1 Introduction

CHAPTER 1

Medical Education in India

Pawankalyan Pinnamaneni

INTRODUCTION

Medical education in India possesses a deep-rooted history characterized by significant transformations that reflect the evolving healthcare requirements of its diverse population. The transition from traditional healing systems to modern medical education represents a complex interplay of socio-political and cultural elements intrinsic to the nation. This chapter delves into the structural intricacies, prevailing challenges, and progressive advancements in medical education across India, offering a comprehensive analysis of its influence on healthcare delivery.

HISTORICAL OVERVIEW

Traditional Systems of Medicine

India's medical landscape is enriched by a formidable legacy of various traditional systems, particularly Ayurveda, Unani, and Siddha. These practices have been integral to the holistic approach to health and wellness for centuries. Ayurveda, the most prominent among them, emphasizes the restoration of balance within the body through the use of natural remedies derived from plants, minerals, and animal products. This system not only addresses physical ailments but also takes into account mental and spiritual well-being, a perspective that profoundly influences health practices in contemporary India.[1]

Colonial Influence

The advent of British colonial rule fundamentally altered India's medical education framework. The establishment of the Calcutta Medical College in 1835 marked a significant turning point, heralding the introduction of formal Western medical training in the country. This institution laid the groundwork for a structured curriculum that mirrored the Western educational model, which has been instrumental in shaping the current landscape of medical education in India. The colonial era ushered in a new paradigm, setting standards and benchmarks that still resonate within the medical education system today.[2,3]

CURRENT STRUCTURE OF MEDICAL EDUCATION

Undergraduate Medical Education

In India, the standard pathway to becoming a physician is through the Bachelor of Medicine and Bachelor of Surgery (MBBS) degree. This rigorous program spans a total of 5.5 years, including a mandatory 1-year rotating internship that provides practical exposure across various departments. The curriculum for the MBBS program was comprehensively formulated by the National Medical Commission (NMC), which succeeded the Medical Council of India (MCI) in 2019, with the intention of modernizing and standardizing medical education across the nation.[4]

Curriculum: The MBBS curriculum integrates a broad spectrum of theoretical and practical subjects that are essential for aspiring medical professionals. Fundamental areas of study encompass anatomy, physiology, biochemistry, pharmacology, microbiology, and community medicine, which foster a well-rounded medical education. The NMC's recent reforms in 2020 put a lot of emphasis on an integrated approach to teaching. This helps students to get more clinical experience early on, which improves their learning and makes them better prepared for working as a doctor in the real world.[4]

Entrance examinations: Gaining admission to MBBS programs is an intensely competitive process driven by the National Eligibility-cum-Entrance Test (NEET). This nationwide examination is the primary means through which students secure placements in undergraduate medical schools, and it is an essential milestone for aspiring doctors.[5]

Postgraduate Medical Education

Postgraduate medical education in India offers a diverse range of specialties and subspecialties, which are crucial for developing expertise in specific areas of medicine. The predominantly sought-after qualifications in this domain include the Doctor of Medicine (MD) and Master of Surgery (MS) degrees, which serve as essential credentials for healthcare professionals aiming to attain advanced training in their respective fields.[5]

Specialization: The rising complexity and demands of modern healthcare necessitate a higher degree of specialization among medical practitioners. In response to this need, the NMC has initiated substantial reforms to enhance the quality of postgraduate training through the adoption of competency-based medical education (CBME). This new way of teaching focuses on developing the basic skills needed for independent practice in various fields, such as pediatrics, obstetrics, gynecology, internal medicine, and general surgery.[5]

Fellowship programs: Besides MD and MS degrees, fellowship programs provide advanced training opportunities that allow medical professionals to further hone their subspecialty skills. Typically lasting 1–3 years, these programs offer in-depth clinical training alongside research experience in cardiology, endocrinology, and neurology. The increasing prevalence of fellowship programs underscores the growing need for specialized healthcare providers in India.[5]

Alternative Medical Education

Besides conventional allopathic medicine, India is also home to a diverse array of alternative medical education systems, prominently featuring Ayurveda, Unani, Siddha, and Homeopathy. These traditional healing practices are regulated by the Central Council of Indian Medicine (CCIM) and the Central Council of Homeopathy (CCH), which oversee the educational standards and professional development of practitioners. Students can pursue undergraduate and postgraduate degrees in these fields, enhancing the richness and diversity of India's healthcare system. This multiplicity of medical education pathways not only fosters a more inclusive approach to health care but also lays the groundwork for a holistic understanding of health and wellness in the country.[5]

CHALLENGES IN MEDICAL EDUCATION: AN IN-DEPTH ANALYSIS

Despite the continuous advancements and innovations in medical education, there are several significant challenges that continue to impact the effectiveness and quality of training for future healthcare professionals.[6]

Quality of Education

The overall quality of medical education can vary widely among institutions, leading to significant disparities in training outcomes. Certain medical colleges struggle with inadequate infrastructure, insufficient faculty recruitment and retention, and a curriculum that is not regularly updated to incorporate the latest medical knowledge and practices. The NMC has undertaken initiatives aimed at bridging these gaps, yet the variation in educational standards across different medical schools remains a pressing concern that warrants continued focus and improvement efforts.

Faculty Development

The growth and enhancement of medical faculty are crucial for delivering a comprehensive educational experience to students.[6] However, many institutions lack structured and effective faculty development programs that can equip educators with the skills and tools needed for high-impact teaching and mentoring. This deficiency can hinder faculty members' ability to foster an engaging learning environment, thereby impacting students' educational experiences and outcomes.

Assessment Methods

Conventional assessment techniques, particularly standardized written examinations, often fall short of accurately gauging students' clinical competencies and practical skills. As a result, there is an increasing push toward adopting competency-based assessment methods that not only evaluate theoretical knowledge but also assess students' hands-on abilities and decision-making skills in clinical settings. This shift is essential for ensuring that graduates emerge fully equipped with the requisite skills and knowledge to provide high-quality patient care.

Mental Health Concerns

The medical profession is precipitating a future where stress, anxiety, and burnout may become increasingly prevalent among medical students. The intense competition for placements, coupled with the demanding nature of medical education, is likely to exacerbate mental health challenges. As these future physicians navigate their training under significant pressure, there is a growing concern that untreated mental health issues could adversely impact their academic performance, professional development, and, ultimately, their ability to provide compassionate and effective patient care.

This multifaceted landscape underscores the urgent need for comprehensive strategies to address these persistent challenges in medical education, ensuring a well-rounded, supportive, and effective training environment for the next generation of healthcare providers.

INNOVATIONS AND REFORMS IN MEDICAL EDUCATION IN INDIA: A COMPREHENSIVE OVERVIEW

Numerous innovative practices and reform initiatives have been thoughtfully implemented in response to the various challenges facing medical education in India. These efforts aim to significantly enhance the quality of educational experiences and adapt to the rapidly changing landscape of healthcare.

Competency-based Medical Education

The shift toward CBME represents a pivotal development in the field of medical training. This groundbreaking approach emphasizes the acquisition of vital competencies, moving away from the traditional model that largely focuses on rote memorization of a fixed curriculum. The NMC has strongly advocated for CBME in undergraduate medical programs, underscoring the necessity for students to demonstrate their knowledge and skills through real-world clinical interactions. This essential transformation is designed to produce graduates who not only possess extensive medical knowledge but are also fully prepared to deliver high-quality patient care effectively and compassionately.[7]

Integrated Curriculum

The integrated curriculum is a holistic educational model that harmoniously combines basic sciences with clinical experiences. By interlinking theoretical knowledge with practical application, this innovative curriculum enables students to comprehend the real-world implications of their studies within clinical contexts. Medical institutions have enthusiastically adopted integrated teaching methodologies, fostering collaboration among various departments. This approach enriches the overall learning experience, ultimately cultivating a more connected and comprehensive understanding of medical practice among students.[7]

Technology-enhanced Learning

The infusion of technology into medical education has revolutionized conventional learning methodologies. The widespread use of e-learning platforms, virtual simulations, and a plethora of online resources has become indispensable in enriching classroom instruction. Medical students now have access to an expansive array of information, coupled with interactive learning experiences that include virtual patient simulations and engaging case-based discussions. These technological innovations not only foster higher levels of engagement but also create valuable opportunities for self-directed learning, empowering students to take charge of their educational journeys.[8,9]

Community-based Education

Community-based education emphasizes the crucial need for medical students to develop a genuine understanding of the diverse healthcare needs present within various populations. Students are increasingly encouraged to participate in community health initiatives and outreach programs that address local health challenges. This hands-on experience not only hones their clinical skills but also instills in them a profound sense of social responsibility and empathy. By engaging directly with communities, students can effectively bridge the gap between their medical training and the real healthcare needs they are likely to encounter in their careers, thereby fostering a healthier society as a whole.

Faculty Development Programs

Recognizing the pivotal role that educators play in molding the next generation of healthcare professionals, numerous medical institutions are prioritizing robust faculty development programs. These initiatives are specifically designed to enhance the teaching capabilities and pedagogical skills of medical faculty. Through comprehensive workshops, interactive seminars, and mentorship opportunities, educators are empowered with essential tools to deliver exceptional instruction. This investment in faculty development ultimately benefits students, producing a higher standard of medical education and training.

Focus on Mental Health and Well-being

In recent years, addressing mental health concerns among medical students has gained increasing recognition as a critical aspect of medical education. Institutions are actively setting up diverse support systems, including counseling services, peer support networks, and wellness programs, all intended to cultivate a nurturing environment that prioritizes mental well-being. These initiatives aim to equip students with the skills to effectively navigate the stressors associated with medical training. Additionally, the integration of mental health education into the curriculum is vital to prepare future healthcare providers to recognize and address mental health issues within their patient populations.

Interprofessional Education

Interprofessional education (IPE) represents a transformative approach that is rapidly gaining traction in medical education. This model facilitates collaborative training among healthcare students from various disciplines, including medicine, nursing, pharmacy, and allied health fields. By participating in joint training sessions, these students learn to appreciate each other's roles and develop essential teamwork and communication skills necessary for providing comprehensive patient care. Preparing future healthcare professionals to work effectively in multidisciplinary teams is crucial for improving overall patient's outcomes across the healthcare system.

Research Opportunities

Encouraging research engagement among medical students is essential for the progress of medical knowledge and the improvement of healthcare practices. Many educational institutions are now embedding research components within the medical curriculum, allowing students to participate actively in research projects, present their findings at conferences, and contribute meaningfully to the body of scientific literature. This involvement not only enhances students' critical thinking and analytical skills but also helps to cultivate a dynamic culture of inquiry, creativity, and innovation within medical education.

Overall, these reforms and innovations in medical education are crucial steps toward cultivating a more competent, empathetic, and skilled future healthcare workforce in India.

THE ROLE OF GOVERNMENT AND REGULATORY BODIES

The government and regulatory bodies play a crucial role in shaping the landscape of medical education in India, acting as guardians of quality and equity. The establishment of the NMC in 2019 represented a watershed moment in the regulatory architecture of medical education. The NMC is charged with the formulation of comprehensive policies, the establishment of rigorous standards for medical institutions, and the assurance of educational quality across the country. A key aim of the NMC is to implement reforms such as CBME, which focuses on developing practical skills that meet healthcare needs, along with promoting transparency in the admissions process. These initiatives are designed not just to enhance the quality of medical education but also to ensure that future healthcare professionals are equipped to navigate the complexities of modern medicine.[4]

ACCREDITATION AND QUALITY ASSURANCE

Accreditation serves as a cornerstone in the quest to maintain and elevate standards in medical education. The NMC has outlined a set of rigorous accreditation criteria for medical colleges, which emphasizes not only faculty qualifications and institutional infrastructure but also the quality of the curriculum and student performance outcomes. Continuous evaluations and audits are conducted to uphold accountability and inspire a culture of ongoing improvement within medical institutions, ensuring they adapt to emerging healthcare challenges.[4]

FUTURE DIRECTIONS

Addressing Healthcare Needs

The dynamic healthcare landscape in India necessitates a shift in medical education to effectively address emergent challenges. With the increasing prevalence of noncommunicable diseases (NCDs), escalating mental health issues, and an urgent call for preventive healthcare approaches, it is critical to realign medical training priorities. Future healthcare professionals must be adept at managing chronic illnesses, promoting health literacy, and engaging in community health advocacy to combat these pressing issues.

Emphasizing Rural Health

A significant portion of India's population resides in rural areas, often grappling with inadequate access to healthcare services. It is essential for medical education programs to target this disparity by prioritizing training focused on rural health issues. Incorporating hands-on initiatives, such as mandatory rural internships and immersive experiences in community health settings, will enable future physicians to understand and address the specific healthcare challenges faced by underserved populations. This approach can cultivate a healthcare workforce that is not only knowledgeable but also empathetic to the unique needs of rural communities.

Integration of Artificial Intelligence and Technology

The rapid advancements in technology, particularly in artificial intelligence (AI), are transforming the healthcare sector in unprecedented ways. To prepare students for this evolution, it is imperative to integrate AI and digital health technologies into the fabric of medical education. Training programs that encompass telemedicine, data analytics, and the ethical considerations surrounding AI will equip future healthcare providers with the skill set necessary to enhance diagnostic accuracy, improve treatment strategies, and ultimately elevate patient's care standards.

Lifelong Learning and Continuous Professional Development

In the fast-paced and ever-evolving field of medicine, maintaining a commitment to lifelong learning is invaluable. Medical education should cultivate a culture that encourages continuous professional development, motivating students to seek further education through workshops, specialized training, and active participation in research throughout their careers. This commitment ensures that healthcare professionals remain informed about the latest advancements, thus delivering the best possible care to patients.

Collaboration with Global Institutions

Forging partnerships with prestigious international medical institutions can substantially enhance the quality and scope of medical education in India. Such collaborations facilitate the exchange of knowledge, the sharing of faculty expertise, and access to resources that embody global best practices. Additionally, these partnerships provide students with invaluable opportunities for international exposure, transforming their educational experience and broadening their understanding of healthcare on a global scale.

CONCLUSION

The realm of medical education in India is at a critical juncture, filled with both formidable challenges and promising opportunities. The proactive reforms initiated by the NMC, alongside efforts from educational institutions, are working tirelessly to elevate the standards of training. By placing a strong emphasis on competency-based education, advancing mental health initiatives, integrating cutting-edge technology, and progressively addressing the diverse healthcare needs of our population, India is poised to nurture a remarkable new generation of healthcare professionals. Together, we have the potential to shape a brighter and more equitable future for healthcare in our nation!

REFERENCES

1. Ravishankar B, Shukla VJ. Indian systems of medicine: a brief profile. African J Traditional Complement Alternat Med. 2007;4(3):319-37.
2. Supe A. Evolution of medical education in India: The impact of colonialism. J Postgrad Med. 2016;62(4):255-9.
3. Robert M. Crafting British medicine in the Empire: the establishment of medical schools in India and Canada, 1763–1837. Med History. 2024;68(2):128-45.
4. NMC. (2019). Rules and Regulations, NMC | NMC [Internet]. Nmc.org.in. 2019. [online] Available from https://www.nmc.org.in/rules-regulations-nmc/ [Last accessed Jan., 2026].
5. Wikipedia. (2024). Medical education in India [Internet]. [online] Available from https://en.wikipedia.org/wiki/Medical_education_in_India [Last accessed Jan., 2026].
6. Supe A, Burdick WP. Challenges and issues in medical education in India. Acad Med. 2006;81(12):1076-80.
7. Kulkarni P, Pushpalatha K, Bhat D. Medical education in India: Past, present, and future. APIK J Internal Med. 2019;7(3):69-73.
8. Ruiz JG, Mintzer MJ, Leipzig RM. The impact of e-learning in medical education. Acad Med. 2006;81(3):207-12.
9. Dhir SK, Verma D, Batta M, et al. E-learning in medical education in India. Indian Pediatr. 2017;54:871-7.

CHAPTER 2

Curriculum and Syllabus

Sanjiv Lewin

INTRODUCTION

In this chapter, we introduce the concept of a curriculum as relevant to medical education while clarifying a syllabus.

Early efforts focused on creating systematic knowledge and texts for medical practices rather than medical education as documented in the ancient Egypt (*c1825 BC:* Kahun Gynecological Papyrus was divided into 34 sections dealt with specific problems, diagnosis, and nonsurgical treatments); ancient India works of Charaka and Sushruta (c 350 BC Charaka Acharya was a physician who edited the medical treatise entitled Charaka Samhita, one of the foundational texts of classical Indian medicine and Ayurveda; c 550 BC: Suśruta was an ancient Indian physician and surgeon, who made significant contributions to the field of plastic and cataract surgery and authored the Suśruta Saṃhitā); ancient Greece (c 250 BC: Hippocratic Corpus is a collection of 60 early medical works associated with Hippocrates that covered many diverse aspects of medicine, medical theories, and ethics); Islamic golden age (C850 AD: Hunayn ibn Ishaq's translations of medical literature); and Europe (c 850 AD: Schola Medica Salernitana was possibly the first medical school). It was finally by the Flexner Report of 1910, with key learnings of the need for clinical instruction through direct patient observation, the integration of scientific research into the curriculum and the establishment of university-affiliated medical schools with full-time faculty began to direct the need for curriculum development.[1]

WHAT IS CURRICULUM?

The word curriculum is derived from the Latin word *currere* which means "to run" and refers originally to a course as in a racecourse. An entire essay entitled "Etymologies, Epistemologies and The Emergence of Curriculum" elaborate on this aspect.[1] The plural are both curricula and curriculums that are considered correct.[2]

Many experts have different definitions for a curriculum, all focused on what happens in a medical education program as listed by Ganet J et al.[3] Prideaux stated that a curriculum is a document that represents the expression of educational ideas in practice.[4] It includes components that guide students, teachers, and educational institutes through a course of study. In the context of medical education, it is usually driven with purpose that reflects population (community) health needs and dependent on the professional roles and responsibilities of the healthcare professional that graduate from the course. The curriculum defines what is to be learnt, why it is required to be learnt, how it will be learnt, who will provide learning opportunities, when will this learning occur, and most importantly how will learning be assessed during the course. Harden defined a curriculum as "....a sophisticated blend of educational strategies, course content, learning outcomes, educational experiences, assessment, the educational environment and the individual students' learning style, personal timetable and program of work."[5] And Green defined it as "a planned educational experience that encompasses behavioral goals, instructional methods and actual experiences of the learners".[6]

Thomas and Kern's chosen definition of a curriculum is probably the simplest defined as a planned educational experience.[7]

WHAT IS A SYLLABUS?

Traditionally, a syllabus is a statement of contents to be taught and to be learnt in an education course.[4] It will be a predetermined specific listing of all within the domains of knowledge, psychomotor skills, and attitudes including communication skills, professional and ethical behaviors, etc. expected to be taught–learnt during a course. Hence, a syllabus is only a component of a curriculum that lists what is to be learnt.

EVOLUTION OF MEDICAL EDUCATION CURRICULUM

Soriano-Estrella describes the evolution of curriculums over time from an information-loaded to an outcome-driven medical education curriculum. This progression now includes defining competencies, entrustable professional activities (EPA), incorporating technology, and the need to recognize the wellbeing of students. This evolution reflects the explosion in medical science, changes in healthcare delivery and patient expectations, and improved understanding of effective learning.

Both competencies and EPAs support outcome-based education though they differ and are not alternatives. EPAs are performed, observed, and measured to decide if a physician student is trustworthy by supervisors. They describe work tasks to enable competencies into practice. The advances in technology in healthcare delivery and education make it vital to evolve education to equip the graduate to deal with these advances. Digital health, artificial intelligence and global access to information make curriculum changes essential. Student mental health issues driven by competition, selection processes, information overload, workloads, parental and peer pressure, and the inadequacy in resilience require consideration in evolving curriculums. Curriculums require to remain dynamic and reviewed more frequently than ever before. Expectations of patients desiring delivery of healthcare and global accessibility to information, even misinformation, make for the need of aspects of curriculum not previously prioritized. Theories of learning have evolved and the generation of students of yesterday, today, and tomorrow differ in how and why they learn.[8]

MODELS OF CURRICULUM DEVELOPMENT

Many models of curriculum development have been described and reviewed by Kwakye et al.[9] However, Prideaux simplifies models into prescriptive and descriptive models. Prescriptive models describe what ideal curriculums should appear like while descriptive models describe what curriculums are.

An example of a prescriptive model is by Ralph Tyler. He described a deductive model argued from the administrator's approach.

It had four steps: (1) Learning objectives, (2) learning experiences, (3) organizing learning experiences, and (4) evaluation. The Tyler model requires the active participation of learners with learning objectives clearly defined in the purposes with a simple linear approach to development of behavioral objectives. However, the defined objectives were usually narrowly interpreted, restricted student's skills and knowledge, and involved time and difficulties in their construction. Another example is the outcome-based curriculum. The descriptive model would be one that focuses on a situational analysis that makes it dependent on the context in which the process takes place.[10]

It was Hilda Taba who described an inductive approach that was a teacher approach simply because she believed that teachers are aware of the students' needs. These needs directed the curriculum. The Hilda Taba model had steps that included the diagnosis of needs, formulation of objectives, selection and organization of content, selection and organizing learning experiences, defining teaching strategies for both knowledge and affective domains, and finally evaluation.

The Kern's curriculum development process described six steps in the process: (1) Problem identification and general needs assessment, (2) targeted needs assessment, (3) goals and objectives, (4) educational strategies, (5) implementation, and (6) evaluation and feedback. This cyclical process is a useful tool toward developing a dynamic curriculum.[7]

TYPES OF CURRICULUM

It is Murray Print[11] that has summarized types of curriculum to be either prescriptive or descriptive; and, either rational-objective-based or dynamic-reactive. Harden reminds us of the need to recognize the declared or planned curriculum, the taught or delivered curriculum, and the learned or experienced curriculum remembering that an informal hidden curriculum exists. The declared curriculum is what our regulatory body, i.e., National Medical Council, prepares and disseminates to all educational institutes. Of that, faculty teach most of what has been declared, and students learn parts of the same. However, students also informally learn from what is not declared, taught, or learnt, that is needed based on observations by students of behavior i.e., hidden. Common among types of curriculum are traditional (information), competency-based (outcome), problem-based, community-based, integrated, and spiral curriculum to name a few. In 1999, Harden described a three-circle for classifying learning objectives in outcome-based education (doing the right thing, doing things right, and the right person to do it).[12]

The traditional curriculum was driven by content that had to be taught and learnt and was teacher-driven. Competency-based curriculum is driven by defined competencies, hence, EPAs are to be achieved through the course of learning, therefore, definitely, student-focused. An excellent guide for a competency-based workplace curriculum development using EPAs is described by ten Cate. The EPAs are defined in a curriculum to guide the faculty in the provision of feedback and entrustment decisions during study.[13,14] A few universities follow a problem-based curriculum where clinical problems drive the learning across all disciplines. Community-based curriculum direct learning to the needs, the resources, and learning settings to be that of the community to enhance authenticity of learning. An integrated curriculum may integrate disciplines horizontally, vertically, and even spirally, with the latter building from early phases to later phases from simple to complex. It was Harden that defined integration as "the organization of teaching matter to interrelate or unify subjects frequently taught in separate academic courses or departments." In the same article, described are six educational strategies: (1) Student-centered/teacher-centered, problem-based/information-gathering, integrated/discipline-based, community-based/hospital-based, elective/uniform, and systematic/apprenticeship-based. Building on the original SPICES model,[15] ten Cate proposed in a 2014 blog and quoted by Yusoff about a SPICES 2.0 model.[16] This stands for simulation-based preparation for practice; portfolio-based monitoring; individualized workplace learning; competency-based education; electronic media support; and structured workplace assessment. This is proposed to be used for curriculum strategy analysis.

COMPONENTS OF CURRICULUM

The World Health Organization's Educational Handbook for Health Personnel first described the educational spiral. It included a cyclic pathway that begins with a population's health needs; professional tasks to fulfil roles and responsibilities; defining educational objectives; planning an evaluation system; implementing the educational program; then implementing the evaluation to restart the cycle.[17] Similar elements of a curriculum are described in order of content; teaching and learning strategies; assessment processes; and evaluation processes. Additional elements in curriculum design —statements of intent (behavioral objectives) and context—are terms mentioned.[3] Purpose, goals, outcomes desired, learning objectives, content, teaching-learning strategies, learning opportunities, learning environment, and assessments are all included in a curriculum. In addition, Janet Grant points to the need to specify processes, feedback, and supervision to the definition.[18] It was Mulder and ten Cate that described in detail a ten-element definition further simplified by ten Cate and Simonia that includes: (1) Mission, (2) objectives, (3) intended learners and admission policy, (4) educational philosophy, (5) curriculum framework, (6) individual units, (7) assessments, (8) governance, (9) funding and (10) quality assurance.[19]

ESSENTIAL LITERATURE ON CURRICULAR DEVELOPMENT

Following a modified Delphi method, Lai S et al.[20] selected 5 of a total of 1,708 articles in English as key literature for curriculum development and renewal, probably essential for all educators involved in curriculum development as shown in **Table 1**.

FUTURE DIRECTIONS

Key challenges in curriculum for the future require one to predict changing trends, especially, in technology and healthcare needs of populations that require changes to adapt to the new generation of learning preferences and balancing skills required of healthcare professionals. Curriculums require reviews periodically to be able to adapt and improve to suite requirements.

CONCLUSION

In essence, the curriculum is the overarching framework for education, while the syllabus is only a detailed outline for a specific course usually content within that framework.

TABLE 1: Curriculum development and renewal.

S. No.	*Citation*	*Brief*
1.	Chen BY et al., 2019[21]	The article illustrates the application of the six-step approach to create effective online curriculum. It also compares blended, instructor-lead, self-paced and massive open online course curriculum
2.	Prideaux D. 2003[4]	Levels and elements of a curriculum are described Prescriptive and descriptive models of curriculum development are simplified The last main section is on curriculum maps, illustrating the relations between elements
3.	Mills DM et al. 2020[22]	*Described are key concepts of educational research:* Plan to publish at the beginning, create the question, construct curriculum, framework, aiming high on Kirkpatrick's pyramid, a structured approach and planning, choosing the journal, and final touches to submit
4.	Schneiderhan J et al. 2019[23]	Describes steps in curriculum development modified from Kern's steps and the University of Michigan Faculty Development Institute's Workshop on Curriculum Development
5.	McLeod P et al. 2015[24]	This article shares 12 steps while it reminds us that curriculum requires regular revision that should be informed by emerging societal trends, healthcare innovations, and education practices It must be an evidence-based curriculum renewal process

KEY POINTS

- A curriculum is defined as a planned educational experience.
- A syllabus is a statement of contents to be taught.
- Curriculum development includes models that are prescriptive and descriptive.
- Types of curriculums include a declared or planned curriculum, the taught or delivered curriculum, and the learned or experienced curriculum. There is an informal hidden curriculum that is neither taught nor declared but learnt.
- The SPICES model to guide curriculum development includes six educational strategies—student-centered, problem-based, integrated, community-based, elective, and systematic. SPICES 2.0 includes simulation-based preparation for practice; portfolio-based monitoring; individualized workplace learning; competency-based education; electronic media support; and structured workplace assessment.

REFERENCES

1. Flexner A. (1910). Medical Education in the United States and Canada: A Report to the Carnegie Foundation for the Advancement of Teaching. [online] Available from http://archive.carnegiefoundation.org/publications/pdfs/elibrary/Carnegie_Flexner_Report.pdf [Last accessed January, 2026].
2. Goodson BF. Etymologies, Epistemologies and The Emergence of Curriculum: A speculative essay in the making of the curriculum, 2nd edition. London, UK: Routledge; 2002. pp. 25-38.
3. Ganet J, Abdelrahman MYH, Zachariah A. Curriculum design in context. In: Walsh K (Ed). Oxford Textbook of Medical Education. Oxford, UK: Oxford University Press; 2013. pp. 13-24.

4. Prideaux D. ABC of learning and teaching in medicine: Curriculum design. BMJ. 2003;326(7383):268-70.
5. Harden RM. AMEE Guide No.21: Curriculum mapping: A tool for transparent and authentic teaching and learning. Med Teach. 2001;23(2):123-37.
6. Green ML. Identifying, appraising and implementing medical education curricula: A guide for medical educators. Ann Intern Med. 2001;135(10): 889-96.
7. Thomas P, Kern DE, Hughes MT, et al. Curriculum development for medical education: A six-step approach, 4th edition. Baltimore: John Hopkins University Press; 2022.
8. Soriano-Estrella AL. The evolution of medical education: From teacher-centered to learner-centered approaches. Acta Med Philipp. 2025;59(6):6-8.
9. Kwakye DO, Susuoroka G, Bashiru A, et al. A review of technical-scientific and nontechnical-scientific curriculum models: Tyler and Walker's model. Int J Develop Res. 2024;14:65341-6.
10. Reynolds J, Skilbeck M. Culture and the classroom. London: Open Books, 1976.
11. Print M. Curriculum development and design. 2nd edition. London: Routledge; 2021.
12. Harden RM, Crosby JR, Davis MH. (1999). AMEE Guide No 14: Outcome-based education: Part 1—an introduction to outcome-based education. [online] Available from https://paeaonline.org/wp-content/uploads/imported-files/19e-Intro-to-Outcome-Based-Education.pdf [Last accessed January, 2026].
13. ten Cate O, Chen HC, Hoff RG, et al. Curriculum development for the workplace using Entrustable Professional Activities (EPAs): AMEE Guide No. 99. Med Teach. 2015;37(11):983-1002.
14. ten Cate O. Nuts and Bolts of Entrustable Professional Activities. J Grad Med Educ. 2013;5(1)157-8.
15. Harden RM, Sowden S, Dunn WR. Educational strategies in curriculum development: The SPICES model. Med Educ.1984;18(4):284-97.
16. Yusoff MSB. The future ready medical curriculum: Personalised medical education and SPICES 2.0. EIMJ. 2019;11(3):1-3.
17. Guilbert JJ. Educational handbook for health personnel, 6th edition. Geneva: World Health Organization; 1998.
18. Grant J. Principles of curriculum design. In: Ed Swanwick T (Ed). Understanding Medical Education: Evidence, Theory and Practice, 2nd edition. New Jersey, USA: Wiley Blackwell; 2014. pp. 31-46
19. ten Cate O, Simonia G. Curriculum, course and faculty development for case based clinical reasoning. In: ten Cate O, Custers EJFM, Durning SJ (Eds). Principles and Practice of Case-based Clinical Reasoning Education: A Method for Preclinical Students. Cham: Springer; 2018. pp. 109-19.
20. Lai S, Buchheit BM, Kitamura K, et al. Five key articles on curriculum development for graduate medical educators. J Grad Med Educ. 2024;16(1):75-9.
21. Chen BY, Kern DE, Kearns RM, et al. From modules to MOOCs: Application of the six-step approach to online curriculum development for medical education. Acad Med. 2019;94(5):678-85.
22. Mills DM, Teufel RJ 2nd. Tools for medical education scholarship: From curricular development to educational research. Hosp Pediatr. 2020;10(5):452-7.
23. Schneiderhan J, Guetterman TC, Dobson ML. Curriculum development: A how to primer. Fam Med Community Health. 2019;7(2):e000046.
24. McLeod P, Steinert Y. Twelve tips for curriculum renewal. Med Teach. 2015;37(3): 232-8.

CHAPTER 3

Competency-based Medical Education

Latha Ravichandran

Learning Objectives

- Present an overview of the concept and principles of Competency-based Medical Education (CBME).
- Explain the rationale for CBME.
- Describe the key elements of National Medical Commission (NMC) CBME.
- Discuss the specific implementing strategies for CBME in India.
- Describe the roles and responsibilities of a teacher in CBME.
- Describe the roles and responsibilities of a student in CBME.
- Recognize the role of Indian Academy of Paediatrics (IAP) Medical Education Chapter (MEC).

INTRODUCTION

Competency-based Medical Education (CBME) is a paradigm shift in medical training, focusing on achieving of learning outcomes rather than time bound training. It emphasized on the development and assessment of competencies required for effective, ethical and patient centered medical practice. This chapter outlines the principles, key elements and implementation strategies of CBME.

WHAT DO YOU MEAN BY CBME?

Competency-based medical education is a transformative approach to medical education, which focuses on the achievement of certain competencies or abilities required for the practice of Medicine.[1] The competencies are otherwise defined as observable abilities or predetermined tasks to run a patient care service. These competencies are defined in alignment with the health needs of the community and the healthcare system existing. The competencies may include clinical skills, communication skills, professionalism, ethical decision making, teamwork, leadership, and life-long learning. The ultimate goal is to produce competent physicians who are able to meet the healthcare needs of the community they serve, providing optimal and safe patient care. This in turn impacts the overall quality of the health care.

The healthcare needs of a community are influenced by the disease patterns, demographic profile, the healthcare systems. The cultural diversities also impact. Hence, there is a local context to the curricular framework designed, which makes any curricular designs to be contextual and at the same time conform to the global competencies.

WHAT WAS THE RATIONALE FOR CBME?

There have been constant calls to reform the medical education since Flexner's report in 1910.[2] The competency approach gained popularity due to the themes that were constantly evolving.

1. *It focused on the outcomes:* The competency-based education shifts focus on observable and measurable outcomes and demonstration of competence or abilities in the predetermined real world tasks for effectively rendering their services from the traditional education that laid emphasis on time-based learning.[3] The traditional curriculum emphasized on the theoretical knowledge, less of skills in the real world experiences, used standardized testing with a gap noticed on the skill assessment, and practice applications. The graduates were less prepared to function as a first contact physician.[3,4]
2. *Learner-centered approach:* The CBME has shifted from the traditional teacher-centered approaches where teachers play an active role toward learner-centered approaches where teachers and learners have shared responsibilities. The self-directed learning, project-based learning, case-based discussions in groups, and self-paced learning are some of the approaches that CBME adopts encouraging autonomy individualized learning and assessment fostering active engagement and a motivating learning environment.[3,4]
3. *Catering to the healthcare changes:* The current healthcare demands a team approach and requires health professionals who can work as a team, embrace and integrate technology, and show adaptability to the continued changes. Competency-based education imparts these abilities in the health professionals.[4,5]
4. *Patient-centered care:* The competency-based education addresses the core domains of attitude, ethics, and communication due to patient demand for physicians who demonstrate empathy, effective communication, and ethical judgment.[4,6]
5. *Adaptation to healthcare changes:* The increasing complexity of healthcare requires professionals who can work in teams, integrate technology, and adapt to ongoing changes. CBME equips learners with these competencies.[2,4]
6. *Quality assurance and accountability:* The patient-centric approach and their demands require that the outcome of the training results in medical practitioners who are prepared for independent practice with capabilities in predetermined tasks as service providers. Hence, CBME training integrates into it a system of continuous assessment and documentation of achievement of competencies for student progression.[7,8]
7. *Individualized learning:* While traditional curriculum was time bound, CBME provided flexibility in the competency acquisition in alignment with the individual learning pace, providing support to students wherever needed progressing them toward competence and mastery of abilities.[3,4]
8. *Global standards and mobility:* Currently, there is global demand for health professionals and their transborder mobility. Frameworks such as those from the World Federation for Medical Education (WFME) standardize competencies and facilitate international equivalence to support student cross-border mobility.[9]
9. *Bridging the gap between theory and practice:* The CBME has integrated clinical exposure, experiential learning, and skill training early, to ensure that the students

are ready to function as first contact physicians at graduation.[1,4,7]

10. *Better assessment and feedback:* The CBME gives greater emphasis on formative, competency-based assessments, and structured feedback that promotes student progression and growth. The gaps in attaining competencies are identified and early remediation initiated, improving the overall competency and student outcomes.[3,5]

KEY ELEMENTS OF NMC CBME IN INDIA

The overall goal of the CBME was to produce an Indian medical graduate who will function effectively as the first contact physician. The key elements include defined roles of the IMG. The IMG is expected to function as a clinician, leader and member of healthcare team, communicator, lifelong learner and a professional.

The competencies under each role have been defined in the NMC UG curriculum.[10]

Outcome-oriented curriculum: The NMC curriculum has defined the learning outcomes to be achieved under each of the departments that will align with the roles. The curriculum has defined learning outcomes under each subject and indicated areas for vertical and horizontal integration.

Newer Elements in Teaching Learning and Assessment

Integrated teaching and learning: Horizontal and vertical integration across subjects to encourage holistic understanding by introducing aligned and integrated teaching modules within the calendar. (a) Early clinical exposure (ECE): These introduce students to clinical settings from the first year itself to build context and relevance. (b) Electives: These provide flexibility and exposure to diverse fields that may allow students to explore more for their future and promote self-directed. (c) Attitude, Ethics, and Communication (AETCOM) module: This element addresses the need for providing structured training and competency building on attitudinal domains such as demonstrating empathy, effective communication, and ethical judgement in clinical practice. (d) Skill-based training: Which puts emphasis on hands-on training through clinical skills lab and simulations. (e) Formative and summative assessments: Continuous internal assessment and competency-based assessments using tools such as Objective Structured Clinical Examination (OSCE) and Direct Observation of Procedural Skills (DOPS)[9] and workplace-based assessments. (f) Self-directed learning (SDL): It encourages students to take responsibility for their own learning, with faculty acting as facilitators. (g) Reflective practice and feedback: Students are trained and encouraged to reflect on their learning, and regular feedback is provided to support improvement.[10]

KEY COMPONENTS OF PEDIATRICS IN CBME (INDIA)[11]

- *Defined competencies:*
  - Assessment of growth and development
  - Nutrition assessment and management
  - Offer immunization services
  - Diagnose and manage common pediatric illnesses (diarrhea, pneumonia, malaria, etc.)
  - Provide primary neonatal care
  - Rational usage of drugs in children
  - Recognize and manage pediatric emergencies including timely referral
  - Promote adolescent health
- *Competency classification:* classified as core and noncore: Core is taught and

assessed both in formative and summative assessments and noncore is taught and assessed in formative assessment only.

- *Early clinical exposure (ECE):* Students are introduced early to pediatric practice through community and hospital visits and visits to primary health centers and immunization clinics.
- *Skill-based learning:*
  - Focus on acquiring practical skills such as:
    - Performing newborn resuscitation
    - Growth chart plotting and interpretation
    - Vaccine Administration techniques
    - Management of dehydration
    - Communication with caregivers
- *AETCOM integration:* Emphasis on ethical issues, empathy, and communication—especially crucial in pediatric care
- *Use of simulation and skills labs:* Skills such as bag-mask ventilation in neonates or assessing malnutrition are taught via simulation.
- *Logbook maintenance:* Students must document clinical encounters, observed procedures, and skills performed.
- *Assessment strategy:*
  - Formative (ongoing feedback, mini clinical evaluation exercise, and case discussions)
  - Summative (OSCEs, DOPS, and theory exams; **Table 1**)

SPECIFIC IMPLEMENTING STRATEGIES FOR CBME IN INDIA

The specific strategies adopted for the implementation of CBME in India. These measures were introduced by the NMC, previously the Medical Council of India (MCI), to bring about a learner-centered, outcomes-oriented medical education system.

- *Faculty development and capacity building:*
  - Basic and advanced courses in medical education were mandated for faculty through medical education units (MEUs).
  - Curriculum implementation and support program (CISP) to support

TABLE 1: Sample pediatric competencies from NMC document.[12]

Competency code	*Competency description*	*Domain*	*Level*	*Core/ noncore*
PE 1.2	Assess a child's growth using growth charts and interpret findings	Skills	SH	Core
PE 3.1	Enumerate vaccine types, schedules, and adverse effects	Knowledge	KH	Core
PE 5.4	Demonstrate the correct technique of administering vaccines	Skills	SH	Core
PE 6.1	Describe the clinical features and management of acute respiratory infections	Knowledge	KH	Core
PE 9.3	Perform neonatal resuscitation using a manikin	Skills	SH	Core
PE 11.4	Discuss ethical issues in pediatric care, including assent and parental consent	Attitude	KH	Core
PE 12.5	Communicate effectively with parents regarding child health and development	Attitude/skill	SH	Core

(Core: mandatory competencies; Domain: knowledge, skill, and attitude; KH: knows how; Noncore: supplemental learning; SH: shows how) faculty in implementing the new curriculum.[13] Training included modern teaching methodologies and assessment tools such as OSCE, mini-CEX, and DOPS. Programs were coordinated through NMC-designated regional and nodal centers.[14] Currently, there are 12 nodal centers and 23 regional centers in India.

- *Curriculum structuring and governance:* Over 2,900 competencies were mapped across all subjects, divided into core and noncore categories. Competencies were distributed phase wise with clearly defined learning objectives and teaching and assessments methods.[14] Curricular governance in NMC CBME curricular governance refers to the formalized structure and processes that ensure the planning, implementation, evaluation, and continuous improvement of the undergraduate medical curriculum, in line with the Graduate Medical Education Regulations (GMER) 2019 laid down by the NMC.[15] Governance structure as per NMC included:
  - *Curriculum committee (CC):* It is mandated by NMC to oversee CBME implementation. It is composed of the dean/principal, heads of departments, MEU coordinator, and nominated faculty. Roles include planning curriculum, mapping competencies, coordinating integration, and ensuring compliance with CBME guidelines.
  - *Medical education unit (MEU):* Responsible for faculty training, ensuring educators understand CBME principles, such as active learning, formative assessment, and feedback. Conducts Curriculum Implementation Support Programs (CISP I & II) under the guidance of NMC's nodal/regional centers.[15]
- Establishment of committees to have an oversight on the implementation of the newer elements such as foundation course committee, skills committee, AETCOM committee, alignment and integration committee, electives committee, and early clinical exposures introduced from the first MBBS year, integrating basic science with clinical relevance. It included hospital visits, patient simulations, and case-based discussions.[16]
- *Establishment of skills laboratories:* Skills labs were mandated in every college with simulation mannequins and audiovisual tools. Training included common procedures and clinical examination skills.[17]
- *AETCOM module implementation:* AETCOM modules were introduced with year-wise progression. Included teaching of empathy, communication, and ethics using case studies and reflective writing.[18]
- *Student-centered learning strategies:* Self-directed learning (SDL) was incorporated with facilitated sessions and student reflections. Electives were introduced to allow personalized learning in selected areas.[14]
- *Integration of subjects:* Horizontal integration linked subjects within the same phase; vertical integration connected preclinical and clinical learning. Encouraged problem-based and case-based learning.[14]
- *Assessment reforms:* Shift to formative assessments with tools such as OSCE, mini-CEX, and logbooks. Blueprint-based summative assessments aligned with competencies.[19]
- *Monitoring and evaluation:* Medical colleges were required to submit implementation progress reports to NMC. Feedback systems for students and faculty were institutionalized.[10]

THE ROLES AND RESPONSIBILITIES OF AN UNDERGRADUATE TEACHER IN CBME IMPLEMENTATION

Roles and responsibilities of a medical teacher in CBME are summarized in **Table 2**.

ROLES AND RESPONSIBILITIES OF STUDENTS IN CBME

Roles and responsibilities of students in CBME are summarized in **Table 3**.

ROLE OF IAP MEC MEDICAL EDUCATION CHAPTER IN COMPETENCY BASED MEDICAL EDUCATION

The Indian Academy of Paediatrics—Medical Education Chapter (IAP-MEC) plays a pivotal role in supporting and advancing CBME, especially in the field of pediatrics. Established in 2021, IAP-MEC provides academic leadership, training, and standardized resources for effective pediatric education.[31] In curriculum development and alignment, IAP-MEC has contributed significantly by translating the NMC's prescribed competencies into specific learning objectives (SLOs) tailored for pediatric undergraduate education. These SLOs help ensure consistent, measurable outcomes across institutions.

The chapter regularly organizes faculty development programs, including webinars, CMEs, and hands-on workshops, to train educators in modern CBME-based teaching-learning strategies.

It promotes the implementation of CBME-aligned assessment tools such as OSCEs, Mini-CEX, and DOPS, emphasizing holistic evaluation of knowledge, skills, and attitudes.

IAP-MEC has developed and shared structured teaching-learning materials, clinical case scenarios, and simulation exercises to support pediatric competency training.[31] The chapter encourages research on medical education and innovation in pediatric training, often publishing in platforms such as IAPMER.[32] IAP-MEC collaborates with national regulatory authorities such as the

TABLE 2: Roles and responsibilities of a medical teacher in CBME.

Role	Responsibilities
1. Facilitator of learning	Encourage active learning strategies (e.g., problem-based learning, case discussions, and flipped classrooms). Guide students in self-directed learning and critical thinking.[3,12]
2. Planner and curriculum implementer	Develop objectives from competencies. Plan lessons for the defined objectives. Align teaching sessions with the competency-based curriculum. Develop integrated lesson plans with clear learning outcomes. Participate in curriculum mapping and implementation.[13,20]
3. Assessor and evaluator	Conduct both formative and summative assessments using valid tools (OSCE, DOPS, mini-CEX, etc.). Provide timely, constructive feedback and maintain documentation of students' achievement of competencies (logbook).[21,22]
4. Mentor and role model	Serve as a mentor, supporting students academically, professionally, and emotionally. Demonstrate ethical behavior, clinical competence, and professionalism.[18,23]
5. Faculty learner	Continuously update teaching skills and clinical knowledge. Participate in faculty development programs and workshops.[13,24]
6. Researcher and innovator	Engage in educational research to improve teaching and assessment. Innovate in teaching tools, e-learning, and curriculum delivery.[25]
7. Collaborator and team member	Work within interdisciplinary teams to ensure effective integration of content. Participate in curriculum committee activities and policy decisions.[3]

TABLE 3: Roles and responsibilities of students in CBME.

Role	Responsibilities
1. Active learner	Take responsibility for their own learning, engage in self-directed learning, reflective practices, and continuous self-assessment. Participate actively in case discussions, practical sessions, and skills training.[3,20]
2. Self-directed and reflective practitioner	Learners should possess ability to identify learning needs and set learning goals. Use learning portfolios and reflective journals to track progress. Regularly reflect on performance and act on feedback.[7,26]
3. Team member and collaborator	Work collaboratively in group tasks, interprofessional learning, and peer-assisted learning. Respect diverse perspectives and contribute to a cooperative learning environment.[27]
4. Ethical and professional individual	Demonstrate professionalism, empathy, integrity, and accountability. Uphold ethical standards in clinical and academic environments. Adhere to codes of conduct and patient confidentiality.[18,28]
5. Competency achiever	Aim to acquire core competencies in knowledge, skills, attitude, communication, and professionalism. Ensure progression by meeting milestones and participating in workplace-based assessments.[4,28]
6. Feedback seeker and adapter	Actively seek and accept feedback from teachers and peers. Modify learning strategies and behaviors based on feedback[29]
7. Lifelong learner	Develop habits of continuous inquiry and staying updated with the latest evidence-based practices. Prepare for lifelong learning beyond graduation and into professional life.[30]

National Medical Commission (NMC) to align pediatric curricula with national health goals (IAP, 2020).

CONCLUSION

In conclusion, CBME provides a structured and an outcome-oriented approach to medical training ensuring readiness to practice in a clinical setting. Sustained faculty training, robust assessment system and continuous curricular refinement are key factors for successful adoption.

REFERENCES

1. Bhattacharya S. Competency-based medical education: An overview. Ann Med Sci Res. 2023;2(3):132-8.
2. Carraccio CL, Englander R. From Flexner to competencies: reflections on a decade and the journey ahead. Acad Med J Assoc Am Med Coll. 2013;88(8):1067-73.
3. Frank JR, Snell LS, Cate OT, et al. Competency-based medical education: theory to practice. Med Teach. 2010;32(8):638-45.
4. Ten Cate O. Competency-Based Postgraduate Medical Education: Past, Present and Future. GMS J Med Educ. 2017;34(5):Doc69.
5. Englander R, Cameron T, Ballard AJ, et al. Toward a Common Taxonomy of Competency Domains for the Health Professions and Competencies for Physicians: Acad Med. 2013;88(8):1088-94.
6. WFME, BME. World Federation for Medical Education. WFME Global Standards for Quality Improvement of Medical Education. [online] Available from https://wfme.org/standards/ [Last accessed January, 2026].
7. Medical Council of India. Competency Based Undergraduate Curriculum for the Indian Medical Graduate. New Delhi: MCI; 2018.
8. Chacko TV. Quality Assurance of Medical Education in India: The Concerns, Available Guiding Frameworks, and the Way Forward to Improve Quality and Patient Safety. Arch Med Health Sci. 2021;9(2).
9. WFME. (2022). WFME Standards - World Federation for Medical Education. [online] Available from https://wfme.org/standards/ [Last accessed January, 2026].
10. National Medical Commission. (2020). UG Curriculum. [online] Available from https://

www.nmc.org.in/information-desk/for-colleges/ug-curriculum/ [Last accessed January, 2026].
11. Singh T, Gupta P. Indian Academy of Pediatrics Releases Uniform Learning Objectives for Competency Based Curriculum in Undergraduate Pediatric Education. Indian Pediatr. 2020;57(2):182-3.
12. National Medical Commission. (2024). UG Curriculum. [online] Available from https://www.nmc.org.in/information-desk/for-colleges/ug-curriculum/ [Last accessed January, 2026].
13. National Medical Commission. (2021). National Faculty development program-Curriculum Implementation and support program 3. [online] Available from https://www.nmc.org.in/wp-content/uploads/2021/06/CISP-II-paper-17-05-2021.pdf [Last accessed January, 2026].
14. Medical Council of India. (2019). Competency Based Undergraduate Curriculum for the Indian Medical Graduate. Available from: https://www.nmc.org.in [Last accessed January, 2026].
15. NMC, FDP. (2020). National Faculty Development Programme. [online] Available from https://www.nmc.org.in/information-desk/national-faculty-development-programme-new/ [Last accessed January, 2026].
16. Sarkar S, Badyal D, Sharma R, et al. Navigating Through the Newer Components of the Indian Competency Based Medical Education. J Med Sci Health. 2022;8(3):236-45.
17. Medical Council of India. (2019). Skills Training Module. [online] Available from https://www.nmc.org.in/wp-content/uploads/2020/08/Skill-Module_23.12.2019.pdf [Last accessed January, 2026].
18. Medical Council of India. AETCOM. [online] Available from https://www.nmc.org.in/wp-content/uploads/2020/01/AETCOM_book.pdf [Last accessed January, 2026].
19. Lee GB, Chiu AM. Assessment and feedback methods in competency-based medical education. Ann Allergy Asthma Immunol. 2022;128(3):256-62.
20. Harden RM. Outcome-Based Education: the future is today. Med Teach. 2007;29(7):625-9.
21. Medical Council of India. (2019). Competency based undergraduate curriculum for Indian Medical Graduate -Assessment Module. [online] Available from: https://www.nmc.org.in/wp-content/uploads/2019/10/Module_Competence_based_02.09.2019.pdf [Last accessed January, 2026].
22. Norcini J, Burch V. Workplace-based assessment as an educational tool: AMEE Guide No. 31. Med Teach. 2007;29(9-10):855-71.
23. Cruess SR, Cruess RL, Steinert Y. Role modelling—making the most of a powerful teaching strategy. BMJ. 2008;336(7646):718-21.
24. McLean M, Cilliers F, Van Wyk JM. Faculty development: Yesterday, today and tomorrow. Med Teach. 2008;30(6):555-84.
25. Steinert Y, Mann K, Centeno A, et al. A systematic review of faculty development initiatives designed to improve teaching effectiveness in medical education: BEME Guide No. 8. Med Teach. 2006;28(6):497-526.
26. Murad MH, Varkey P. Self-directed learning in health professions education. Ann Acad Med Singap. 2008;37(7):580-90.
27. Frenk J, Chen L, Bhutta ZA, et al. Health professionals for a new century: transforming education to strengthen health systems in an interdependent world. Lancet. 2010;376(9756):1923-58.
28. Cruess RL, Cruess SR. Teaching professionalism: general principles. Med Teach. 2006;28(3):205-8.
29. Nicol DJ, Macfarlane-Dick D. Formative assessment and self-regulated learning: a model and seven principles of good feedback practice. Stud High Educ. 2006;31(2):199-218.
30. Greiner AC, Knebel E (Eds). Health Professions Education: A Bridge to Quality. Washington (DC): National Academies Press (US); 2003.
31. Indian Academy of Pediatrics. Medical Education Chapter (IAP-MEC). [online] Available from https://www.iapmec.com [Last accessed January, 2026].
32. Advanced Research Publications. Indian J Med Educ Res (IAPMER). [online] Available from https://www.advancedresearchpublications.com/publish-iapmer [Last accessed January, 2026].

CHAPTER 4

Medical Education Unit

Anil Gurtoo, Madhulika Monga

INTRODUCTION

If you are reading this book, you surely are a medical educator, and are likely to have encountered medical education unit (MEU) in your academic career. The essential term here is, academic career, which has a very different scope as compared to clinical career. Within the realm of this academic career, lies embedded the functional core: The MEU.

Contemplating on the functional role of MEU, a question inevitably arises: How is it that a unit which was largely unheard of some 30 years back in our country (apart from a few institutes), has garnered such a place of importance in the current times so as to have been included under the National Medical Commission's mandate? To understand this, lets delve a little into the background of MEUs as we see them today, the triggers which led to establishment of worlds first MEU and further into the history of MEUs in our country in the context of evolving global scenario.

MEDICAL EDUCATION UNIT: THROUGH THE EYES OF HISTORY

In early days, medical education was taught on the basis of "see one, teach one, do one" and it was believed to be an effective way of teaching. However, by early 1950s, the ever-expanding universe of medical knowledge led to the realization of the need to organize the vast and growing medical knowledge into a coherent curriculum of teaching, learning, and assessment. The traditional methods of teaching were being questioned for utility and effectiveness. As the challenges mounted, newer methods such as problem-based learning and task-based learning were being introduced. Assessment methods were facing the same challenge of contested validity, objectivity, and standardization. Moreover, principles from educational psychology, cognitive science, and methodologies from the social sciences were beginning to be seen as applicable to medical education. A firm belief that teaching in itself is a skill which could be developed through study and research and could be applied to medical education was setting in. Challenging the perception that a good doctor would automatically be a good teacher, it was now thought essential to train faculty in educational technology.

In response to these mounting challenges, which were increasingly being recognized, different institutes started their own units to address these. With each institute having its own scope and hence names such as Office of Medical Education, Division of Research in Medical Education, Audiovisual department, and Department of MEU. Whereas, the nations of the Western world such as USA, UK, Germany, and Canada started such units in some colleges, the WHO played an important role in establishing such units across the rest of the world by creating and funding a system of the Regional Teacher

Training Centers (RTTCs) backed up by a network of National Teacher Training Centers (NTTCs) under such RTTCs. In Southeast Asia, RTTCs were established at the Chulalongkorn University in Thailand and the University of Sri Lanka, which further led to the creation of the first NTTCs in India. Though the funding by WHO to NTTCs was later withdrawn, a spark had been ignited. Over the next many decades, several colleges in our country successfully started their MEUs, which though not mandatory, were purely voluntary and diverse efforts of dedicated and passionate medical educators. However, a more concrete shape to MEUs was provided by the Vision 2015 document of the erstwhile Medical Council of India. This document underlined systematic capacity building of medical teachers through Faculty Development Programmes as a platform for training medical teachers into the newer teaching practices. The final push came with the implementation of Competency-based Medical Education (CBME), which not only mandated the presence of MEU, but also clearly outlined its structure, administrative support and role.

SO, WHY DO WE NEED AN MEU?

Accountability to Society

Medical education does not exist in a vacuum, it owes an accountability to the society to produce doctors who are not just grounded in scholastic excellence, but are also competent clinicians, rooted in ethics, effective communicators, empathetic, culturally competent and socially responsive healthcare professionals. The societal expectations are great and even more critical in our country with its diverse demography, population and healthcare challenges defined by the dual epidemiological burdens of communicable and non-communicable diseases and marked social inequities. This accountability is increasingly being acknowledged by the society and hence is also being reflected in the laws of the land. MEUs can help the medical institutions to fulfil this societal accountability by aligning the curricula, teaching methods and practices to needs of the society.

Patient-centric Approach

With increasing awareness, it is now realized that patients are not merely at the receiving end of the healthcare system but are seen as active and equal partners in the system. Increasingly, the healthcare system is now transitioning toward patient centric approaches emphasizing their health belief models, safety, autonomy, cultural sensitivities, dignity, and respect. The education of our healthcare professionals needs to be tailored to include such patient centric approaches. Without a paradigm shift in our educational training, true shift toward patient centric healthcare delivery would not be possible. The challenge is to bring this change amidst the diversity of the contextual realities of patients with varied literacy, cultures, and languages.

Student-centric Approach

The student profile has changed drastically over the years. Not only has the number of students in each institute increased manifold, the diversity has also increased. We encounter diversity of socioeconomic status, educational background, culture, language, learning mediums, learning styles, career aspirations, digital literacy, and access. A singular method of teaching, learning, and assessment would obviously not be suitable for all. One size fits all approach can no longer be applicable. Apart from the educational challenge, this diversity also more often than not leads to many socio-emotional adjustment challenges in adaptation leading to stress and mental health issues among students. This poses an additional challenge of student welfare for the institute. The educational curricula as well as the educational atmosphere has to be made student centric with capacity to cater the diverse needs and harnessing potential of each individual. There is a need to make students active stakeholders in their own education rather than passive learners.

Knowledge Explosion

Given the explosion of knowledge and an inability to keep pace with it, it has become imperative to develop systems of just-in-time access to knowledge combined with educational processes that shift focus from knowledge delivery and acquisition, to conceptual learning, knowledge application, critical thinking, problem solving, and most importantly strategies for lifelong learning by "learning how to learn". This change will have to be brought about in all spheres of medical education: Curriculum, teaching-learning methods, and assessment.

Technological Revolution

Technology has embedded itself in all aspects of our lives, including healthcare and medical education. Convergence and integration of AI, VR with IT and biotechnology is transforming the very context of healthcare delivery and education. This convergence poses unique challenges to traditional delivery models of healthcare and medical education as personalized healthcare and medical education delivered by these platforms becomes reality of the coming times. New medical education models will need to be aligned to these realities and the new skills will need to be structured within the new curricula.

There is also an urgent need to address the challenges emerging from the application of newer cyber-digital technologies: Ethics, cyber security, data privacy, and inequity of access to technological resources.

Advances in Cognitive Sciences

We have progressed a lot in our understanding of how we learn and how can we improve learning. With a large body of evidence for concepts such as differentiated cognitive learning schemas, cognitive restructuring, Dreyfus model of skill acquisition, spaced repetition systems, and interleaved practice, it has today become an imperative necessity to incorporate all these new and emerging concepts into the design of medical curriculum.

Globalization of Medical Education Standards and Benchmarks

The world is no longer the same, nations no longer can exist as silos, unaccountable to each other. The borders are no longer sacrosanct for healthcare and medical education. In both these sectors, the best practices, the standards, and benchmarks cannot exist in isolation, rather these transcend borders in a way never imagined before. We see an ever increase in the number of Indian students who seek medical education outside India and as many international students who aspire to study in India. There is also growing medical tourism in the country with high quality healthcare available at affordable cost.

But meeting international standards cannot happen at the cost of neglecting our local healthcare and educational needs, thus bringing in the concept of having local relevance to the process of globalization, often referred to as "glocalization". Keeping in mind the diversity of our country, this glocalization is rather a huge challenge that we healthcare professional educators have ahead of us: Reconciling global benchmarks with local needs and interests.

Professionalization of Medical Education

Teaching or medical education can no longer be considered as an optional accessory to clinical practice. It is not something that we can afford to learn on the way through hits and misses. It is now getting increasingly professionalized by processes driven by external standards, benchmarks, accreditation, and codes of conduct. It has thus emerged as a discipline in its own right with an identity based on evidence, science, and research.

Shift to Outcome-based Educational Approaches

In recent times we have seen and experienced firsthand the paradigm shift from traditional teach and test approaches to outcome-based model of medical education. We are still grappling to adjust with this culture shift in most of the institutions. The focus is now to see "what should student be able to do" rather than "what should be taught to the student". Though seemingly subtle, this is a huge shift in the way content is taught, learnt, and assessed. Moreover, the outcome is not just of desirable knowledge or clinical skills, but also creating a doctor capable of responding to varying primary healthcare needs and contexts of our country.

SO, WHAT IS MEU?: THE STRUCTURE AND PROCESSES OF MEU

Following the imperative need of having MEUs, we now turn to understanding the functional architecture of MEUs. As per the mandate of the National Medical Commission, each medical college must have a MEU headed by the Dean/Principal/Vice chancellor of the university/college and comprising a coordinator with a minimum of eight to a maximum 14 members. These mandates have seen, and will continue to see changes from time to time; but it is pertinent to discuss some key aspects regarding the composition of the MEU.

- *Link with the top administrative leadership*: The importance of having the academic and administrative head involved in a supportive role with the MEU cannot be emphasized enough. The MEU can fulfil the various roles only when it has the authority to make decisions, implement them and take necessary feedback to evaluate the programs. Absence of this would reduce the MEU to a very restrictive role of exclusively training the teachers.
- *The MEU team*: The major criterion for membership of the MEU is a faculty member who is passionately engaged in medical education who has been trained through NMC accredited courses in medical education.
- *Full-time or part-time MEU*: This is an ongoing debate since a long time, whether MEU faculty should be full-time educators or part-time, drawn from existing departments.

  Part-time is the common model seen across the country where the members primarily are in their respective departments, and the team up for MEU activities. This model keeps the MEU faculty grounded in their respective clinical disciplines on the one hand, and remain connected with the field of Medical education, on the other. It is a cost-effective model that allows for a greater participation of a greater number of motivated faculty in the activities of MEU. However, the disadvantage is that the educator is burdened with dual tasks of the MEU and parent departmental/clinical work, which adds to the existing multiple roles that a healthcare professional is expected to fulfil, often leading to burn out and draining away of the motivation. This also might compromise on the expertise in the field of education of the part-time faculty. Some institutes follow the full-time model, usually seen in large institutes with ample resources. Such full-time faculty would for obvious reasons be more focused, dedicated, invest time in developing expertise in the field of medical education, have energy and time for innovative research in medical education, would be able to contribute more to the institutional educational environment. But, such dedicated medical educators over time would be disconnected from the evolving clinical and medical field specific realities. A model where the faculty is given daily or weekly protected time for contributing toward MEU may be a more practical, economical, and feasible option.

- *Administrative staff*: A dedicated team of administrative staff attached exclusively to the MEU is very important.

SO, WHAT IS MEU SUPPOSED DO?: ROLES OF MEU

In a rapidly changing world of education driven by forces of globalization, technology and new cognitive science, MEUs have a larger role to play in adapting medical education to the changing world and its emergent realities. To play across such a large and varied canvas, newer leadership models are required that are at once capable of fulfilling the core NMC mandate and responding to other emergent challenges as well. Let us now discuss the multifaceted roles that MEU can fulfil.

Faculty Development

Faculty development and building the education capacity of the institute is the most important role of a MEU. In India, MEU has been involved in training faculty in basic and advanced courses in medical education technology. NMC has designed a basic course in medical education which the MEU of each college is expected to conduct for their faculty in the presence of an NMC observer from the regional center. The cascading model of a Nodal Center, which trains the faculty of Regional Center, who in turn trains the MEU faculty of individual institutions has proven to be a very cost and time effective method of faculty development across the country. With the implementation of CBME, using the cascading model and workshops on Curriculum Implementation Support Program (CISP) were also initiated. This model was also utilized for introducing, training, and implementing the AETCOM (Attitude, Ethics and Communication) module as a part of undergraduate curriculum.

MEU played a pivotal role in spearheading the CBME implementation across the country and without this cascading model it would not been possible at such a large scale within limited time and restricted resources.

Faculty development is not restricted to just training; it involves mentoring faculty in educational innovations and research. As per the new postgraduate guidelines by NMC, MEU is also responsible for training the postgraduate students in medical education technology.

Curriculum Implementation

Designing, planning, mapping the outcomes with teaching, and assessment strategies and curriculum evaluation are the integral roles of MEU. Globally MEU has been instrumental in incorporating need-based regular timely curricular changes keeping abreast with evolving medical knowledge. As per the latest NMC guidelines regarding faculty development program, the task of curriculum implementation has been assigned to curriculum committee and it has been mandated to have curriculum committee separate from the MEU, except for the MEU coordinator who is a part of both of them. This requires MEU and curriculum committee to closely coordinate with each other for various overlapping roles. Before these recent guidelines, across the country it was usual practice to have members of MEU to constitute the curriculum committee too. Many institutes consider curriculum committee as a subset of MEU dedicated for curricular implementation. Each setup has its respective pros and cons; separate bodies would face the challenge of coordination and appropriate task division. If both the tasks are looked into by MEU members it is overburdening the already burdened MEU faculty.

Assessment Reforms

From merely taking a decision to promote the undergraduate student to the next level, assessment has come to represent the newer thinking: Assessment drives learning. Besides it has developed into a multifaceted construct incorporating domains such as formative assessment, feedback of assessment, assessment of skills beyond theory, newer valid reliable, and context specific repertoire of assessment tools. With a move toward competency assessments, for the large number of undergraduate students, within limited resources of time, human resources and finance; necessitates an imperative of designing and using newer assessment techniques. MEU needs to train the faculty in the newer assessment methods and also develop contextually appropriate solutions while maintaining quality standards.

Educational Research

With ever changing milieu of medical education; innovating, evaluating the innovations, and sharing successful innovations is imperative. MEU can actively encourage faculty to pursue such educational scholarships. It can also play a lead role in evaluating new programs or curricular changes implemented in the institute. Keeping abreast with latest research or innovations around the world, sharing these and look into feasibility of its implementation in the local context.

Technology Integration

MEU should take the lead in integrating medical education with the evolving technology. Exploring and recommending new technologies, training faculty in technology enhanced teaching methods, implementing learning management systems, developing E-learning modules and digital resources, establishing simulation laboratories, and creating innovative gamification platforms are some of the areas that MEU can work with. Most importantly using technology to tailor teaching, learning, assessment, and remedial measures to the needs of an individual student should now be the goal of the MEU. MEU can ensure that the use of technology is instructionally sound and value adding to education, and not merely blindly used for technology's sake. Integration with technology, if not translated to better learning, better quality of Indian Medical Graduate and better healthcare, will be waste of precious resources.

Student Support and Mentoring

MEU can play a vital role in improving the quality of education and thus the quality of doctors by mentoring the students and have an active student support system in place. Remedial teaching for struggling learners, providing a robust and transparent feedback system, learning strategy workshops, peer study and mentor groups, career guidance sessions, time and stress management programs, and leadership skill development can be some of the activities that can be taken up by the MEU.

Quality of Medical Education

Role of MEU goes over and above the process of quality assurance and accreditation. It involves an endeavor to build a system of improving all aspects of education from curricular development to assessment reforms, based on active feedback from students, faculty, and in sync with national policies. Developing a culture of quality improvement in the institute can be the crucial task of MEU.

SO, WHAT ARE THE CHALLENGES FOR MEU

The goals and roles of MEU cannot be achieved overnight by the mere wave of a magic wand of decree and mandate. The road for MEU is long and arduous. Let us try to dissect and discuss the various hurdles that any MEU is bound to face:

- *Resource constraints*: To fully realize the role of being an active innovation and technology integration hub requires funds, space, and manpower. Unfortunately, most MEUs run on restricted funds, inadequate dedicated space, and limited administrative staff.
- *Faculty development and engagement*: There is a continuing shortage of faculty in medical education, with many faculty members not having undergone formal training in various aspects like curriculum design or assessment, which seriously hampers the effectiveness of MEU initiatives. Faculty engagement also differs with many faculty undertaking the BCME course only because it is mandatory with little scope of its application in the classroom settings. Many believe the older established methods to be of value and are either resistant to change or reluctant to adopt newer methodologies.
- *Institutional support and sustaining motivation*: Many institutes have established MEUs just as a mere token presence to meet the regulatory requirements, rather than a functional asset of long-term value. With limited institutional and administrative support, the scope and role of MEU is largely constricted. Even in institutes where MEU is strong, MEU faculty still suffers from limited recognition of their efforts. Contributions to medical education are often undervalued in academic promotions and awards. Protected time for medical education initiatives is unheard of. MEU members juggle clinical, teaching, and administrative responsibilities, leaving limited time for educational research and innovation initiatives. It is difficult for such an overburdened faculty with inadequate recognition of their efforts to sustain motivation and is also a deterrent for interested faculty to join MEU.
- *Constantly changing regulations*: With a paradigm shift from traditional to CBME, the regulatory authorities are continually upgrading the new guidelines. It is a challenge for MEU to keep pace and navigate through new

and evolving regulations. Every change involves fresh administrative approvals, training, dissemination, implementation, evaluation and appropriate corrective measures. Such repeated and rapid changes, along with limited resources can be very daunting for any setup.

- *Lacking educational scholarship*: Under the given constraints of paucity of resources, inadequate institutional support, lack of training in medical education research, mentorship, and dedicated time for work in medical education, the educational scholarship is affected both in quality and quantity. This limits the innovation for local context specific educational methods and practices.
- *Technology adoption*: Adopting to new technology faces challenge not only because of lack of funds and space, but also because of lack of technical know-how and support, insufficient training and inability to keep pace with the rapidly changing technology. Moreover, there is huge disparity in the digital access and infrastructure across the country. This digital gap prevents MEU to fully adopt and utilize the technological advances.

SO, WHERE DO WE GO FROM HERE?

MEU has seen a paradigm shift in its role. From being a basic administrative support system to a driver of medical education innovations, MEU has changed tremendously in the short span of its life. However, currently medical knowledge, health scenario, student awareness, technology, and societal consciousness is changing at a never seen before pace. The threat of irrelevance in the face of newer challenges is looming large on the horizon. It is now time for MEU and its members to take the lead and make anticipatory visionary changes. Some key roles that the MEU should move toward are:

- *Educational innovation centers*: In the future, MEUs should become the nucleus of educational innovation, revolutionizing medical education with a focus on local institutional context which is replicable in different setups. It is time to move beyond mandated faculty development programs to developing educational leadership for a constantly changing field of medical education.
- *Leadership role*: Proactive leadership by the MEU to steer medical education toward newer directions and pathways across the emerging landscapes of undergraduate, postgraduate, and interprofessional education is an imperative. Medical education should be made more relevant to the student, with the aim of serving the patient and society at large.
- *Change management*: MEU faculty have the huge responsibility of being the agents of change. Futuristic thinking, cognitive flexibility, skills to bring people into effective teams, and motivate them to adapt, change, and persevere with a passion for medical education would be the strengths needed to function at the institutional level.
- *Interprofessional education*: Health is not a singular domain of doctors, but rather a pluralistic concept involving multiple sectors such as nursing, allied medicine, pharmacy, information technology, digital technology, and many more fields. Future of health hinges on the well-coordinated working of all such professional domains. MEU can play a role in bridging gaps and building bridges among such professional domains by designing and implementing Inter Professional Educational initiatives

where students of different streams learn with, from, and about each other. This will help them to understand the high interdependence of their work leading to mutual respect, improved teamwork, better patient care, and relevant research.

- *Networking and collaboration*: Sharing resources, best practices, collaborating on research and innovation between MEUs at local, national, and international level ought to be the strategic direction forward. This would also significantly contribute toward developing communities of practice and narrowing the global north-south divide internationally; and urban-rural divide at the national level.
- *Faculty welfare and professional identity formation*: Moving forward from its mentoring and supportive role to students, MEU can engage itself in faculty welfare and their professional identity formation as medical educators. Capacity building, identifying and nurturing faculty with a passion for education and raising them to become capable torch bearers of medical education in future should be a natural instinct of the MEU. Such an approach would be of substantial benefit to the overall educational and collaborative environment of the institute and thus indirectly to student welfare and their learning.
- *Integrating artificial intelligence*: The limitless potential of artificial intelligence has the capacity to change the very foundation of medical education. Integrating artificial intelligence for personalized learning, with learning analytics to optimize teaching by precisely identifying the specific topic and domain that a student is struggling in and designing tailored learning strategies. Other promising uses can be virtual reality for immersive clinical skills training, blockchain-based credential verification systems, and customized analytical based feedback.
- *Student, faculty, and patient partnership for cocreation of knowledge*: To keep medical education student and patient centric, MEU should lead by developing avenues for student patient faculty partnership. Student involvement in curriculum design or for feedback of educational methods would give the student the ownership of their learning and assessment. Patients can be involved in programmatic assessment, 360° feedback, and in various community programs.

CONCLUSION

With humble beginnings in a purely administrative role of the MEU to being the central driving force of medical education institute in current times, the role of MEU in the future would be more dynamic than ever imagined. However, the distance that MEU can cover depends on institutional support, investment in faculty development for MEU members themselves, and a culture that genuinely values educational scholarship and leadership.

SUGGESTED READINGS

1. Al Shawwa LA. The establishment and roles of the medical education department in the faculty of medicine, King Abdul Aziz University, Jeddah Saudi Arabia. Oman Med J. 2012;27(1):4-9.
2. AlSheikh MH, Zaini R, Abdalla ME. The wicked role of the medical education department. Health Prof Educ. 2022;8(1):3-8.
3. Al-Wardy NM. Medical education units: History, functions, and organisation. Sultan Qaboos Univ Med J. 2008;8(2):149-55.
4. Batool S, Raza MA, Khan RA. Roles of medical education department: What are

expectations of the faculty? Pak J Med Sci. 2018;34(4):864-8.
5. Benor DE. Faculty development, teacher training and teacher accreditation in medical education: twenty years from now. Med Teach. 2000;22(5):503-12.
6. Bhuiyan PS, Rege NN. Evolution of medical education technology unit in India. J Postgrad Med. 2001;47(1):42-4.
7. Davis MH, Karunathilake I, Harden RM. AMEE Education Guide no. 28: The development and role of departments of medical education. Med Teach. 2005;27(8):665-75.
8. Faghihi A, Hoseini Moghadam M, Yamani N. Analysis of the key factors affecting the future of medical education discipline in 2025 based on STEPV model: A qualitative study. Adv Med Educ Pract. 2020;11:191-201.
9. Glicken AD, Merenstein GB. Addressing the hidden curriculum: Understanding educator professionalism. Med Teach. 2007;29(1):54-7.
10. Gruppen L. Creating and sustaining centres for medical education research and development. Med Educ. 2008;42(2):102-3.
11. Hamdy H. Medical college of the future: From informative to transformative. Med Teach. 2018;40(10):986-9.
12. Hu WC, Nguyen VA, Nguyen NT, et al. Becoming agents of change: Contextual influences on medical educator professionalization and practice in a LMIC context. Teach Learn Med. 2023;35(3):323-34.
13. Hu WC, Thistlethwaite JE, Weller J, et al. 'It was serendipity': a qualitative study of academic careers in medical education. Med Educ. 2015;49(11):1124-36.
14. Kiguli-Malwadde E, Talib ZM, Wohltjen H, et al. Medical education departments: A study of four medical schools in Sub-Saharan Africa. BMC Med Educ. 2015;15(1):1-9.
15. Lindberg MA. The process of change: Stories of the journey. Acad Med. 1998;73(9 Suppl):S4-10.
16. Qureshi SN, Khan RA. Challenges faced by faculty of medical education due to the structural variation in its departments across medical colleges. Pak J Med Health Sci. 2023;17(1):148.
17. Rahman S, Talukder MH, Alam KK. Activities of Medical Education Unit (MEU) in medical colleges of Bangladesh and some challenges faced. Bangladesh J Med Educ. 2019;10(2):12-18.
18. Shrivastava SR, Shrivastava PS. Fulfillment of the expected roles of a medical teacher: Role of the medical education department. South-East Asian J Med Educ. 2020;14(2):83-5.
19. Singh T, Bansal P, Sharma M. A need and necessity for faculty development: The role of medical education units in the Indian context. South-East Asian J Med Educ. 2008;2(1):1-3.
20. Srinivas DK, Adkoli BV. Faculty development in medical education in India: The need of the day. Al Ameen J Med Sci. 2009;2(1):6-13.
21. Tassoni D, Kent F, Simpson J, et al. Supporting health professional educators in the workplace: A scoping review. Med Teach. 2023;45(1):49-57.
22. Thammasitboon S, Ligon BL, Singhal G, et al. Creating a medical education enterprise: Leveling the playing fields of medical education vs. medical science research within core missions. Med Educ Online. 2017;22(1):1377038.
23. Varpio L, Bidlake E, Humphrey-Murto S, et al. Key considerations for the success of Medical Education Research and Innovation units in Canada: Unit director perceptions. Adv Health Sci Educ Throry Pract. 2014;19(3):361-77.

CHAPTER 5

Group Dynamics

Vishnu Mohan PT

INTRODUCTION

Medical education, by its very nature, is a social enterprise. Students, faculty, patients, and healthcare teams interact continuously in clinical and nonclinical settings. These interactions are rarely isolated; rather, they occur in groups—be they problem-based learning (PBL) tutorials, ward rounds, interprofessional teams, or research collaborations. Understanding group dynamics is therefore fundamental for both teachers and learners in medical education. Group dynamics refer to the forces, processes, and behaviors that emerge when individuals interact in a group setting.[1]

The study of group dynamics provides insights into how learning occurs in small groups, how collaboration improves clinical care, and how team-based approaches can either enhance or hinder outcomes. For medical educators, the ability to recognize, analyze, and influence group processes can determine whether educational activities are effective, equitable, and sustainable.

This chapter explores the theoretical underpinnings of group dynamics, its relevance in medical education, the stages of group development, roles and leadership, team learning, and practical strategies for fostering positive group dynamics in teaching and clinical practice.

THEORETICAL FOUNDATIONS OF GROUP DYNAMICS

The concept of group dynamics originated with Kurt Lewin, who argued that behavior is a function of both the individual and the social environment.[2] His field theory emphasized that individuals are best understood within the context of their group interactions. Lewin coined the term "group dynamics" to highlight the shifting psychological processes that emerge when people interact collectively.

Several educational theories intersect with group dynamics:

- *Constructivism*: Learning is socially constructed; group dialogue helps learners build knowledge collaboratively.[3]
- *Social Interdependence Theory*: Positive interdependence—where individuals perceive that their success depends on others' success—enhances cooperation and achievement.[4]
- *Communities of Practice (Lave and Wenger)*: Groups of learners develop shared practices and identity through participation.[5]
- *Transformative Learning*: Group discussions can challenge assumptions, promoting critical reflection and professional growth.[6]

Medicine is both a science and a profession grounded in teamwork. Clinical practice requires collaboration among doctors, nurses, technicians, and patients. Similarly, medical students learn in small groups through PBL, case-based learning, and simulation-based teamwork exercises. These activities depend on well-managed group dynamics for success.[7]

STAGES OF GROUP DEVELOPMENT

Groups rarely function optimally from the outset. Psychologists have described predictable stages of group development, the most influential being Tuckman's model: Forming, storming, norming, performing, and adjourning.[8]

1. *Forming*: Group members are polite, roles are unclear, and anxiety about acceptance is high. In medical education, this might be the first meeting of a PBL tutorial group.
2. *Storming*: Conflicts emerge as individuals assert opinions. Learners may challenge facilitators or clash over approaches.
3. *Norming*: Members establish shared norms, trust, and role clarity. Group discussions become more productive.
4. *Performing*: The group functions efficiently toward learning or clinical goals, with high collaboration and trust.
5. *Adjourning*: Groups disband, often with mixed emotions. Reflection on learning and relationships is key.

Understanding these stages helps facilitators anticipate challenges and support groups through transitions. For example, a faculty member may normalize early conflict (storming) as part of group growth, preventing premature judgments of group failure.[9]

ROLES WITHIN GROUPS

Groups are shaped by the roles individuals assume. Roles may be explicit (leader, recorder, and timekeeper) or implicit (innovator, harmonizer, and critic). Belbin's team role theory identifies categories such as coordinator, implementer, completer-finisher, and resource investigator, each contributing uniquely.[10]

In medical education:

- Students may oscillate between active participation and passive observation depending on confidence.
- Facilitators often act as guides rather than content experts, especially in PBL.
- Clinical team leaders must balance authority with inclusivity to promote learning.

Unbalanced roles can hinder progress. For instance, a dominant student may silence peers, reducing diversity of thought. Conversely, absence of leadership may create diffusion of responsibility.

LEADERSHIP AND GROUP DYNAMICS

Leadership profoundly shapes group dynamics. Theories relevant to medical education include Trait Theory, Situational Leadership, and Distributed Leadership.[11,12] Facilitators in PBL must often model adaptive leadership, balancing structure with learner autonomy. In clinical teams, leadership oscillates: A medical student may lead a case presentation, while the consultant steers management decisions. Good leaders foster psychological safety, allowing learners to voice uncertainties without fear.[13]

COMMUNICATION IN GROUPS

Communication patterns define group effectiveness. Open, respectful communication enhances trust, while hidden agendas, interruptions, or judgmental remarks undermine learning.[14]

Barriers include hierarchy, cultural differences, language barriers, and time pressure. Tools like closed-loop communication,[15] Situation, Background, Assessment, Recommendation (SBAR),[16] and active listening can improve effectiveness.

CONFLICT IN GROUPS

Conflict is inevitable, particularly in diverse medical groups. It can be constructive (stimulating critical thinking) or destructive (causing disengagement). Sources of conflict include differing learning styles, power dynamics, interprofessional tensions, and resource competition. Resolution strategies include acknowledging differences openly, encouraging evidence-based reasoning, mediating structured dialogue, and faculty training.[17]

GROUP DYNAMICS IN LEARNING MODALITIES

Problem-based learning depends heavily on group processes.[18] Effective PBL groups show trust, distributed participation, and accountability. Dysfunctional groups show dominance or disengagement.

In simulation-based education, group dynamics mirror real teams. Debriefing allows reflection on teamwork, leadership, and communication.[19]

Interprofessional education (IPE) adds complexity, requiring negotiation of roles across professions. Successful IPE enhances respect and collaboration.[20]

GROUP DYNAMICS IN CLINICAL TEAMS

In clinical settings, group dynamics directly impact patient safety. TeamSTEPPS emphasizes communication, leadership, and mutual support.[21] Poor dynamics contribute to errors, while well-functioning teams enhance outcomes.

ASSESSMENT OF GROUP DYNAMICS

Assessment tools include group observational assessment of learning (GOAL),[22] anaesthetists' non-technical skills (ANTS),[23] and peer/self-assessments. Faculty must be trained to observe subtle dynamics.[24]

CHALLENGES AND PITFALLS

Common issues include free riders, dominance, hidden curriculum, and cultural influences.[25] Educators must actively mitigate these with structured facilitation.

STRATEGIES FOR EDUCATORS

Practical strategies include establishing psychological safety, balancing participation, fostering reflection, training faculty, and leveraging technology in online groups.[26]

FUTURE DIRECTIONS

Group dynamics in medical education are evolving with digital platforms, global collaborations, and emphasis on IPE. AI may support analysis of group interactions. Research into cultural influences and patient involvement remains important.[27]

CONCLUSION

Group dynamics are central to medical education. Whether in tutorial rooms, clinical wards, or virtual classrooms, learning occurs in groups, and the quality of interactions determines success. By understanding theories, stages, communication, leadership, and conflict, educators can harness group processes to improve both learning and healthcare outcomes.

REFERENCES

1. Forsyth DR (Ed). Group Dynamics, 7th edition. Belmont: Cengage Learning; 2018.
2. Lewin K (Ed). Field Theory in Social Science. New York: Harper & Row; 1951.
3. Vygotsky LS (Ed). Mind in Society: The Development of Higher Psychological Processes. Cambridge: Harvard University Press; 1978.
4. Johnson DW, Johnson RT. Cooperative learning and social interdependence theory. In: Gillies R, Ashman A (Eds). Cooperative Learning. New York: Routledge; 2003. pp. 9-35.
5. Lave J, Wenger E (Eds). Situated Learning: Legitimate Peripheral Participation. Cambridge: Cambridge University Press; 1991.
6. Mezirow J. Transformative learning: Theory to practice. New Directions for Adult and Continuing Education. 1997;74:5-12.
7. Harden RM, Laidlaw JM (Eds). Essential Skills for a Medical Teacher, 3rd edition. Edinburgh: Elsevier; 2022.
8. Tuckman BW. Developmental sequence in small groups. Psychol Bull. 1965;63(6):384-99.
9. Wheelan SA (Ed). Creating Effective Teams, 6th edition. Thousand Oaks: Sage; 2020.
10. Belbin RM (Ed). Management Teams: Why They Succeed or Fail, 3rd edition. Oxford: Butterworth-Heinemann; 2010.
11. Hersey P, Blanchard KH, Johnson DE (Eds). Management of Organizational Behavior, 10th edition. Upper Saddle River: Prentice Hall; 2012.
12. Spillane JP. Distributed leadership. Educational Forum. 2005;69(2):143-50.
13. Edmondson AC. Psychological safety and learning behavior in work teams. Admin Sci Quart. 1999;44(2):350-83.
14. Gibb J. Defensive communication. J Commun. 1961;11(3):141-8.
15. Salas E, Sims DE, Burke CS. Is there a "big five" in teamwork? Small Group Research. 2005;36(5):555-99.
16. Haig KM, Sutton S, Whittington J. SBAR: A shared mental model for improving communication between clinicians. Jt Comm J Qual Patient Saf. 2006;32(3):167-75.
17. Thomas KW. Conflict and conflict management. In: Dunnette MD (Ed). Handbook of Industrial and Organizational Psychology. Chicago: Rand McNally; 1976. pp. 889-935.
18. Dolmans DH, De Grave W, Wolfhagen IH, et al. Problem-based learning: Future challenges. Med Educ. 2005;39(7):732-41.
19. Rudolph JW, Simon R, Dufresne RL, et al. There's no such thing as "nonjudgmental" debriefing: a theory and method for debriefing with good judgment. Simul Healthc. 2006 spring;1(1):49-55.
20. Reeves S, Fletcher S, Barr H, et al. A BEME systematic review of interprofessional education. Med Teach. 2016;38(7):656-68.
21. Agency for Healthcare Research and Quality. TeamSTEPPS® 2.0 Core Curriculum. Rockville: AHRQ; 2019.
22. Edmonson KM, Roloff KS. Assessing group learning in PBL: The GOAL instrument. Med Educ. 2009;43(1):77-83.
23. Fletcher G, Flin R, McGeorge P, et al. Rating non-technical skills: Developing ANTS. Cogn Technol Work. 2004;6(3):165-71.
24. Steinert Y. Faculty development in the health professions. Med Teach. 2010;32(5):425-31.
25. Hafferty FW. Beyond curriculum reform: Hidden curriculum. Acad Med. 1998;73(4):403-7.
26. Salmon G (Ed). E-Moderating: The Key to Online Teaching and Learning, 4th edition. New York: Routledge; 2011.
27. Frenk J, Chen L, Bhutta ZA, et al. Health professionals for a new century. Lancet. 2010;376(9756):1923-58.

CHAPTER 6

Systems Approach to Medical Education

Roosy Aulakh

INTRODUCTION: THE POWER OF PERSPECTIVE

Medical education is a dynamic field. It is affected not only by the scientific and technological advancements but also by the evolving needs of society. To produce competent medical professionals well-adapted to these societal needs, medical education must be delivered via a holistic, open framework based on a problem-solving approach that ensures quality assurance through a continuous feedback mechanism. This chapter introduces one such approach—"the systems approach"—that can help us transform how we plan, implement, and evaluate medical education to ensure our students are competent and well-adapted to the changing needs of our society.[1]

UNDERSTANDING "THE SYSTEM:" A HOLISTIC VIEW

In its simplest form, a system is a collection of organized things working together. It can be understood as a conglomeration of interacting, interrelated, and interdependent components (subsystems), whose functioning is synergistic, orderly, and harmonious, all working together to achieve a common goal. The major benefit of systems thinking is in maximizing outputs while utilizing minimum inputs, which is achieved by optimizing the process based on a continuous feedback mechanism. The human body is a perfect example of a system wherein various organs work interdependently to achieve homeostasis. Similarly, a medical college is a conglomeration of units that work interdependently towards the common goal of producing competent medical professionals.

Thus, at its core, any system operates with four broad components:

- *Input*: The resources used in the system.
- *Process:* The activities that convert the input into the output.
- *Output*: The modified form of the input with the achieved objectives.
- *Environment*: The external factors that can affect a system, which can be conducive or non-conducive.
- *Feedback*: An inbuilt mechanism wherein the outcome is compared to the desired objectives at regular intervals, and suggestions for modifications are made to achieve the desired output.

THE SYSTEMS APPROACH IN MEDICAL EDUCATION

The application of a systems approach to medical education is crucial for quality assurance in healthcare, as it employs a problem-solving approach to manage the ever-emerging issues by addressing the interconnectedness of its sub-components to achieve the desired objectives.

Components of the Medical Education System[3,4]

- *Input*: This is what we feed into the system to achieve our desired outcomes.

- *The learner*: Primarily, the novice medical student entering the medical college, equipped with some basic knowledge in foundational sciences. The quality of admitted students may influence the graduate output and thus emphasizes the importance of student selection criteria.
- *Teaching-learning resources*: These are the essential requirements for the educational journey.
  - *Human resources*: Our faculty members, administrators, and support staff. The quality of human resources is thus a crucial input.
  - *Hardware and software*: Infrastructure like wards, operation theatres, laboratories, libraries, medical equipment, the curriculum being adopted, the duration of the course, technological aids, and teaching-learning materials.

- *Process*: This is the transformative phase where inputs are acted upon. The educational process involves three interconnected steps:
  1. *Defining aims and objectives*: These define the expected characteristics of a medical graduate, which are always learner-oriented.
  2. *Planning and implementing the teaching-learning process*: This involves the actual delivery of education across various settings, such as via didactic lectures, small group discussions, demonstrations, field postings, skill labs, or workplace-based teachings.
  3. *Assessment of the outcome of learning*: This involves assessing the learners' achievement of objectives, whether through summative or formative assessments.
- *Output:* The primary output aimed for is a qualified, certified, competent health professional suited to provide healthcare to the community. Other important outputs include the quality of service rendered to the patients, research output, and service provided to society. The medical graduate's competency is continually evaluated by the patients and the society, providing crucial feedback to the system.

The Educational Spiral and Continuous Improvement

Systems can be broadly categorized as closed or open. A closed system has predetermined inputs, processes, and outputs that are not meant to change based on any external input, like a Diwali rocket, which fires once ignited. In contrast, an open system continuously monitors itself and uses feedback-based, timely modification to ensure the desired outcome. Medical education is unequivocally an open system, constantly influenced by external factors, such as scientific and technological advances and the evolving societal needs. Regular modifications based on feedback from these ensure continuous quality improvement (CQI). The relationship between objectives, teaching-learning processes, and evaluation is best described as an "educational spiral" rather than a closed circle. For instance, it was realized based on multisource feedback that medical graduates, being knowledgeable, often still lack competence to work in community settings. Hence, many countries, including India, introduced competency-based medical education. Many new teaching-learning methodologies were introduced under competency-based medical education, the feasibility and impact of these were evaluated and analyzed, and thereafter, multiple modifications were introduced based on a continuous feedback mechanism.

Measuring Success: Yardsticks of a Good Medical Education System

To ensure CQI, the following yardsticks are used:

- *Effectiveness*: This gauges the extent to which the actual outcome aligns with the desired output specifications. Effectiveness is essentially a measurement of the quality of the output. If graduates are competent to practice as primary healthcare physicians, the process has been effective.
- *Efficiency*: This relates to the cost, time, and resources expended to achieve the output. Efficiency, therefore, relates to the quantity of the outcome to the inputs utilized. A college that produces better-qualified doctors with optimal resource utilization is considered more efficient.
- *Openness*: As an open system, a good medical college responds dynamically to its environment and the feedback on its outcome. If effectiveness or efficiency is unsatisfactory, an open system should revise the necessary educational process (objectives, activities, and evaluation) to perform better in subsequent cycles. This responsive, self-correcting nature is crucial for success.

ROLE OF A MEDICAL TEACHER IN A SYSTEMS APPROACH[2]

In the context of a systems approach, a teacher is fundamentally one who facilitates learning by:

- Contributing to the planning and implementation of the curriculum.
- Planning a blueprint of topics, classes, and assessments.
- Implementing various teaching-learning methodologies, such as theory classes, seminars, tutorials, and case presentations.
- Establishing rapport with learners during teaching-learning activities.
- Acting as a mentor, committed to the overall development of their students.
- Guiding learners to become self-directed and lifelong learners
- Keeping abreast of newer developments in their specialty.
- Ensuring continuous personal and professional development.

IMPLEMENTING THE SYSTEMS APPROACH: A STEP-BY-STEP GUIDE

Below is a pragmatic approach to integrating systems thinking into one's teaching practice:

- *Define objectives (what is the desired outcome?)*:
  - *Identify stakeholders' needs*: Ensure the desired graduate competencies align with the needs of patients, the public, and society.
  - *Frame objectives:* Clearly state the specific, measurable, achievable, relevant, and time-bound (SMART) objectives and learning outcomes that students are expected to acquire at the end of a course based on the needs of society.
- *Analyze the current scenario (where are we now?)*:
  - *Identify input characteristics*: Understand the backgrounds, prior knowledge, attitudes, and skills of the students. Consider any common challenges or limitations that may be addressed during the foundation course.

- *Select curricular content*: Analyze the content to ensure the imparting of essential knowledge and skills.
- *Rationalize the available resources*: human, technological, environmental, and financial resources need to be rationally used.
- *Anticipate challenges and limitations*: Consider constraints, such as time, money, and facilities.

- *Design the process (how will we get there?)*:
  - *Select appropriate curriculum*: Based on your defined objectives and learner characteristics, choose effective teaching-learning methods and strategies like competency-based medical education, recently adopted in numerous countries.
  - *Select teaching aids and media*: Determine suitable supportive media and materials to facilitate learning.
  - *Determine and define system elements*: Clarify the functions and responsibilities of all components involved, teacher, student, and administration.
  - *Construct a comprehensive program*: Develop a curriculum, including overall structuring, pacing, and sequencing of content, such that it is learner-paced.
- *Operate and implement the program (do it!)*: Put the planned program into action.
- *Assess and evaluate outcomes (did it work?)*: Continuously evaluate and compare the outcomes achieved against the specified objectives.
- *Analyze results and collect feedback (why or why not?)*: Analyze the outcomes and gather feedback from all the stakeholders, and check whether or not the desired goals have been achieved.
- *Course-correct and improvise (how can we do better?)*: Based on continuous evaluation and feedback, identify areas for improvement. This could involve reframing objectives, revising the teaching-learning methods, or even reassessing students' prior knowledge. Less effective practices need to be abandoned, and better ones need to be incorporated.
- *Quality assurance (keep it going!)*: Continuously monitor the executed method and their utility over time. This continuous quality improvement process ensures that the educational system remains dynamic, responsive, and constantly striving for excellence.

POWER OF WHOLENESS: ADVANTAGES OF THE SYSTEMS APPROACH

Embracing a systems approach offers numerous advantages for medical educators and institutions:

- *Apt goal setting*: It encourages looking at the medical institution as a system with various interconnected units, such that common goals can be set and teamwork and cooperation can be emphasized.
- *Systematic planning, implementation, and evaluation*: It provides a clear framework for planning, implementing, and modifying educational initiatives.
- *Problem identification and resolution*: Helps in identifying issues early, course-correcting, and ensuring the desired outcome.
- *Enhanced efficiency and effectiveness*: It brings better alignment between desired and achieved outcomes via better coordination of various departments and ensures efficiency by rational utilization of resources.
- *Quality assurance (QA)*: By integrating continuous evaluation and feedback

at every step, it allows for necessary modifications.

NAVIGATING COMPLEXITY: SYSTEMS APPROACH IN A "STICKY" WORLD[5]

While the systems approach is a powerful tool for optimizing medical education, we must acknowledge the challenges and limitations when dealing with realistic, complex scenarios or what some call "sticky issues" in medical education. Not all such issues have a clear correct and wrong answer, but rather some common patterns can be identified by introspection. These arise from multiple stakeholders holding diverse perceptions of real issues and challenges. Some commonly encountered issues include agreeing on the need and ways to enhance the quality of medical education, designing and implementing curricular reforms, and overcoming resistance to changes being adopted or implemented.

Such complex scenarios require a pragmatic approach. Instead of simply attempting to find ready-made, easy solutions to such problems, focus on creating a supportive environment where all the stakeholders are free to discuss and give suggestions. This helps tackle the issue collectively and move forward by consensus. One suggested approach is outlined below:

- Ask "What?": Identify the core issue and inquire deeply into what is happening by understanding the perceptions of all stakeholders (students, teachers, patients, and administrators) without being judgmental.
- Ask "So, what?": This is a call for introspection and reflection—what is the impact of the current issue if left unattended? This encourages contemplation and planning for adaptive action, allowing us to implement short- or long-term measures within our sphere of influence, such as serving as a role model or fostering a hidden curriculum.
- Ask "Now, what?": This step prioritizes the action that needs to be taken. The ultimate resolution in complex systems often comes not from hierarchical control, but from the ability to introspect, discuss in a free environment, adapt, and take the best course of action amidst the pressures and limitations.

CONCLUSION: TOWARD A RESPONSIVE AND RESILIENT MEDICAL EDUCATION

The systems approach is a time-tested, powerful framework that helps us systematically plan, implement, evaluate, and refine our teaching-learning processes to produce competent health professionals suited to the evolving needs of society. By understanding inputs, the process, and outputs, and harnessing the power of continuous feedback, we can not only significantly enhance the effectiveness and efficiency of medical training in India but also ensure continuous quality improvement.

REFERENCES

1. Adkoli BV, Parija SC. Systems approach in medical education: The thesis, antithesis, and synthesis. Trop Parasitol. 2019;9(1):3-6.
2. Bhaskar V, Lajwanti. Role of Systems Approach in Education. J Educ Pract. 2019;10(23):104-110.
3. Dilara K. Systems approach in medical education. Nat J Physiol. 2016;4(1):39-42.
4. Oparaji IC, Eziamaka CN. The role of systems approach in educational management. UNIZIK J Educ Res Pol Stud. 2024;17(1), 102-110.
5. Patil VA. Systems approach to Medical Education. In: Vallabha T (Ed.). Being a Competent Medical Teacher. Ahmedabad: Mahi Publication; 2020. pp. 5-10.

SECTION 2

Teaching and Learning

CHAPTER 7

Teaching–Learning Methods for Undergraduates: Overview

Anurag Tomar

INTRODUCTION

Effective teaching–learning methods are crucial for undergraduate medical students to acquire the necessary knowledge, skills, and attitudes to become competent healthcare professionals. Traditional didactic lectures alone are no longer sufficient to meet the demands of modern medical education. This chapter will explore various teaching–learning methods that can be used to engage undergraduate medical students and promote active learning.

TRADITIONAL TEACHING METHODS

Lectures: Lectures are a common teaching method in medical education, where a faculty member delivers a presentation to a large group of students. While lectures can be useful for conveying information, they can be passive and may not promote active learning.[1]

Didactic teaching: Didactic teaching involves a teacher-centered approach, where the instructor lectures or talks to the students without much interaction.

INNOVATIVE TEACHING–LEARNING METHODS

Problem-based Learning

Problem-based learning (PBL) is a student-centered approach that involves presenting students with a real-life scenario or problem to solve. Students work in small groups to identify learning objectives, gather information, and develop solutions **(Box 1)**.

BOX 1: Problem-based learning.

- Small group learning
- Real-life scenarios
- Encourages critical-thinking and problem-solving

Example: PBL scenario:

- *Scenario*: A 45-year-old diabetic patient presents with chest pain.
- *Learning objectives*: Diagnose and manage acute coronary syndrome.
- *Process*:
  - Students read scenario and identify learning objectives.
  - Group discussion allows to brainstorm possible diagnoses and management.
  - Students research and present findings.
  - Facilitator guides discussion and provides feedback.[2]

Case-based Learning

Case-based learning (CBL) is similar to PBL, but it focuses on a specific case or scenario. Students analyze the case, identify key issues, and develop a management plan.

- Real-life cases
- Group discussions
- Develops clinical reasoning and decision-making

BOX 2: Tips for case-based learning.

- *Use real-life cases*: Authentic cases with complex medical issues
- *Encourage critical thinking*: Ask open-ended questions and encourage discussion.
- *Foster collaboration*: Encourage students to work together to solve problems.

BOX 3: Bedside teaching.

- Clinical setting
- Real-time learning
- Develops clinical skills and professionalism

Example: CBL case:

- *Case*: A 25-year-old woman with sudden onset weakness and numbness in her arm
- *Learning objectives*: Diagnose and manage stroke
- *Process*:
  - Students read case and identify key issues.
  - Group discussion allows to analyze case and develop management plan.
  - Students present findings and discuss outcomes.[3]

  Tips for CBL are mentioned in **Box 2**.
  Bedside teaching is mentioned in **Box 3**.

Example: Bedside teaching plan:
Topic: Neurological examination

- *Presession*:
  - Review of anatomy and physiology.
  - Demonstration of examination techniques
- *Bedside*:
  - Student practice with patient
  - Feedback and guidance from faculty
- *Post-session*:
  - Reflection and feedback
  - Further practice and reinforcement

Team-based Learning

Team-based learning (TBL) involves dividing students into small groups to work on a specific task or project. Each team member is responsible for contributing to the team's efforts and learning from one another.[4]

Self-directed learning is given in **Box 4**.

BOX 4: Self-directed learning (SDL).

- Independent learning
- Online resources and modules
- Encourages lifelong learning

Simulation-based Education

Simulation-based learning (SBE) involves using simulated patients, mannequins, or virtual reality to recreate real-life clinical scenarios. This method allows students to practice clinical skills in a safe and controlled environment **(Box 5)**.

Example: Simulation scenario:

- *Scenario*: A patient with anaphylaxis
- *Learning objectives*: Recognize and manage anaphylaxis.
- *Process*:
  - Students assess patient and identify symptoms.
  - Students administer treatment and manage patient.
  - Debriefing and feedback on performance is given.

Flipped Classroom

In a flipped classroom, students learn basic concepts through online lectures or readings before class. Class time is then used for active learning activities, such as discussions, group work, or problem-solving **(Box 6)**.

Example: Flipped classroom plan:
Topic: Cardiovascular physiology

BOX 5: Simulation-based education (SBE).

- Simulated patients or scenarios
- Develops clinical skills and confidence
- Safe and controlled environment

BOX 6: Flipped classroom.

- Preclass preparation
- In-class discussions and activities
- Enhances engagement and understanding

- *Preclass*:
  - Online lectures and readings
  - Quizzes and discussion questions
- *In-class*:
  - Group discussions and case studies
  - Hands-on activities and simulations
- *Post-class*: Reflection and feedback

Competency-based Education

- *Clear competencies*: Define specific competencies for students to achieve.
- *Entrustable professional activities (EPAs)*: Students demonstrate competence in specific tasks.
- *Milestones*: Students progress through milestones and achieve competencies.[5]

Peer-led Team Learning

Peer-led team learning (PLTL) involves training students to lead small group discussions or activities. This method promotes peer-to-peer learning and develops leadership skills.

Interprofessional Education

- *Collaborative learning*: Students learn with and from other healthcare professionals.
- *Case-based learning*: Interprofessional teams work together to solve cases.
- *Simulation-based learning*: Interprofessional teams practice together.

Example: Interprofessional education scenario:

- *Scenario*: A patient with diabetes mellitus and hypertension
- *Learning objectives*: Manage patient with interprofessional team.
- *Process*:
  - Students from different professions work together to develop plan.
  - Students present plan and discuss outcomes.
  - Feedback and reflection on teamwork and communication are given.

Gamification

Gamification involves using game design elements to engage students and promote learning. This method can be used to teach complex concepts or reinforce learning **(Table 1)**.

TABLE 1: Comparison of teaching–learning methods.

Method	*Description*	*Advantages*	*Disadvantages*
Lectures	Traditional teaching method	Efficient, informative	Passive learning, limited interaction
PBL	Student-centered approach	Promotes active learning, develops problem-solving skills	Resource-intensive, may not cover all topics
CBL	Case-based learning	Develops critical thinking, clinical decision-making	May not be suitable for all topics
TBL	Team-based learning	Promotes teamwork, communication skills	Can be challenging to implement
SBE	Simulation-based education	Develops clinical skills, safe environment	Resource-intensive, may not replicate real-life scenarios

TECHNOLOGY-ENHANCED LEARNING

E-Learning

E-learning involves using digital platforms to deliver educational content. This method can be used to provide students with flexible learning opportunities and access to resources.

Virtual Reality and Augmented Reality

Virtuality reality (VR) and augmented reality (AR) can be used to create immersive learning experiences that simulate real-life clinical scenarios.

Mobile Learning

Mobile learning involves using mobile devices to access educational content or participate in learning activities.

ASSESSMENT AND FEEDBACK

Assessing Clinical Competence

Objective structured clinical examinations (OSCES): Standardized examinations with simulated patients

- Short, focused clinical examinations
- *Direct observation of procedural skills (DOPS)*: Assessment of practical skills

Formative Assessment

Formative assessment involves ongoing evaluation of student learning to provide feedback and guide instruction with regular quizzes and feedback.

Summative Assessment

Summative and regular assessment involves evaluating student learning at the end of a course or program to determine whether learning objectives have been met. It identifies areas for improvement, and includes end-of-block examinations and evaluations.

Feedback

Feedback is an essential component of the learning process. It should be timely, specific, and constructive to help students improve their performance.

360-degree feedback: It includes feedback from peers, faculty, and self-assessment.

OVERVIEW OF METHODS

Table 2 provides overview of teaching methods and their advantages.

CREATING A SUPPORTIVE LEARNING ENVIRONMENT

- *Respect and inclusivity* foster a positive and respectful atmosphere.
- *Emotional support*: It provides resources and support for students' well-being.
- *Role modeling*: It demonstrates professionalism and empathy.

CONCLUSION

Effective teaching-learning methods for undergraduate medical students involve a combination of traditional and innovative approaches. By incorporating active learning strategies, technology-enhanced learning, and ongoing assessment and feedback, educators can promote student engagement, motivation, and learning outcomes. As medical education continues to evolve, it is essential to stay up to date with best practices in teaching and learning to provide students with the best possible education.

TABLE 2: Overview of teaching methods and their advantages.

Method	*Description*	*Advantages*
Problem-based learning (PBL)	Small group learning with real-life scenarios	Develops critical thinking and problem-solving
Case-based learning (CBL)	Real-life cases with group discussions	Develops clinical reasoning and decision-making
Flipped classroom	Preclass preparation with in-class discussions	Enhances engagement and understanding
Simulation-based learning	Simulated patients or scenarios	Develops clinical skills and confidence
Small group discussions (SGDs)	Interactive topic-specific discussions	Encourages active participation
Lectures	Didactic teaching with overview of topics	Provides foundation for further learning
Bedside teaching	Clinical setting with real-time learning	Develops clinical skills and professionalism
Self-directed learning (SDL)	Independent learning with online resources	Encourages lifelong learning

REFERENCES

1. Harden RM. Developments in outcome-based education. Med Teach. 2002;24(2): 117-23.
2. Thomas PA, Kern DE, Hughes MT, et al. Curriculum Development for Medical Education: A Six-Step Approach. Baltimore: Johns Hopkins University Press; 2015.
3. McGaghie WC, Issenberg SB. Simulation-based medical education. Med Educ. 2003;37(11):1003-11.
4. Dent JA, Harden RM. A Practical Guide for Medical Teachers. Philadelphia: Elsevier; 2013.
5. Swanwick T. Understanding Medical Education: Evidence, Theory, and Practice. Chichester: Wiley-Blackwell; 2013.

CHAPTER 8

Teaching–Learning Methods for PG: Overview

Sahil Saini, Richa Ambey, Ravi Ambey

INTRODUCTION

Postgraduate medical education represents a demanding and specialized stage of learning, designed to develop advanced clinical expertise, empathetic attitude, critical thinking, research proficiency, and leadership abilities. The implementation of effective teaching and learning methods is crucial to ensure that postgraduate trainees not only gain knowledge but also apply it effectively within practical healthcare environments.

Postgraduate students, being adult learners, have unique learning preferences compared to undergraduates. Malcolm Knowles' principles[1] of adult learning suggest they typically:

- Prefer to take control of their own learning.
- Rely on their past experiences to shape new knowledge.
- Emphasize problem-solving and practical, real-world applications.
- Are motivated by the pursuit of professional advancement and skill mastery.

In the context of medical education, applying these principles leads to more effective learning experiences. Educators should incorporate active, experiential learning approaches to improve both knowledge retention and a critical thinking approach for practical application.

The earlier medical education system in India was structured around a rigid, subject-based curriculum with a fixed timeline. In a teacher-centered classroom, students focus entirely on the teacher, who leads the discussion while they listen. The environment is typically quiet and well-organized. In this setup, the teacher plays a central role, responsible for imparting knowledge and guiding the learning process. The competency-based medical education (CBME) system was introduced to address its shortcomings. This transition has shifted the focus from a teacher-led approach to a more learner-centered model,[2] emphasizing practical skills and competency development not only for undergraduate students but also for postgraduate programs.

This chapter explores various contemporary teaching-learning methods that enhance the educational experience for postgraduate medical students. It emphasizes the importance of adapting to the changing landscape of medical education. It highlights the benefits of implementing innovative strategies that cater to diverse learning styles and promote lifelong learning.

THE NEED FOR CHANGE IN TEACHING-LEARNING METHODS

Evolving Healthcare Landscape

The healthcare environment is rapidly evolving, characterized by advancements in medical technology, an increase in patient complexity, and a shift toward patient-centered care. As healthcare systems strive to improve outcomes and efficiency, the role of healthcare professionals is becoming increasingly multifaceted. Postgraduate medical education must respond to these changes by equipping students with the skills necessary to navigate this dynamic landscape.

The introduction of new technologies, such as telemedicine, artificial intelligence, and electronic health records, has transformed the way healthcare is delivered. Medical professionals are now required to be proficient not only in clinical skills but also in the use of technology to enhance patient care. This necessitates a curriculum that integrates these competencies into the training of postgraduate students.

Limitations of Traditional Methods

Traditional teaching methods, while effective in specific contexts, often fail to engage students actively. Didactic lectures, for instance, can lead to passive learning, where students absorb information without fully understanding or applying it. This approach can lead to knowledge retention issues and inadequate preparedness for real-world clinical situations. Furthermore, the one-size-fits-all nature of traditional methods does not accommodate the diverse learning styles and preferences of postgraduate students.

Research has shown that students often struggle to retain information presented in a purely lecture-based format. A study conducted by Zinski et al. (2017),[3] found that medical students who engaged in active learning techniques demonstrated significantly better retention of knowledge compared to those who relied solely on traditional lectures. This highlights the need for a more interactive and engaging approach to teaching.

The Importance of Active Learning

Active learning strategies have been shown to enhance student engagement, critical thinking, and retention of knowledge. By involving students in the learning process, educators can foster a deeper understanding of complex concepts and encourage the application of knowledge in practical settings. Methods such as problem-based learning (PBL), case-based learning (CBL), and simulation-based learning (SBL) promote active participation and collaboration, allowing students to develop essential skills for their future practice. These methods have proven effective in several reputable educational programs, including advanced life support (ALS) and the neonatal resuscitation program (NRP).

Active learning not only improves knowledge retention but also encourages the development of critical thinking skills. According to a meta-analysis by Freeman et al. (2014),[4] active learning techniques lead to improved academic performance across various disciplines, including medical education. This underscores the necessity of incorporating active learning into postgraduate curricula.

Embracing Technological Advancements

The integration of technology in medical education presents new opportunities for enhancing teaching and learning. E-learning platforms, virtual simulations, and online resources can supplement traditional methods, providing students with flexible and accessible learning options. The COVID-19 pandemic has accelerated the adoption of digital tools, highlighting the importance of incorporating technology into the educational framework. By leveraging these advancements, educators can create a more engaging and effective learning environment.

E-learning has become a vital component of medical education, allowing for asynchronous learning and access to a wealth of resources. Platforms such as Coursera, Khan Academy, and specialized medical education websites offer courses and materials that can enhance the learning experience. A study by Al-Balas et al. (2020),[5] demonstrated that students who engaged in e-learning during the pandemic reported high levels of satisfaction and perceived effectiveness in their learning.

Preparing for Lifelong Learning

In an era of rapid change, the ability to engage in lifelong learning is crucial for healthcare professionals. Postgraduate medical education should not only focus on imparting knowledge but also on instilling a mindset of continuous improvement and self-directed learning. By employing diverse teaching methods that encourage critical thinking and reflection, educators can prepare students to adapt to new challenges and advancements throughout their careers.

The concept of lifelong learning is essential in the medical field, where new research, technologies, and treatment modalities are constantly emerging. Medical professionals must be equipped with the skills to seek out new information, evaluate its relevance, and apply it in practice. This requires a shift in educational philosophy, where the focus is on developing independent learners who are capable of self-assessment and continuous growth.

TYPES OF TEACHING METHODS

Traditional Teaching Methods

Didactic Lectures

Traditional lectures offer structured learning, but they can be somewhat passive. Enhancing engagement through multimedia, interactive discussions, and case-based teaching can improve learning outcomes. To maximize effectiveness, lectures should be concise, interactive, and supplemented with digital resources. Incorporating audience response systems and short quizzes can help maintain student engagement. This approach offers the advantage of efficiently covering a broad range of content and can be delivered to large groups. However, it also has its drawbacks, such as limited student engagement and fewer opportunities for interaction and feedback.

Chalk and Talk

The "chalk and talk" method includes the instructor presenting information using a chalkboard or whiteboard. While this method allows for real-time illustration of concepts, it often lacks interactivity. This method provides the advantage of offering an immediate visual representation of ideas and allows for flexibility in adapting content on the spot. However, creating complex diagrams can be time-consuming and may not effectively cater to all learning styles.

Bedside Teaching

Traditional teaching methods often overlook the invaluable experiences gained at the patient's bedside, which serve as the soul of medical teaching. It offers postgraduate students a unique opportunity to interact with patients, observe clinical signs, and apply theoretical knowledge in real-life scenarios. Unlike classroom learning, bedside teaching allows students to refine their diagnostic and communication skills under the direct supervision of experienced physicians.[6] It fosters clinical reasoning, empathy, and professionalism, ensuring that students develop both technical expertise and a patient-centered approach. This hands-on method not only strengthens their medical knowledge but also prepares them to handle real-world challenges with confidence.

Modern Teaching Methods

Problem-based Learning

Problem-based learning (PBL) is an instructional method that encourages students to learn through the exploration of complex, real-world problems. This approach fosters critical thinking, teamwork, and self-directed learning. In this approach, small groups of students engage in discussions around case studies, with facilitators guiding the learning process without offering direct answers. The benefits include enhanced problem-solving skills and the promotion of collaborative learning.

Case-based Learning

Case-based learning (CBL) utilizes clinical cases to bridge the gap between theory and practice. Students analyze real patient scenarios, which enhances their clinical reasoning and decision-making skills. In this structure, students work in groups to discuss cases, with a strong emphasis on applying theoretical knowledge to practical situations. The outcomes include improved clinical skills, enhanced teamwork, and greater retention of knowledge through contextual learning.

Simulation-based Learning

Simulation-based learning (SBL) involves the use of high-fidelity simulations to replicate clinical scenarios. This method allows students to practice skills in a safe environment without risking patient safety. There are various types of simulation, including mannequins for procedural training and virtual reality for immersive experiences. The advantages of simulation include providing a safe practice environment and offering immediate feedback on performance.

Flipped Classroom

In the flipped classroom model, traditional lecture content is delivered outside of class (e.g., through video lectures), while class time is dedicated to interactive activities and discussions. In this process, students review materials at their own pace, while class time is devoted to problem-solving and the application of knowledge. The benefits include encouraging active participation and allowing for personalized learning experiences.

E-learning and Blended Learning

E-learning incorporates digital resources and online platforms to facilitate learning. Blended learning combines traditional face-to-face instruction with online components. The tools used include learning management systems (LMS) for course materials and video conferencing for remote learning. These tools offer the advantages of flexibility in learning and access to a wide range of resources.

Peer-assisted Learning

Peer-assisted learning (PAL) involves students teaching and supporting each other in their learning process. This method fosters collaboration and reinforces knowledge through teaching. In this structure, more experienced students mentor their peers, with a focus on collaborative study sessions. The outcomes include an enhanced understanding of the material as well as the development of communication and leadership skills.

Observational Learning

Observational learning is a method where students learn by watching experienced practitioners perform clinical tasks. This approach is instrumental in developing procedural skills. In this implementation, students observe surgeries or clinical procedures, with reflection on the observed practices enhancing their learning. The benefits include real-time learning from experts, as well as the opportunity to ask questions and clarify any doubts.

Interactive Teaching Methods

Interactive teaching methods engage students actively in the learning process. These methods can include role-playing, group discussions, and case analyses. The techniques involve role-playing to simulate patient interactions and group discussions to explore diverse perspectives. The advantages include increased student engagement and the development of critical thinking and interpersonal skills.

MENTORSHIP AND COACHING

Mentorship involves a more experienced clinician guiding a less experienced student. This relationship can significantly impact the professional development of postgraduate students. The structure includes one-on-one mentoring sessions as well as group mentoring for broader discussions. The benefits are personalized guidance and support, along with valuable networking opportunities within the medical community.

Assessment and Feedback

Effective formative assessments and feedback mechanisms are crucial in postgraduate education. They help students identify their strengths and areas for improvement.

Formative Assessment

Formative assessments are ongoing evaluations that offer feedback throughout the learning process, including quizzes, peer assessments, and reflective journals. The purpose of these assessments is to monitor student progress and to guide the development of future learning strategies. Regular formative assessments help identify gaps in knowledge and provide opportunities for improvement. Examples are case-based discussion (CBD), direct observation of procedural skills (DOPS), and mini clinical evaluation exercise (Mini-CEX).

Summative Assessment

Summative assessments evaluate student learning at the end of an instructional unit. These can include written exams, practical assessments, and objective structured clinical examinations (OSCEs). The importance of assessments lies in their ability to measure overall competency and ensure students are fully prepared for clinical practice.

Objective structured clinical examinations serve as pivotal assessments in medical education, simulating real-world clinical scenarios to evaluate students' preparedness for practice. The authenticity of these assessments is crucial, as it influences the validity of the judgments made about candidates' competencies. Research indicates that OSCEs designed with realistic, complete cases and minimal examiner intervention enhance students' immersion and ability to demonstrate their clinical skills naturally.[7] However, challenges such as anxiety and incongruities in scenarios can disrupt this authenticity, highlighting the need for thoughtful design to ensure OSCEs effectively reflect the complexities of actual clinical practice.

NOVEL TEACHING-LEARNING AND ASSESSMENT TOOLS

In the evolving landscape of medical education, the integration of innovative teaching strategies is essential to enhance learning outcomes and prepare students for the complexities of modern healthcare. Among these strategies, virtual teaching, serious gaming, role plays, and the use of portfolios stand out as effective methods that cater to diverse learning needs.[8]

VIRTUAL TEACHING

Virtual teaching has emerged as a transformative approach, particularly in the wake of the COVID-19 pandemic. This method leverages digital platforms to facilitate learning beyond traditional classroom settings. It allows for greater flexibility, enabling students to engage with educational content at their convenience. The interactive nature of virtual teaching fosters a collaborative learning environment where students can participate in discussions, access a wealth of resources, and connect with experts from around the globe.

The effectiveness of virtual teaching lies in its ability to accommodate various learning styles. For instance, students can benefit from multimedia presentations, online quizzes, and interactive discussions that enhance their understanding of complex medical concepts. Moreover, incorporating virtual teaching into the curriculum can lead to improved engagement and retention of knowledge, as students are more likely to participate actively in their learning process.

SERIOUS GAMING

Serious gaming represents another innovative educational tool that has gained traction in medical training. These games are designed not merely for entertainment but to impart knowledge and develop critical skills in a simulated environment. By engaging in serious gaming, students can practice clinical decision-making, enhance their problem-solving abilities, and experience real-world scenarios in a risk-free setting. The interactive nature of serious games promotes active learning, allowing students to experiment with different strategies and receive immediate feedback on their performance. This instant feedback loop is crucial in medical education, where timely decision-making can significantly impact patient outcomes. Furthermore, serious gaming can foster teamwork and communication skills, as many games require collaboration among players to achieve common goals. Virtual reality (VR) surgical simulators—platforms simulate surgical procedures, allowing trainees to practice operations in a risk-free virtual environment. *Body interact*: An interactive platform that simulates patient cases, allowing users to diagnose and manage virtual patients.

ROLE PLAYS

Role plays are a dynamic teaching method that encourages students to step into the shoes of various healthcare professionals or patients. This experiential learning technique allows students to practice communication skills, empathy, and ethical decision-making in realistic scenarios. By simulating real-life situations, role plays to help students understand the complexities of patient interactions and the importance of a patient-centered approach to care. Incorporating role plays into the curriculum can enhance students' confidence and competence in handling challenging situations. For example, students can practice obtaining informed consent, delivering bad news, or managing difficult conversations with patients and families. The reflective nature of role plays also encourages students to analyze their performance and identify areas for improvement, fostering a culture of continuous learning.

PORTFOLIOS

The use of portfolios in medical education serves as a powerful tool for self-reflection and assessment. A portfolio is a curated collection of a student's work, experiences, and reflections that demonstrate their learning journey and professional development. This method encourages students to take ownership of their learning by documenting their achievements, challenges, and growth over time. Portfolios facilitate a deeper understanding of the competencies required in medical practice. By reflecting on their experiences, students can identify their strengths and weaknesses, set personal learning goals, and develop a plan for continuous improvement. Additionally, portfolios provide a comprehensive view of a student's capabilities, which can be valuable during evaluations and residency applications.

Reflective diary is also a key method of teaching and learning for postgraduate students.

CONCLUSION

The landscape of postgraduate medical education is evolving rapidly, necessitating the adoption of diverse teaching-learning methods. By integrating traditional and modern approaches, educators can create a rich learning environment that fosters critical thinking, clinical skills, and lifelong learning. The emphasis on student-centered learning, collaboration, and practical application of knowledge is essential in preparing competent healthcare professionals for the challenges of modern medicine, enabling them to perform at their best in a diverse working environment.

Summary points

- Postgraduate medical education is a demanding and specialized stage of adult learning.
- The objective of postgraduate medical education is to prepare competent, expert healthcare professionals for the challenges of modern medicine.
- Traditional techniques provide essential knowledge and personal connections, while modern methods, such as digital tools and group work, offer flexibility and greater engagement.
- Modern teaching methods in postgraduate medical education prioritize active engagement and collaboration. Approaches such as problem-based learning, simulation-based learning, and the flipped classroom foster critical thinking and practical skills. Additionally, e-learning and mentorship cater to various learning preferences, equipping students to navigate the complexities of today's healthcare landscape while promoting lifelong learning.
- Novel teaching methods in postgraduate medical education emphasize innovative approaches that enhance student engagement and learning outcomes. Techniques such as gamification, virtual reality simulations, and interprofessional education encourage active participation and collaboration. These methods not only foster critical thinking and problem-solving skills but also prepare students to address the challenges of modern healthcare effectively.
- Continuous feedback through formative assessments helps track student progress, identify improvement areas, and guide learning. This ongoing process fosters growth, enhances outcomes, and supports academic success.

REFERENCES

1. Knowles M. Adult Learning. In: Craig RL (Ed). The ASTD Training and Development Handbook. NY: McGraw-Hill; 1996. pp. 253-64.
2. Pannala DR, Shyamala R. Evolution of Teaching Methods in Medical Education Over the Years. Int J Curr Microbiol App Sci. 2021;10(11):362-8.
3. Zinski A, Blackwell KTCPW, Belue FM, Brooks WS. Is lecture dead? A preliminary study of medical students' evaluation of teaching methods in the preclinical curriculum. Int J Med Educ. 2017;8:326-333.
4. Freeman S, Eddy SL, McDonough M, et al. Active learning increases student performance in science, engineering, and mathematics. Proc Natl Acad Sci USA. 2014;111(23): 8410-5.
5. Al-Balas M, Al-Balas HI, Jaber HM, et al. Distance learning in clinical medical education amid COVID-19 pandemic in Jordan: current situation, challenges, and perspectives. BMC Med Educ. 2020;20:341.
6. Hennus MP, Ramani S, van Dam M. Giving the patient a leading role in bedside teaching; a truly collaborative and inclusive effort. Med Teach. 2025;3:375-6.
7. Yeates P, Maluf A, Kinston R, et al. A realist evaluation of how, why and when objective structured clinical exams (OSCEs) are experienced as an authentic assessment of clinical preparedness. Med Teach. 2025;3:458-66.
8. Joshi MK. Novel teaching-learning and assessment tools to complement competency-based medical education in postgraduate training. Indian J Anaesth. 2024;68:11-6.

FURTHER READINGS

1. Harden RM, Laidlaw JM. Essential Skills for a Medical Teacher: An Introduction to Teaching and Learning in Medicine. Elsevier; 2017.
2. Spencer J, Jordan R. Learner centred approaches in medical education. BMJ. 1999;318(7193):1280-83.
3. Swanwick T (Ed). Understanding Medical Education: Evidence, Theory and Practice. Wiley-Blackwell; 2019.
4. Dent JA, Harden RM. A Practical Guide for Medical Teachers. Elsevier; 2021.
5. Ramani S, Konings KD, Mann KV, et al. Twelve tips for implementing a mentorship program. Med Teach. 2018;40(2):146-9.

CHAPTER 9

Teaching Skills

Sharmila Banerjee Mukherjee

Learning Objectives

By the end of this chapter, the learner should be able to:

- Explain the evolving role of the medical teacher and the need to align teaching with contemporary learners' needs and alternative learning resources.
- Apply key principles of adult learning and learner analysis to plan teaching appropriate to learner level, motivation, and context.
- Describe essential elements of prelesson, lesson, and postlesson planning required for effective, engaging teaching sessions.
- Identify and describe core individual attributes and competencies that characterize an effective medical teacher, including subject expertise, communication, classroom management, empathy, use of technology, mentorship, and professionalism.
- Reflect on one's own teaching practices, including openness to feedback and self-evaluation, to support ongoing professional growth as a teacher.

The mediocre teacher tells. The good teacher explains. The superior teacher demonstrates. The great teacher inspires.

William A Ward

INTRODUCTION

Let me start by asking you to reflect on two pertinent questions, dear reader. First, do you agree with the above description? Second, do you think that a teacher is great intrinsically (someone described as being a "born teacher");[1] or can be trained to a level of excellence by employing specific strategies and cultivating certain skills? Hopefully, by the end of this chapter, we will be able to answer these queries with conviction.

Now we all know that learning is defined as the acquisition of new or the reinforcement of existing knowledge, skills, or behaviors that lead to an increase in depth and proficiency of the same. This can be achieved through exposure to various experiences or by being taught by an expert. In contrast, teaching is a form of engagement with learners to enable their understanding and application of knowledge, concepts, and processes. So, it stands to reason that we, the medical faculty, are not the only teaching-learning resource that our undergraduate and postgraduate learners need for them to learn and attain various competencies in the medical profession. We have all observed that student attendance in theory, practical, and clinical classes has been dwindling over the years. In fact, it would likely be even less than the current state if a specific cut-off was not being mandated for the summative examinations by the medical council. All medical teachers should remember that with the easy availability and accessibility of a variety of teaching-learning resources at their fingertips—such as scientific texts, offline and online training courses, YouTube videos, and generative artificial intelligence chatbots—the role and importance of medical faculty in students' learning is, from the learner's perspective, gradually waning. We know that this is far from the truth. Our wisdom, garnered from the ability to discriminate between junk and gold, and years of experience, is neither redundant nor irrelevant in the teaching process. Although their perspective is incorrect, we must still establish a connection with our present-day learners. This can be achieved by proactively modifying our teaching-learning approaches to help our audience realize the importance of our experience through our sessions in their journey to becoming competent medical professionals.

First, I will discuss the strategies that one can use to make the content that you intend to teach and its delivery meaningful. That will be followed by practices that can be incorporated into one's teaching style so that the engagement and attention of the learner is sustained. When used in combination, both should make the learner want to attend your teaching session, even if other resources are available.

REALIZE THAT OUR LEARNERS ARE ADULTS

An adult is a person who has reached a certain age defined by law, in which they are entitled to the roles and responsibilities of adulthood.

TABLE 1: Principles of adult learning.

Individual principle	*Learner's perspective*	*Faculty's role to foster this*
Adults need to know why they need to learn something	Why do I need to know this?	Identify objectives at the onset and link them with something familiar and of interest
Adults are independent and responsible for their own learning	I am responsible for my own decisions	Actively involve learners in the learning process. Treat with respect, allow voicing opinions
Adults have different levels of experience that help in the learning process by serving as an educational resource	I have experiences which I value, and you should respect them	Draw out learners' experience and knowledge which is relevant to the topic
Adults are ready to learn things they feel they should know or be able to do to cope effectively with their real-life situations	I need to learn because of the changing circumstances	Respect the reasons for their participation and use them to reinforce learning
Adults are focused on learning information or skills that will help to solve problems with respect to the learner's context	Learning this particular aspect will help me deal with situations I often find myself in	Tell the learners explicitly how the lesson will be of use to them in their work or life
Adults have different types of motivation: cognitive interest, social relationships, social welfare, personal advancement, external expectations, and to escape a situation	I learn because I want to	Recognize the underlying motivation and use it to reinforce learning

In India, the majority of our undergraduate and all our postgraduate learners are 18 years and above. That means we will need to stop treating them like school going students, so that they become as responsible, consistent, and invested in their medical learning while pursuing the course, as they are in cracking their entrance examinations. This can be achieved by applying the principles of adult learning (andragogy) whenever we engage with them **(Table 1)**. The first step in practicing these is to stop referring to them as children and/or addressing them with terms that are usually used for the younger population (something that we all do as a manner of speech). An essential thing for us to realize is that turning 18 years old does not necessarily magically convert a person into someone who has developed the capacity to think maturely. So, we will need to match our style of teaching to their level of motivation and stage of learning. A dependent learner (early in the course or in the phase of understanding a subject) will require an authoritative teacher. An interested learner will need to be taught in a style that motivates them to push himself/herself further and deeper. An involved learner will require someone who can facilitate or help when he/she face challenges while learning. And last but not least, a self-directed learner will need someone who can delegate tasks that will promote and enhance learning.

KNOW YOUR LEARNERS

Before taking a teaching session, you must determine the learning objectives in relation to the content and your target audience.[2] This will obviously differ depending upon whether these are undergraduate students (preclinical, paraclinical, or clinical), postgraduate students (1st year, 2nd year, or 3rd year), professional colleagues, or others; and the phase of learning (early, intermediate, or advanced). The next important factor will be the size of the group (large or small), which is not really determined by a cut-off number. However, the teacher has the opportunity to interact one-on-one with all audience members and clarify their doubts in-depth. The various modalities that should be used for either is beyond the scope of this chapter, but can be found in any standard textbook on medical education.

PRELESSON PLANNING

Be familiar with the setting in which the teaching session will be take place: the venue (classroom, lecture hall, laboratory, skills lab, out-patient department room, ward, etc.) and whether the space will be able to accommodate the number of learners comfortably; the audiovisual equipment that you will be using and connectivity; if any additional props are required (personnel, real life or simulated patients, mannikins, instruments, etc.), and; whether the environment is conducive for learning (lighting, sound proofing, ventilation, air-conditioning, etc.). If the session is online, check the following at your end and the hosts beforehand: audio-video connection, how to share screen, whether your videos run properly or not, who will check and when you will respond to comments in the chat box, the view that will be used while broadcasting, recording facilities, translation facilities, time management, etc.

LESSON PLANNING

Obviously, one must be thoroughly prepared. You need to be familiar with the domain that is being addressed [cognitive, psychomotor, or affective (communication)]; the learning objectives and the teaching-lesson activity or activities intended to deliver each one of these; the ice-breaker/set-induction that will generate inquisitiveness within the learner for the topic and highlight its relevance in a real-life setting.[3] Time management and self-recognition of running at the correct pace so that you do not have to rush at the end because you took extra time at the onset; the strategies that you will use in-between to make it interactive, change the pace and break the monotony (asking questions, using a pop quiz, a crossword, buzz groups to discuss a point, a poll, etc.).[4] The introduction of props at the right time and place in the session content should be arranged in advance. Additionally, the session closure should be planned, possibly by emphasizing key messages, outlining what participants need to cover independently for completion, and providing additional resources for their use. You must also be familiar with the way attendance is being taken.

POSTLESSON PLANNING

This can include a short Google survey comprising a few well-crafted multiple choice questions or short answer questions that will check the understanding of the lesson; any assignments to be completed (deadline and who will check it), and if you want to audit your teaching an anonymized strategy to obtain critical appraisal of the session from the learners regarding the content, and the delivery of the content. The lesson plan can be reviewed by receiving formal and/or informal feedback from learners, colleagues, and self. After all, the best reviewer of the quality of a teaching session is the learner.

INDIVIDUAL ATTRIBUTES

These are a list of attributes and competencies that I believe high-quality teachers should possess or cultivate to enable them to make learning engaging, effective, and impactful; as well as create a positive and safe classroom environment. This has been compiled from a literature search, my recollections as a learner of being exposed to "good teachers" and "not-so-good teachers", the feedback (learn to recognize honesty from sycophancy and focus on the former) that I have received from my learners, and self-reflection (what seemed to work in the session and what did not).

Be a subject expert: Familiarize yourself with the content you will teach and tailor it to meet the learners' needs. The presentation should focus on aspects that learners typically struggle to understand without additional explanations or real-life examples, such as what is relevant in the field and for their examinations. The addition of personal experience and wisdom (always ensuring that it is evidence-based) makes it interesting and appropriate to the learner. This is what will attract learners to attend your teaching sessions despite the easy availability and accessibility of other resources on the same topic.

Good communication skills: This involves both verbal and nonverbal attitudes, starting from having good oratorical skills so that one can deliver content effectively and simplify complex concepts, active listening and the ability to encourage learners to get their doubts clarified, and give constructive feedback after formative evaluation (that does not focus on what the learner failed to do, but identifies the means for course correction so that the likelihood of repetition of the same errors is avoided). Having a good sense of humor helps in building rapport. Along with excellent nonverbal communication, being mindful of facial expressions and body language during the session is crucial, especially when tackling additional issues or stresses.

Classroom management skills: This includes the ability to read the room by recognizing the body language and facial expressions of the majority of the learners (are they bored, confused, getting restless, inattentive, etc.) and adjusting accordingly to keep the learners engaged. You must be able to promote an inclusive learning environment that accommodates all levels of ability. One must be patient and take time to accommodate the slowest learners' needs, who are, in reality, the ones who need you. The smarter ones can learn with or without you. In addition, one should be able to handle disruptors in the classroom respectfully (without humiliation), but firmly.

Empathy: Having a positive, nonintimidating attitude helps to create a positive learning environment that makes the learner feel safe and comfortable enough to express their difficulties. They should feel valued and confident, knowing their doubts will be addressed without judgment. In addition, recognizing that a large proportion of our students are also facing the stress of studies and may not be able to cope appropriately with these, being approachable can be extremely helpful in providing support, giving direction, and averting catastrophes.

Remaining updated with medical education and faculty development programs: This includes knowledge of specific dimensions required as one ascends the teaching hierarchy (curriculum design, exam paper drafting, examiner roles, etc.). It also involves developing leadership qualities that assist in situational analysis, critical thinking, problem solving, and troubleshooting.

Research skills: This includes inculcating a basic knowledge of research in the learners by helping them draft their protocols, supervising the execution of the collection of data and finally completing their theses (including presentation of a paper at a conference and getting their work published); as well as teaching your students how to appraise research papers for journal clubs critically.

Familiarity with technology: This includes the use of educational apps, online research tools, interactive whiteboards, or high-impact digital methods for teaching, grading assignments, and tracking progress.

Mentorship skills: This includes the ability to motivate and inspire your learners to exceed their learning potential. Recognizing the potential in others and guiding them without appearing partial so that they can learn and evolve through self-direction. You can support them in building their curriculum vitae by identifying additional opportunities for academic learning, if they are interested. One may also help in their personal development by teaching your learners to become focused, motivated, and productive.

Organizational and planning skills: Being mentally prepared and able to handle and balance the parallel theory and practical/clinical teaching sessions and assessment of multiple batches.

Being adaptable and flexible: Adjusting to the diverse backgrounds, languages, and learning styles of the learners. It also encompasses environmental issues and technical glitches that may occur during a session. Additionally, it involves the ability to adapt and respond to such situations with dignity, ensuring the session is delivered effectively, either immediately or later.

Commitment and dedication: This is the most challenging aspect because learners absorb values and behavior by observing you, including what to do and what to avoid. Therefore, one must lead by example.

Ability to handle constructive criticism, self-evaluate and reflect: At the end of the day, a teacher is only a not-so-perfect human and, therefore, will commit mistakes. The ability to learn from these experiences and proceed forward is a key trait of any successful individual.

As to the two questions that were asked at the onset, I hope I have created enough curiosity in you regarding this topic, dear reader, that you will now be able to answer both by yourself. In addition, you will be able to rate yourself as a teacher as well. Enjoy the reflections!

KEY POINTS

- Teaching is an active engagement with learners that must go beyond information delivery to enable understanding, application, and professional growth.
- Learners in medical education are adults; applying principles of andragogy and matching teaching style to their stage and motivation improves responsibility and investment in learning.
- Effective teaching requires systematic prelesson, lesson, and postlesson planning, including clear objectives, appropriate methods, logistics, inter-activity, and follow-up.
- High-quality teachers cultivate multiple attributes: subject expertise, clear communication, classroom management, empathy, familiarity with technology, mentoring ability, organizational skills, adaptability, and professional commitment.
- Continuous self-reflection, willingness to accept constructive criticism, and engagement with faculty development are central to evolving from a "good" to a truly inspiring teacher.

REFERENCES

1. Malikow M. Are Teachers Born or Made? The Necessity of Teacher Training Programs. Forum Edu Stud. 2006;16(3):1-3.
2. Burgess A, van Diggele C, Roberts C, et al. Key tips for teaching in the clinical setting. BMC Med Edu. 2020;20(Suppl 2):463.
3. Schwartzstein RM, Roberts DH. Saying Goodbye to Lectures in Medical School — Paradigm Shift or Passing Fad? NEJM. 2017;377(7):605-7.
4. Steinhert Y, Snell LS. Interactive lecturing: strategies for increasing participation in large group presentations. Medical Teacher. 1999;21(1):37-42.

CHAPTER

10 Large Group Teaching

Joseph John

INTRODUCTION

Large-group teaching is a cornerstone of education in many disciplines, particularly in higher education settings such as medicine, law, and engineering. With the growing demands on educational institutions to accommodate large cohorts of students, the traditional lecture remains a prevalent teaching format. Despite the challenges associated with extensive group teaching—such as maintaining engagement and ensuring comprehension—numerous strategies can be employed to enhance learning outcomes. Over the past three decades, significant advancements in pedagogical techniques and technology have transformed how large groups are taught, moving away from purely didactic lectures to more interactive and student-centered learning experiences.[1,2]

This chapter explores the various dimensions of large-group teaching, including its characteristics, advantages, and challenges. It also provides practical strategies for enhancing the effectiveness of large-group instruction by incorporating active learning, technology integration, and innovative classroom models such as the flipped classroom. Finally, we look at the future trends in large-group teaching, considering the rise of digital tools and online platforms that enable more personalized and interactive learning even in large settings.

CHARACTERISTICS OF LARGE GROUP TEACHING

Definition and Context

Large-group teaching is typically characterized by a lecture format, where a single instructor delivers content to a large audience, often ranging from 50 to several hundred students. This format is widespread in foundational courses within disciplines such as science, engineering, and medicine, where a standardized body of knowledge is essential for all students.[3] Despite criticisms that large group lectures are passive and lack interaction, recent innovations have sought to make this format more engaging.[4] Developing active learning strategies and integrating digital tools have helped shift the focus from a purely teacher-centered approach to a more interactive and collaborative one.

LEARNING ENVIRONMENTS

Large lecture halls' physical and social dynamics often characterize the learning environment in large group settings. Large class sizes make it difficult for instructors to personalize their teaching or gauge individual student understanding. This can result in a more passive learning experience, where students listen and take notes without active engagement.[5] However, educators have recognized these limitations and have increasingly focused on creating environments that support interaction through technology and structured group activities.[6] For instance, large lecture halls are being redesigned to include flexible seating arrangements, allowing small group discussions among the learners. Many classrooms are now equipped with technology such as clickers and interactive whiteboards to facilitate student participation.[7]

ADVANTAGES OF LARGE GROUP TEACHING

Efficiency and Accessibility

One of the primary advantages of large-group teaching is its efficiency. A single lecture can reach hundreds of students at once, making it a time- and cost-effective method for disseminating information. This is particularly beneficial for institutions with limited resources, where offering smaller, more personalized classes may not be feasible.[8] Large-group teaching also ensures that all students receive similar core content, contributing to educational consistency and standardization. This is especially important in professional fields where students must master a specific body of knowledge.[9]

Moreover, large-group teaching promotes accessibility by allowing more students to access quality instruction simultaneously. High-demand courses must often accommodate large enrolments, making large-group teaching the only practical option. This format can also enable students from diverse backgrounds to engage with the content at the same level from the same instructor, helping to level the playing field.[10,11]

Standardization of Content and Teaching Quality

Using standardized materials, such as recorded lectures, slides, and readings, can enhance the quality of teaching, ensuring that all students are exposed to the same high-quality resources.[12]

Additionally, the standardization of content in large-group settings allows for aligning learning outcomes with assessments, which is critical in fields where students must demonstrate proficiency in specific competencies.[13] Large-group teaching also supports using technology to deliver preprepared, high-quality lectures, ensuring that instructors deliver consistent content to all students.[14]

Cost-effectiveness

From an institutional perspective, large-group teaching is often more cost-effective than smaller, seminar-based formats. It requires fewer instructors and a single classroom space, which can significantly reduce the overall cost of education.[15] This is especially important in public institutions or large universities where funding may be limited. In addition, large-group teaching often allows institutions to make better use of their facilities by scheduling multiple large lectures in the same space throughout the day.[16]

CHALLENGES OF LARGE GROUP TEACHING

Student Engagement and Attention

One of the most significant challenges of large-group teaching is keeping students engaged. Research shows that attention spans in lectures wane after 10–15 minutes, making it difficult for students to retain information during a typical 60- to 90-minute session.[17] The passive nature of traditional lectures can further exacerbate this issue, as students may struggle to maintain focus without opportunities for active participation.[18]

Many instructors use interactive learning techniques to address this challenge, such as incorporating discussions, polls, and problem-solving activities into their lectures. These strategies help reengage students regularly, increasing their focus and retention.[19] For example, audience response systems, or "clickers," have improved student engagement by allowing them to answer questions and participate in real-time discussions during the lecture.[20]

Lack of Interaction

Another challenge of large-group teaching is the limited opportunity for interaction between students and instructors. In smaller classes, students can ask questions, engage in discussions, and receive personalized feedback. However, these opportunities are often scarce in large groups, leaving students to navigate the material independently.[21] This lack of interaction can hinder students' understanding of the content, as they may not have the chance to clarify concepts or ask for help.[22]

Many educators have begun incorporating peer learning strategies into large-group settings to overcome this issue. For example, students may be asked to discuss questions or problems in small groups before sharing their answers with the larger class.[23] This approach fosters interaction and encourages students to take responsibility for their learning.

Diverse Learning Styles

In large-group settings, instructors often struggle to accommodate their students' diverse learning styles. While some students thrive in lecture-based environments, others may struggle to absorb information without more interactive or hands-on learning experiences.[24] In addition, large-group lectures often rely heavily on auditory learning, which may not suit visual or kinesthetic learners.[25]

To address this challenge, many instructors incorporate various teaching methods into their lectures, such as using visuals, videos, and hands-on demonstrations to supplement traditional lectures.[26] This approach helps cater to students' diverse learning preferences and ensures that all students can engage with the material in a way that suits their needs.

Assessment and Feedback

Assessing student learning in large group settings is challenging, particularly when providing personalized feedback. In large classes, instructors may struggle to keep track of individual students' progress, making it difficult to provide timely and meaningful feedback.[27] In addition, traditional assessment methods, such as multiple-choice exams, may not fully capture students' understanding of the material.[28]

To address these challenges, many educators use technology to facilitate assessment and feedback in large group settings. For example, online quizzes and assignments can provide immediate feedback to students, allowing them to assess their understanding of the material in real time.[29] In addition, automated grading systems can help instructors manage the workload of large classes while still providing valuable feedback to students.[30]

STRATEGIES FOR ENHANCING LARGE GROUP TEACHING

Active Learning Techniques

Active learning techniques have improved student engagement and learning outcomes in large group settings. These techniques encourage students to actively participate in learning rather than passively absorbing information.[31] Examples of active learning techniques include think-pair-share activities, in-class problem-solving exercises, and audience response systems.[32]

Research has shown active learning techniques can lead to better learning outcomes than traditional lecture-based approaches. For example, a study by Freeman et al. (2014) found that active learning increased student performance in science, technology, engineering, and mathematics (STEM) courses by as much as 6%.[33] This is particularly important in large group settings, where keeping students engaged and motivated can be challenging.

Technology Integration

Technology plays a crucial role in enhancing the effectiveness of large-group teaching. Tools such as audience response systems, learning management systems (LMS), and lecture capture technologies have become increasingly popular in large-group settings.[34] These tools facilitate interaction and engagement and allow students to review content at their own pace, reinforcing learning outside the classroom.[35]

For instance, audience response systems (e.g., clickers) allow students to answer questions during the lecture, providing immediate feedback to both the instructor and the students.[36] This helps instructors gauge students' understanding of the material in real time and adjust their teaching accordingly. Similarly, lecture capture technology enables students to review lectures after class, which is particularly helpful for students who may have difficulty keeping up with the pace of the lecture.[37]

Flipped Classroom Model

The flipped classroom model has recently gained popularity as an alternative to traditional lecture-based teaching. This model introduces students to the course material before the lecture through prerecorded videos, readings, or other resources.[38] The lecture time is then used for more interactive activities, such as discussions, problem-solving, or Q&A sessions. This approach shifts the focus from passive learning to active engagement, allowing students to apply what they have learned meaningfully.[39]

The flipped classroom model has improved student engagement and learning outcomes in large group settings. For example, a study by O'Flaherty and Phillips (2015) found that students in flipped classrooms performed better on assessments and reported higher satisfaction levels than traditional lecture-based courses.[40]

FUTURE TRENDS IN LARGE GROUP TEACHING

As technology continues to evolve, the future of large-group teaching will likely be shaped by new digital tools and platforms that enable more personalized and interactive learning experiences. For example, adaptive learning technologies, which use data to tailor instruction to individual students' needs, can transform large-group teaching by providing personalized learning pathways for each student.[41] Similarly, the rise of online learning platforms, such as massive open online courses (MOOCs), has made it possible to reach even larger audiences while providing interactive and engaging learning experiences.[42]

In addition, there is growing interest in using artificial intelligence (AI) in education. AI-powered tools, such as chatbots and virtual tutors, can provide personalized feedback and support to students in large group settings, helping to bridge the gap between students and instructors.[43] As these technologies continue to develop, they have the potential to revolutionize large-group teaching by making it more efficient, interactive, and personalized.

However, every new tool has pros and cons. The introduction of AI for large-group sessions can upgrade the academic connection between instructor and learner, but it will also limit human engagement and linking, so a word of caution. We need to think more in this context, too.

CONCLUSION

Large-group teaching remains a key component of higher education, particularly in fields where large cohorts of students must master a standardized body of knowledge. While this teaching format presents challenges, such as maintaining student engagement and providing personalized feedback, numerous strategies can enhance its effectiveness. By incorporating active learning techniques, leveraging technology, and adopting innovative teaching models like the flipped classroom, educators can create more interactive and engaging learning experiences in large group settings. As technology continues to evolve, the future of large-group teaching will likely be shaped by new digital tools that enable more personalized and adaptive learning.

KEY POINTS

- Large group teaching is critical in higher education for disseminating standardized knowledge to large cohorts but faces challenges such as student engagement and personalized feedback.
- Active learning techniques (e.g., think-pair-share, peer instruction, and flipped classroom) foster interaction and student participation.
- Tools such as clickers, multimedia, and learning management systems enable dynamic and inclusive learning experiences.
- Innovations such as adaptive learning and artificial intelligence promise personalized and efficient teaching in large group settings.
- Evidence-based strategies and technological advancements ensure engaging and impactful large group instruction.

REFERENCES

1. Bligh DA. What's the Use of Lectures? San Francisco: Jossey-Bass Publishers; 2000.
2. Gibbs G, Habeshaw T. Preparing to Teach: An Introduction to Effective Teaching in Higher Education. USA: Technical & Educational Services Ltd; 1992.
3. Biggs J, Tang C. Teaching for Quality Learning at University. Philadelphia: Open University Press; 2011.
4. Race P. The Lecturer's Toolkit: A Practical Guide to Learning, Teaching & Assessment. England, UK: Routledge; 2014.
5. Prince M. Does Active Learning Work? A Review of the Research. J Engineering Edu. 2004;93(3):223-31.
6. Freeman S, Eddy SL, McDonough M, et al. Active Learning Increases Student Performance in Science, Engineering, and Mathematics. Proc Natl Acad Sci. 2014;111(23):8410-5.
7. Nicol DJ, Macfarlane-Dick D. Formative Assessment and Self-Regulated Learning: A Model and Seven Principles of Good Feedback Practice. Studies High Edu. 2006;31(2):199-218.
8. Michaelsen LK, Knight AB, Fink LD. Team-Based Learning: A Transformative Use of Small Groups. Philadelphia: Praeger; 2004.
9. Bonwell CC, Eison JA. Active Learning: Creating Excitement in the Classroom. ASHE-ERIC Higher Education Report No. 1. Washington: The George Washington University; 1991.

10. Chickering AW, Gamson ZF. Seven Principles for Good Practice in Undergraduate Education. Am Assoc High Edu Bull. 1987;39(7):3-7.
11. Smith KA, Sheppard SD, Johnson DW, et al. "Pedagogies of Engagement: Classroom-Based Practices." J Engineer Edu. 2005;94(1):87-101.
12. Mazur E. Peer Instruction: A User's Manual. New Jersey, U.S.: Prentice Hall; 1997.
13. Bates AW, Sangrà A. Managing Technology in Higher Education: Strategies for Transforming Teaching and Learning. San Francisco: Jossey-Bass Publishers; 2011.
14. O'Flaherty J, Phillips C. The Use of Flipped Classrooms in Higher Education: A Scoping Review. Inter High Edu. 2015;25:85-95.
15. Barkley EF, Cross KP, Major CH. Collaborative Learning Techniques: A Handbook for College Faculty. San Francisco: Jossey-Bass Publishers; 2005.
16. Felder RM, Brent, R. Active Learning: An Introduction. ASQ High Edu Brief. 2009;2(4):1-5.
17. McKeachie WJ, Svinicki M. McKeachie's Teaching Tips: Strategies, Research, and Theory for College and University Teachers. California: Wadsworth Publishing; 2013.
18. Terenzini PT, Pascarella ET. Living with Myths: Undergraduate Education in America. Change. 1994;26(1):28-32.
19. Lyman F. Think-Pair-Share: An Expanding Teaching Technique." MAACIE Cooperative News. 1981;1(1):1-2.
20. Caldwell JE. Clickers in the Large Classroom: Current Research and Best-Practice Tips. CBE Life Sci Edu. 2007;6(1):9-20.
21. Biggs JB. "What the Student Does: Teaching for Enhanced Learning." High Edu Res Dev. 1999;18(1):57-75.
22. Light G, Cox R. Learning and Teaching in Higher Education: The Reflective Professional. Philadelphia: Sage; 2005.
23. Bonwell CC, Sutherland TE. The Active Learning Continuum: Choosing Activities to Engage Students in the Classroom. N Direct Teach Learn. 1996(67):3-16.
24. Armstrong N, Chang SM, Brickman M. Cooperative Learning in Industrial-Sized Biology Classes. CBE Life Sci Edu. 2007;6(2):163-71.
25. Herrington J, Reeves TC, Oliver R. A Guide to Authentic e-Learning. England, UK: Routledge; 2010.
26. Pashler H, McDaniel M, Rohrer D, et al. Learning Styles: Concepts and Evidence." Psychol Sci Pub Inter. 2008;9(3):105-19.
27. Hattie J, Timperley H. The Power of Feedback. Rev Edu Res. 2007;77(1):81-112.
28. Wiggins G. Educative Assessment: Designing Assessments to Inform and Improve Student Performance. San Francisco: Jossey-Bass Publishers; 1998.
29. Nicol DJ. Assessment for Learner Self-Regulation: Enhancing Achievement in the First Year Using Learning Technologies. Assess Eval High Edu. 2009;34(3):335-52.
30. Mayer RE. Multimedia Learning, 2nd edition Cambridge: Cambridge University Press; 2009.
31. Kuh GD. The National Survey of Student Engagement: Conceptual and Empirical Foundations. New Direct Institut Res. 2009(141):5-20.
32. Felder RM, Brent R. Understanding Student Differences. J Engineer Edu. 2005;94(1):57-72.
33. Garrison DR, Vaughan ND. Blended Learning in Higher Education: Framework, Principles, and Guidelines. San Francisco: Jossey-Bass Publishers; 2008.
34. Hake RR. Interactive-Engagement vs. Traditional Methods: A Six-Thousand-Student Survey of Mechanics Test Data for Introductory Physics Courses. Am J Phys. 1998;66(1):64-74.
35. Weimer M. Learner-Centered Teaching: Five Key Changes to Practice. San Francisco: Jossey-Bass Publishers; 2013.
36. Novak GM, Patterson ET, Gavrin AD, et al. Just-in-Time Teaching: Blending Active Learning with Web Technology. New Jersey, U.S.: Prentice Hall; 1999.
37. Laurillard D. Rethinking University Teaching: A Conversational Framework for the Effective

Use of Learning Technologies. England, UK: Routledge; 2013.

38. Lage MJ, Platt GJ, Treglia M. Inverting the Classroom: A Gateway to Creating an Inclusive Learning Environment. J Economic Edu. 2000;31(1):30-43.
39. Bishop JL, Verleger MA. The Flipped Classroom: A Survey of the Research. Proceed ASEE Natl Conf. 2013;30(9):1-18.
40. Chen F, Lui AM, Martinelli SM. A Systematic Review of the Effectiveness of Flipped Classrooms in Medical Education. Med Edu. 2017;51(6):585-97.
41. Kavanagh M, Reidsema C, McCredden J, et al. Designing Adaptive Feedback for Student Engagement in the Flipped Classroom. ASCILITE 2017 Conf Proceed. 2017; 47(12):212-20.
42. Siemens G, Gasevic D, Dawson S. Learning Analytics and Knowledge. Philadelphia: Springer; 2013.
43. Baker RS, Yacef K. The State of Educational Data Mining in 2009: A Review and Future Visions. J Edu Data Mining. 2009;1(1): 3-17.

CHAPTER 11

Small Group Teaching

Prashanth SN, Deepti Thandaveshwara, Prabha B Khaire (More), Abhishek Ramesh Jain, Sonali Suresh Purhe

INTRODUCTION

Small group teaching (SGT) has been practiced since ancient times in Indian education systems, including medical education. Historical learning was based on discussions and debates in Pathashalas, Gurukuls and Viharas, where small groups of 8–10 students worked together under the mentorship of learned teachers who were often assisted by advanced students.[1] This pedagogical approach fostered increased student interest, deepened understanding of concepts, improved knowledge retention, and facilitated the development of communication skills and teamwork. SGT inherently develops critical thinking skills, self-directed learning, and robust student-faculty as well as peer-to-peer interactions, providing opportunities for diverse thoughts and the formation of informed opinions.

Over the past few decades, medical education has undergone a fundamental paradigm shift from a teacher-centered to a learner-centered approach, with greater emphasis placed on the learning component than the teaching component. Large-group teaching, the traditional method of delivering content to large student audiences, hasits own limitations. Although didactic lectures can convey content efficiently within a short period, they often result in passive learning and can be monotonous. Large-group teaching presents several challenges, including difficulty in maintaining student attention, limited opportunities for meaningful student participation, and reduced knowledge retention.[2]

Medical education has evolved substantially from merely recalling facts to developing higher-order cognitive skills. Contemporary medical education emphasizes on cultivating critical thinking, effective communication, and the practical application of knowledge in complex clinical settings.[3] The modern concept of SGT as a structured and deliberate teaching methodology emerged in the 19th century. During the 19th and early 20th centuries, medical education remained primarily didactic, relying heavily on lectures and clinical demonstrations.

The evolution of SGT was significantly influenced by the Flexner Report, a landmark study of medical education in the United States and Canada published in 1910, which emphasized the importance of clinical experience and the need for more active learning methods. Subsequently, problem-based learning (PBL) and case-based learning (CBL) were developed and gained widespread adoption in medical education during the 1960s–1970s. This period marked a pivotal shift toward active learning, as educators increasingly recognized the limitations of traditional didactic teaching methods.[4]

The introduction of competency-based medical education (CBME) has shifted the medical curriculum from knowledge-based to skill-based teaching and learning. Incorporating SGT as a deliberate teaching-learning method within the CBME curriculum aims to enhance medical graduates' psychomotor skills and AETCOM (attitude, ethics, and communication) competencies. Medical education now emphasizes effective communication at every level of patient care and throughout the professional career.

Small group teaching is a learner-centered approach that has become a suitable alternative for imparting knowledge and higher-order cognitive skills to medical and other health professional students. The three key elements of SGT are active participation, face-to-face contact between participants (on-site or online via virtual platforms), and purposeful, structured activities.[5] Curriculum and lesson designs must be carefully aligned to achieve intended learning outcomes; however, this dynamic and participatory approach requires extensive planning and preparation.

Small group teaching focuses on active student participation and fosters a social and interactive learning environment. Rather than engaging in traditional one-way teaching, students collaborate, discuss, reflect, and apply knowledge to transfer it meaningfully. SGT plays a vital role in motivating students, boosting their confidence, and encouraging self-directed learning. Additionally, it enhances problem-solving skills, leadership abilities, and collaborative working among students.[5]

The primary highlights of SGT include students' active engagement through discussions, case studies, and problem-solving tasks. SGT fosters interactive learning where students and facilitators collaborate to explore and solve clinical problems, thereby preparing students for real-world clinical settings.[6] Despite challenges such as resource demands and the complexities of group facilitation, SGT has proven to be an effective tool for enhancing both cognitive and communication skills among medical trainees. It is particularly effective in enabling deeper understanding and improved knowledge retention. SGT aligns with contemporary educational theories emphasizing the value of social interaction and experiential learning.[7]

THEORETICAL FRAMEWORK OF SMALL GROUP TEACHING

Small group teaching is grounded in several educational theories that provide a robust theoretical foundation for its implementation and effectiveness:

Constructivism: Learners actively construct and gain knowledge and skills through practical and interactive methods, making SGT an effective framework for active engagement.[8] SGT provides students with opportunities to engage with real-world problems and create their understanding through collaborative discussions, enabling learners to move beyond passive reception of information to active knowledge construction.

Social learning theory: Learning is characterized by interactions with peers and facilitators. SGT fosters role modeling, peer-to-peer teaching, and collaborative learning opportunities.[9] This theory emphasizes the role of observation, imitation, and reinforcement in learning, all of which are inherent elements of small group interactions. SGT facilitates peer learning and allows students to observe and learn from each other's experiences and perspectives.

Experiential learning: Critical thinking and decision-making are paramount in medical practice. Small groups often simulate real-life scenarios and allow students to apply acquired knowledge to handle actual clinical situations.[10] Experiential learning theory posits that concrete experience, reflective observation, abstract conceptualization, and active experimentation are essential components of the learning cycle.

Cognitive load theory: This theory focuses on the limited capacity of working memory compared with the significantly greater bandwidth of sensory and long-term memory. Learners have limited cognitive capacity and overloading them with excessive information can hinder learning. SGT can help to reduce cognitive load by breaking down complex information into smaller, more manageable components and providing opportunities for practice and constructive feedback.[11]

PRINCIPLES OF EFFECTIVE SMALL GROUP TEACHING

Based on these theoretical frameworks, the following principles should guide the effective implementation of SGT:

- **Active learning:** The facilitator should encourage students to be actively involved in the learning process through discussions, problem-solving exercises, and hands-on activities, ensuring that students are not passive recipients of information.
- **Student-centered learning:** The focus should be on the needs and interests of students, creating a learning environment that empowers them to take ownership of their education and fosters autonomous learning.
- **Collaborative learning:** It fosters a collaborative and supportive learning environment where students work together to achieve common goals, recognizing that teamwork is essential in clinical practice.
- **Scaffolding:** It provides students with appropriate support and guidance to help them progress systematically toward learning objectives, gradually reducing support as competence increases.
- **Constructive feedback:** It provides timely and specific constructive feedback to help students identify areas for improvement and reinforce their learning achievements.
- **Assessment and evaluation:** Incorporate peer feedback, self-assessment, and formative assessment to evaluate SGT effectiveness and student learning outcomes.

By adhering to these principles, educators can create effective SGT sessions that promote deep learning, critical thinking, and problem-solving skills essential for medical practice.

GROUP SIZE AND COMPOSITION

The success of SGT depends significantly on optimal group size. The ideal size of a group ranges from 5 to 8 participants, with six frequently considered optimal.[5] This size allows for fruitful interaction while ensuring that individual contributions are meaningful and can be recognized. A varied group composition, including students with different backgrounds, perspectives, and experience levels, leads to more in-depth and higher-quality discussions. Diversity in the group enhances learning through exposure to varied viewpoints and problem-solving approaches.

TEACHING AND LEARNING METHODS IN SMALL GROUP TEACHING

Small group teaching offers a variety of methods to facilitate effective learning in medical education. These methods can be categorized into several distinct approaches:

Problem-based learning: PBL is a form of active learning stimulated by clinical, community, or scientific problems.[12] Here, students work collaboratively in small groups to solve real-world problems or analyze clinical cases. Information related to the case is typically provided to students sequentially (weekly), allowing them to think critically and formulate probable diagnoses with justified reasoning. PBL emphasizes self-directed learning, critical thinking, and problem-solving skills. It is structured to encourage an approach enabling students to understand and practice problem-solving as a team, developing not only cognitive skills but also interpersonal competencies.

Case-based learning: The goal of CBL is to prepare students for real-life clinical practice through systematic exposure to clinical cases.[13] It effectively links theory to practice by applying knowledge to cases using inquiry-based learning methods. CBL emphasizes the improvement of clinical reasoning, problem-solving ability, and informed decision-making by providing repeated experiences in class and focusing on the complexities of actual clinical care. Students analyze patient cases, discuss diagnostic and treatment strategies, and explore the underlying scientific principles.

Team-based learning (TBL): This is an active form of learning in which students apply conceptual knowledge through activities that include individual work, collaborative teamwork, and immediate feedback.[14] TBL develops teamwork, critical thinking, and peer learning—competencies essential in the medical field. Students prepare individually and then engage in team discussions, ensuring accountability while promoting collaborative learning.

Simulation-based learning: This method combines medical simulation technology with simulated patients and clinical scenarios, enabling learners to practice skills before engaging with real patients.[15] This approach has proven effective in reducing risks to real patients while teaching clinical skills and allows for more focused experiential education, leading to improved learning experiences without fear of patient harm. During simulation-based learning, students have the opportunity to repeat clinical skills until achieving competency levels. This method is also effective for developing affective attributes such as communication skills, teamwork, and leadership capabilities.

Role-playing: Role-play is used as a teaching method to impart knowledge, attitudes, and skills across various disciplines and with learners of different ages and settings.[16] It is a form of simulation that focuses on human interactions. A teacher may ask students to imagine themselves in particular situations and encourage them to behave as they believe the person would. As a result, students gain insights about the person and/or situation being portrayed, enhancing their empathetic understanding and communication skills.

Peer teaching: Peer teaching involves a person of similar age or capabilities teaching colleagues.[17] Research has consistently demonstrated that students learn as effectively from peers as from expert teachers, particularly when the peer teacher is recently removed from the same learning challenges as the peer learner. This method builds confidence in both the teacher and learner.

Small group tutorials: Small group tutorials represent a teaching-learning method that is rapidly gaining popularity in medical education.[18] This method is indicative of a deliberate shift from traditional teacher-centered approaches to more student-centered pedagogy, characterized by active participation and autonomous learning. Topics are typically assigned in advance, allowing students to prepare, and in-depth discussions are conducted by the facilitator with students in the classroom.

Online collaborative teaching: With technological advancement, there has been a substantial increase in using online platforms and tools to facilitate teamwork, support learning, and enhance communication.[19] Virtual learning environments provide collaborative online learning experiences and active learning methods that enhance interaction between students and facilitators. These platforms boost student interest and motivation. Students can achieve higher levels of engagement in online environments and learn at their own pace. Social media tools can facilitate team discussions and enable students to share experiences with peers asynchronously.

Discussion-based learning (DBL): Compared with lecture-based learning, DBL facilitates open-ended discussions on a range of topics in medical education.[20] DBL encourages critical thinking, communication skills, and the exchange of diverse ideas, creating an environment where multiple perspectives are valued.

COMMON TECHNIQUES AND SPECIFIC METHODS

Various structured techniques offer unique advantages and customized learning approaches for SGT.

Brainstorming

A tool used to generate numerous ideas uncritically, fostering creativity and broad exploration of topics without premature judgment. This technique is particularly useful at the initiation of group work to encourage divergent thinking.

Buzz Groups

The intensive small group discussion, typically lasting 5–10 minutes, followed by plenary feedback to the larger audience. This technique effectively engages all participants and provides rapid feedback on group thinking.

Think-Pair-Share

Students are paired with colearners and assigned topics or problems. The two discuss among themselves and develop ideas. The ideas from each pair are posted on a blackboard, chart, or digital platform for the rest of the class to view, enabling rapid knowledge sharing.

Snowball/Pyramid

The snowball technique extends the buzz group method. Initially, students pair up to discuss their ideas. These pairs progressively combine to form groups of four and eight, eventually merging into a single larger group. Throughout this process, participants share and refine their ideas. This method systematically builds student confidence and enhances critical thinking through iterative discussion. During the larger group session, each participant is allocated a brief time (20 seconds to 1 minute) to contribute, ensuring inclusive and structured participation.

Fishbowl

Students are arranged in the formation of two concentric circles. Initially, students in the inner circle begin discussing the assigned task or problem while the outer circle observes silently, noting discussion patterns, argument validity, and active participation quality. Subsequently, the roles are reversed, providing the observer group with the opportunity to engage in substantive discussion while others observe their approaches and reasoning.

Jigsaw or Crossover Method

To begin, students are divided into subgroups, each assigned to explore a specific aspect of the topic. Subsequently, new groups are formed, each including one representative from each of the original subgroups. This approach facilitates the exchange of diverse ideas and ensures that information from all subgroups is shared effectively. By rearranging groups systematically, substantial content can be covered efficiently and comprehensively.

Circular Questioning

Students sit in a circle, and each student poses a question to the student sitting next to them. The questioned student answers within approximately 1 or 2 minutes. This cycle continues until the topic is comprehensively covered and all students have participated equally, ensuring equitable engagement.

Horseshoe Arrangement

This configuration combines lecture and discussion formats and is frequently used in workshops. In a horseshoe arrangement, each small group sits facing the front, which allows seamless transitions between formal presentations and interactive group work. Reports, posters, or fishbowl discussions can be used to engage students during group activities, ensuring dynamic interaction and reducing monotony.

Seminars

An interactive experience led by one or two presenters, followed by substantive discussion on a specific topic, combining presentation with interactive dialog.

Workshops

Hands-on experiential learning is incorporated through several methods, directed at developing specific skills or positive attitudes and dispositions.

Mini-projects and Practical Applications

These methods emphasize hands-on learning in real-world contexts, providing students with experience in applying theoretical knowledge to practical problems.

ROLE OF THE FACILITATOR IN SMALL GROUP TEACHING

Facilitators have multiple critical responsibilities in SGT: managing the group dynamics, orchestrating the activities, and promoting learning **(Fig. 1)**. The facilitator in SGT functions as a guide and catalyst rather than a traditional lecturer.

Key Responsibilities of the Facilitator

The teacher in SGT acts as a facilitator, providing set induction and framing for the SGT, and skillfully navigating discussions

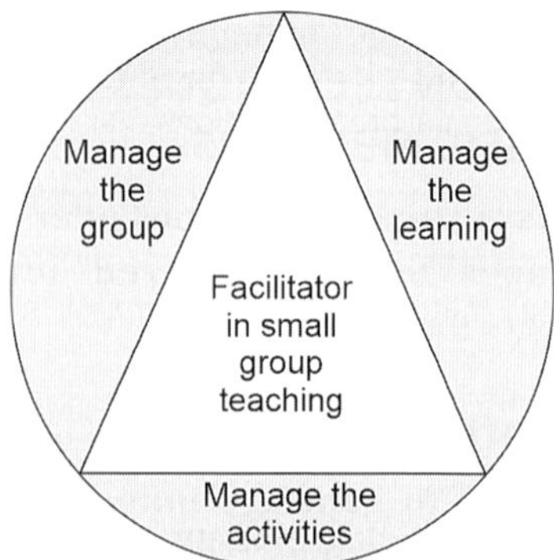

Fig. 1: Responsibilities of a facilitator.

TABLE 1: The TEACHER model: roles of the facilitator in SGT.

T	Task-focused and maintains learner interest
E	Engaged as a facilitator in teaching-learning
A	Adheres to the objectives of SGT
C	Creates a motivating environment
H	Handles group dynamics, time, and process
E	Evaluates learner performance and provides feedback
R	Resource person with subject matter expertise

to sustain focus and productivity. Rather than adopting an orthodox teaching role, facilitators must promote analytical thinking by posing thoughtful, open-ended questions, providing constructive feedback, and cultivating a supportive learning atmosphere. The facilitator should ensure that sessions run on schedule and maintain the flow of content without dominating discussions.

The facilitator is responsible for checking student understanding by asking clarifying questions and addressing doubts in real-time. Facilitators must demonstrate robust interpersonal skills, active listening capacity, and adaptability to varying group dynamics and diverse teaching methods **(Table 1)**. The TEACHER model effectively captures the multifaceted role of facilitators in SGT **(Box 1)**.

BOX 1: Specific facilitator competencies.

- Asking higher-order questions that promote critical thinking
- Active listening to student responses and building upon them
- Managing time effectively while ensuring comprehensive coverage
- Providing balanced and constructive feedback
- Recognizing and addressing nonparticipation
- Mediating conflicts respectfully
- Creating psychological safety for risk-taking and questioning

LOGISTICS AND PHYSICAL ENVIRONMENT

It is essential to plan effectively and allocate appropriate resources to maintain consistent engagement and meaningful participation **(Flowchart 1)**. The physical environment is indispensable for successful SGT. Comfort, adequate lighting, minimal noise levels, and appropriate room layout significantly impact interaction quality and engagement. Small classrooms and simulation laboratories are ideal spaces for group interactions.

Seating Arrangements

Seating arrangements should align carefully with the session's objectives and the type of activity being conducted:

Lecture style arrangement: This formal seating configuration is suitable for lecture delivery. All chairs face the facilitator, who leads the group discussion. While this arrangement facilitates information

Flowchart 1: Workflow of SGT.

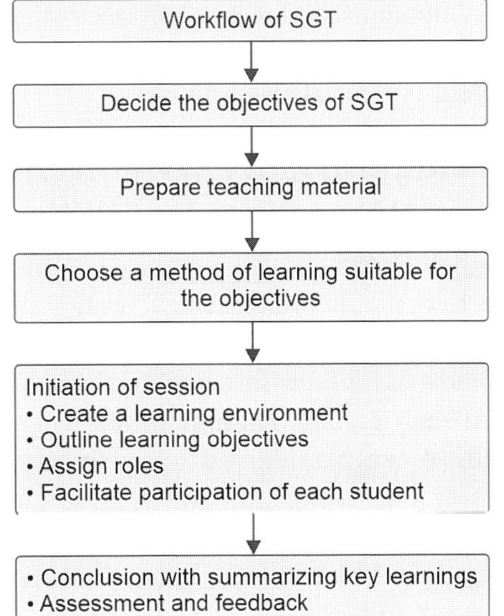

transmission, it limits group interaction and is least conducive to interactive learning.

Group discussion/circle arrangement: This arrangement encourages participation by positioning the facilitator as part of the group rather than as an authority figure, thereby promoting equality and active engagement through enhanced mutual eye contact and opportunities for peer interaction.

Discussion table arrangement: The facilitator and students sit around a table with provision for consulting reference materials and resources. While this arrangement allows for relaxed discussions and consultation of materials, limited eye contact due to seating positions may affect the inclusivity of interactions if not carefully managed.

U-shape or horseshoe arrangement: This configuration facilitates both presentation and interactive discussion, allowing the facilitator to maintain visibility while enabling group members to see each other.

The physical environment, including temperature control can be deleted, acoustic considerations, and technology accessibility, should be optimized to minimize distractions and support focused learning.

PLANNING AND PREPARATION OF SMALL GROUP TEACHING SESSIONS

Teachers should establish clear, well-defined learning objectives before planning SGT sessions (aligned with competencies as per CBME curriculum). The appropriate teaching method can be selected based on group size and learning objectives. Systematic preparation ensures that sessions are effective and aligned with broader educational goals **(Boxes 2 and 3)**.

BOX 2: Presession planning.

- Define clear and measurable learning outcomes
- Select appropriate SGT methods matching learning objectives
- Prepare resource materials and teaching aids
- Arrange the physical environment appropriately
- Brief facilitators on their specific roles
- Prepare student instructions and materials

BOX 3: Workflow of small group teaching sessions.

Initiation of session:

- Create a welcoming and nonthreatening learning environment
- Outline clear learning objectives and expectations
- Assign specific roles to students if needed
- Establish ground rules for respectful participation
- Facilitate active participation from all students

During the session:

- Pose thought-provoking questions
- Monitor group dynamics and address dominance or silence
- Provide guidance while allowing student autonomy
- Encourage peer interaction and learning
- Maintain focus on learning objectives

Conclusion of session:

- Summarize key learnings and concepts covered
- Connect session content to previous and future learning
- Assessment through formative evaluation
- Provide constructive feedback to students
- Assign self-directed learning tasks (e.g., "educational prescription")

Postsession activities:

- Reflective evaluation by both students and facilitators
- Documentation of learning outcomes
- Planning for follow-up or reinforcement

ASSESSMENT IN SMALL GROUP TEACHING

Assessment should evaluate both individual contributions and group efficiency. A balanced approach to evaluation offers constructive feedback for improvement while achieving educational objectives. Formative assessments such as quizzes, group presentations, reflective diaries, and direct observation provide students with ongoing feedback, so they can monitor their progress and make necessary modifications. This continuous feedback is essential for learning and improvement.

Assessment methods in SGT should include:

- *Peer assessment:* Students evaluate each other's contributions, promoting accountability and constructive feedback.
- *Self-assessment:* Students reflect on their own learning and contributions.
- *Facilitator observation:* Direct assessment of participation, reasoning, and collaboration.
- *Performance tasks:* Completion of specific assignments or problems.
- *Reflective diaries:* Written reflection on learning experiences and insights.
- *Group projects:* Collaborative completion of substantive tasks.

While summative assessments can provide overall evaluation of learning outcomes, they should complement rather than replace formative assessment in SGT, which is more aligned with the learner-centered philosophy of SGT.

BENEFITS OF SMALL GROUP TEACHING

Small group teaching has increasingly gained prominence in medical education as it offers numerous significant advantages:

- **Enhances critical thinking:** SGT promotes analytical reasoning by encouraging students to approach problems systematically and think deeply about complex issues. It enables learners to utilize self-directed learning to bridge knowledge gaps. It transforms the learner into a knowledgeable and confident individual capable of independent thought and decision-making.[21]
- **Nurtures communication and teamwork:** Small group teaching enables students to develop communication skills through substantial interaction between learners and educators. The collaboration in groups simulates the team-based approach essential for clinical practice, preparing students for the collaborative challenges of contemporary healthcare delivery.[22]
- **Encourages active participation:** SGT provides intensive learning opportunities with specific learning objectives leading to superior knowledge retention compared to passive lecture-based learning. It enables students to articulate their ideas and perspectives with peers in a safe environment. Learners have meaningful opportunities to provide feedback during discussions, fostering a culture of constructive dialog.
- **Provides personalized feedback:** Based on individual strengths and weaknesses, facilitators can provide immediate and targeted feedback for improvement. This individualized attention boosts student confidence and encourages more effective learning strategies.
- **Develops leadership abilities:** SGT helps students to develop leadership skills as they engage in substantive discussions, take responsibility for group tasks, and support peer learning.[4] Students experience various leadership roles and develop the interpersonal skills necessary for effective leadership in clinical settings.
- **Improves knowledge retention:** Active engagement and meaningful discussion lead to deeper processing of information and better long-term retention compared to passive learning modalities.[5]

- **Builds confidence and self-efficacy:** In supportive small group environments, students are more willing to express ideas, ask questions, and take intellectual risks, leading to enhanced confidence in their knowledge and abilities.

CHALLENGES IN SMALL GROUP TEACHING

Despite its proven benefits, several significant hurdles exist in implementing effective SGT:

- **Resource intensity:** SGT requires substantially more facilitators and appropriate space compared to traditional lectures. SGT sessions can be time-consuming as they require thorough preparation by both facilitators and learners. Sessions may extend beyond allocated time if facilitators struggle to maintain focus on learning objectives. Resource constraints—such as inadequate space, insufficient infrastructure, limited technology, and insufficient trained staff—can substantially hinder desired learning outcomes.[23]
- **Group dynamics challenges:** The responsibility of facilitators to maintain positive group dynamics is of paramount importance. Several specific challenges may emerge:
  - Off-topic discussions that divert conversation from the learning objectives.
  - Dominant participants who overshadow quieter members, restricting diverse contributions
  - Insufficient participation due to member hesitancy to express opinions
  - Interpersonal conflicts requiring skillful mediation
  - Unequal contribution and uneven engagement across group members

  Managing these dynamics requires facilitator skill, experience, and sensitivity.
- **Facilitator training requirements:** Effective SGT requires facilitators skilled in guiding discussions without dominating them and in providing constructive feedback. Teachers must facilitate interactive sessions rather than deliver lectures, requiring a substantial shift in pedagogical approach. Ongoing faculty development is necessary to adapt to different teaching styles, handle diverse group dynamics effectively, and remain current with emerging educational technologies and best practices.[23]
- **Assessment complexity:** The process of evaluating individual contributions and learning outcomes in a group setting is complex and time-consuming. Clear and reliable assessment criteria that are applied equitably must be carefully defined. Both facilitators and students require training in the assessment process to ensure consistency and fairness.[23] Valid and reliable assessment in group settings presents ongoing challenges.
- **Infrastructure and logistic constraints:** Not all institutions have access to appropriately designed spaces for SGT, limiting implementation opportunities.

INNOVATIONS IN SMALL GROUP TEACHING

Technological advancements have introduced promising possibilities for enhancing SGT:

- **Virtual simulations:** Online platforms and virtual patients now allow remote and interactive learning experiences that overcome geographical constraints.[15] High-fidelity simulations can provide safe, controlled environments for skill development and error-free learning.

- **Hybrid models:** Combining SGT with traditional lectures or online asynchronous modules enhances flexibility and accessibility for diverse learners. This blended approach can optimize the strengths of different modalities.
- **Digital collaboration tools:** Learning management systems and collaborative platforms enable real-time communication, document sharing, and asynchronous discussion, extending SGT possibilities beyond physical classroom boundaries.
- **Interprofessional education:** Small groups comprising students from various healthcare disciplines (medicine, nursing, pharmacy, and allied health) foster collaborative skills essential for modern multidisciplinary clinical practice.[15]
- **Artificial intelligence and adaptive learning:** AI-powered systems can provide personalized feedback, adapt content to individual learning needs, and support data-driven improvement of SGT implementation.

RECOMMENDATIONS FOR IMPLEMENTATION

Small group teaching can be made substantially more engaging and effective through careful design and systematic planning. SGT should be integrated thoughtfully and strategically into the curriculum rather than implemented in isolation. Specific recommendations for successful implementation include:

- **Clear curricular alignment:** Integrate SGT deliberately into curriculum design to address specific competencies and learning outcomes aligned with CBME frameworks.
- **Comprehensive faculty development:** Implement ongoing, evidence-based faculty development programs that train facilitators in:
  - Questioning techniques that promote critical thinking
  - Active listening and empathetic communication
  - Group dynamics management
  - Constructive feedback provision
  - Assessment strategies aligned with learning objectives
- **Methodological variety:** Use diverse SGT methods to prevent monotony and accommodate varied learning styles and preferences. Rotating between PBL, CBL, role-plays, and discussions maintains student engagement.
- **Resource allocation:** Ensure adequate provision of space, technology, and human resources to enable effective implementation without compromising educational quality.
- **Student preparation:** Provides clear pre-session materials and orients students on expectations, enhancing their readiness and engagement.
- **Feedback systems:** Establish mechanisms for regular feedback from both students and facilitators to identify challenges and implement continuous improvement.
- **Technology integration:** Thoughtfully incorporates appropriate educational technology to enhance accessibility, flexibility, and engagement while maintaining the fundamental interpersonal elements central to SGTs effectiveness.
- **Attentive facilitation:** Facilitators should listen attentively, question efficiently, and bolster student contributions effectively, rather than merely asking for learner input. Active engagement and responsive facilitation are essential.[24]

CONCLUSION

Small group teaching, through various approaches such as PBL, CBL, TBL, and DBL, has become an indispensable component of contemporary medical education. These methods encourage active participation, develop critical thinking skills, enhance communication abilities, and promote practical application of theory into clinical practice. SGT prepares students to be confident, competent, and collaborative practitioners ready to meet the challenges of modern healthcare delivery.

However, implementing effective SGT requires well-prepared and supported faculty, adequate institutional resources, careful curriculum integration, and a systematic assessment plan to achieve optimal educational outcomes. The investment required to implement quality SGT is substantial but justified by the demonstrated improvements in student learning, engagement, and preparedness for clinical practice.

Future research should identify the most effective strategies for implementing and assessing small group discussions, further enhancing student engagement and knowledge retention. As medical education continues to evolve, SGT remains a cornerstone methodology for developing the competent, compassionate, and collaborative physicians that contemporary healthcare systems require.

REFERENCES

1. Flexner A. Medical Education in the United States and Canada. From the Carnegie Foundation for the Advancement of Teaching, Bulletin Number Four, 1910. Bull World Health Organ. 2002;80(7):594-602.
2. Wartman SA. The empirical challenge of 21st-century medical education. Acad Med. 2019;94(10):1412-5.
3. Sellars M, Fakirmohammad R, Bui L, et al. Conversations on critical thinking: Can critical thinking find its way forward as the skill set and mindset of the century? Educ Sci. 2018;8(4):205.
4. Harden RM, Crosby J. AMEE Guide No. 20: The good teacher is more than a lecturer—the twelve roles of the teacher. Med Teach. 2000;22(4):334-47.
5. van Diggele C, Burgess A, Mellis C. Planning, preparing and structuring a small group teaching session. BMC Med Educ. 2020;20(Suppl 2):462.
6. Burgess A, van Diggele C, Roberts C, et al. Facilitating small group learning in the health professions. BMC Med Educ. 2020;20(2):457.
7. Meo SA. Basic steps in establishing effective small group teaching sessions in medical schools. Pak J Med Sci. 2013;29(4):1071-6.
8. Piaget J. The Psychology of Intelligence. NJ, Totowa: Littlefield Adams; 1972.
9. Bandura A. Social Learning Theory. New York: General Learning Press; 1977.
10. Schmidt HG, Loyens SMM, Van Gog T, et al. Problem-based learning is compatible with human cognitive architecture: Commentary on Kirschner, Sweller, and Clark (2006). Educ Psychol. 2007;42(2):91-7.
11. Young JQ, Van Merrienboer J, Durning S, et al. Cognitive load theory: implications for medical education: AMEE Guide no. 86. Med Teach. 2014;36(5):371-84.
12. Wood DF. Problem-based learning. BMJ. 2003;326(7384):328-30.
13. Thistlethwaite JE, Davies D, Ekeocha S, et al. The effectiveness of case-based learning in health professional education. A BEME systematic review: BEME Guide No. 23. Med Teach. 2012;34(6):e421-44.
14. Michaelsen L, Sweet M, Parmelee D. Team-Based Learning: Small-Group Learning's Next Big Step: New Directions for Teaching and Learning. New York: Wiley; 2011.
15. Silk H, Agresta T, Weber CM. A new way to integrate clinically relevant technology into small-group teaching. Acad Med. 2006;81(3):239-44.
16. Dewey J. Experience and Education. The Kappa Delta Pi Lecture Series. Lonmdon: Collier Books; 1998.
17. Rawekar A, Choudhari SG, Mishra V, et al. Formative assessment in practical for Indian postgraduates in health professions education: A strategic initiative towards

competency-based education. J Fam Med Prim Care. 2020;9(7):3399-404.
18. Jaques D. Teaching small groups. BMJ. 2003;326(7387):492-4.
19. Mir MM, Jeelani M, Alshahrani MS. A practical approach for successful small group teaching in medical schools with student-centred curricula. J Adv Med Educ Prof. 2019;7(3):149-53.
20. Badge A, Chandankhede M, Gajbe U, et al. Employment of small-group discussions to ensure the effective delivery of medical education. Cureus. 2024;16(1):e52655.
21. Jones RW. Learning and teaching in small groups: characteristics, benefits, problems and approaches. Anaesth Intensive Care. 2007;35(4):587-92.
22. McKimm J, Morris C. Small group teaching. Br J Hosp Med. 2009;70(11):654-7.
23. Dornan T, Scherpbier A, Boshuizen H. Supporting medical students' workplace learning: Experience-based learning (ExBL). Clin Teach. 2009;6(3):167-71.
24. Steinert Y. Twelve tips for effective small-group teaching in the health professions. Med Teach. 1996;18(3):203-7.

CHAPTER 12

Competencies and Teaching–Learning Methods

Prabha B Khaire (More), Abhishek Ramesh Jain, Aniket Sarwade

INTRODUCTION

Teaching MBBS undergraduates is a major responsibility which leads in shaping the future of healthcare delivery. The undergraduate phase lays the foundation for clinical knowledge, essential skills, and the right professional attitudes. In India, the Competency-Based Medical Education (CBME) curriculum has brought a major shift from traditional knowledge based teaching to a more skill-oriented, outcome-based approach. The purpose of CBME is to ensure that every learner becomes a safe, confident, and competent medical graduate capable of providing holistic patient care.[1]

This chapter focuses on various teaching-learning methods that can be applied to teach MBBS undergraduates. It highlights principles, strategies, tools, and the importance of student engagement in building competence. Examples of competencies on breastfeeding are taken for easy understanding of aligning competencies with teaching learning methods.

The CBME curriculum for MBBS includes clear, measurable competencies in pediatrics, especially related to newborn feeding and breastfeeding support.[2]

Enlisted competencies on breastfeeding include:[2]

- PE 7.1—Awareness on the cultural beliefs and practices of breastfeeding
- PE 7.2—Explain the physiology of lactation
- PE 7.3—Describe the composition and types of breast milk and discuss the differences between cow's milk and human milk
- PE 7.4—Discuss the advantages of breast milk
- PE 7.5—Observe the correct technique of breastfeeding and distinguish right from wrong technique
- PE 7.6—Enumerate the baby friendly hospital initiatives
- PE 7.7—Perform breast examination and identify common problems during lactation such as retracted nipples, cracked nipples, breast engorgement, breast abscess
- PE 7.8—Educate mothers on ante natal breast care and prepare mothers for lactation
- PE 7.9—Educate and counsel mothers for best practices in Breastfeeding
- PE 7.10—Respects patient privacy
- PE 7.11—Participate in breastfeeding week celebration
- PE 18.6—Perform postnatal assessment of newborn and mother, provide advice on breastfeeding, weaning and on family planning
- PE 18.7—Educate and counsel caregivers of children
- PE 20.6—Explain the follow-up care for neonates including breastfeeding, temperature maintenance, immunization, importance of growth monitoring, and red flags

Each competency should be aligned and integrated with teaching learning method by preparing and selecting specific learning objectives for that competency.

PRINCIPLES OF EFFECTIVE TEACHING–LEARNING FOR MEDICAL STUDENTS

Effective medical teaching follows a few core principles:

- *Active learning*:[3] Active learning emphasizes the learner's participation through discussion, problem-solving, case analysis, and hands-on tasks rather than passive listening. It promotes deeper processing of information, which enhances comprehension and retention. By engaging learners cognitively and behaviorally, it develops critical thinking and clinical reasoning skills. In medical education, active methods also prepare students to apply knowledge effectively in real patient situations.
- *Integration of knowledge and skills*: Learning should combine cognitive knowledge, psychomotor skills, and communication skills. The knowledge gained through theory lectures, books and tutorials should be correlated with clinical findings in patient. This will ensure comprehensive learning of medicine. This also includes horizontal as well as vertical integration while teaching students.
- *Context-based and patient-centered learning*: Context-based learning situates concepts within real or simulated clinical scenarios, helping students to understand application of theoretical knowledge in clinical practice. Patient-centered learning further emphasizes empathy, communication, and decision-making tailored for need of the patient. These approaches develop strong clinical reasoning and foster professional attitude essential for safe patient care. It also increases motivation of student by making learning relevant and meaningful.
- *Feedback-oriented teaching*:[4] Constructive, timely feedback is essential for helping learners identify strengths, correct mistakes, and improve performance. Effective feedback is specific, objective, and focused on behaviors rather than personal attributes. It promotes self-reflection, guiding students toward self-regulated learning. In medical training, feedback also plays a key role in developing clinical competence and professional growth.
- *Multiple teaching strategies*: Every student has specific learning style and he/she learns through different methods. Combining various methods—lectures, simulations, small-group discussions, TBL/PBL, and bedside teaching—helps address this diversity. Multiple strategies stimulate interest and reinforce learning through repeated exposure in varied formats. Blended approaches enhance long-term retention and allow students to develop a range of competencies. In pediatrics, this flexibility is particularly useful to teach both theoretical knowledge and practical clinical skills.
- *Assessment drives learning*:[5] Assessments influence students learning methods, prioritization of study, and the depth of their learning. When assessments emphasize understanding, application, and skill-based competencies, students naturally shift their preparation toward deeper learning strategies. This encourages them to engage with concepts meaningfully, integrate knowledge across topics, and develop the ability to apply what they learn in real clinical situations.

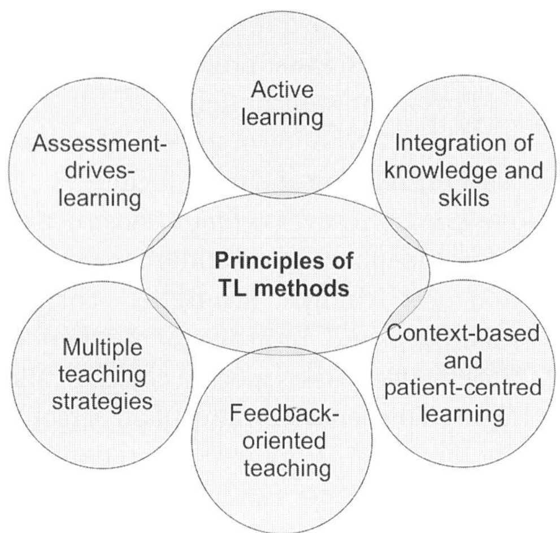

Fig. 1: Principals of teaching learning methods.

Flowchart 1: Methods of teaching.

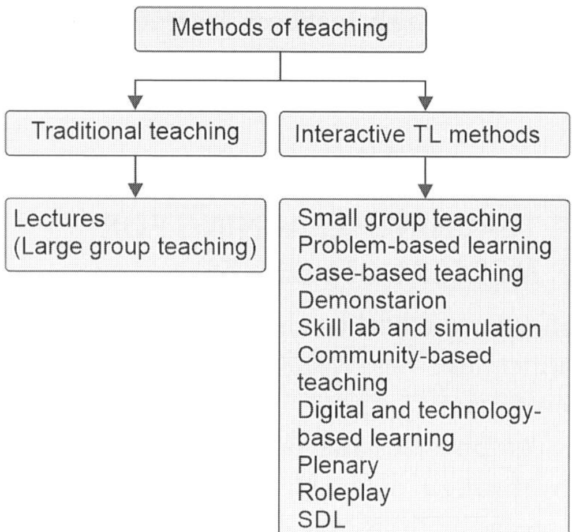

Well-aligned assessment systems thus guide learners toward achieving intended educational outcomes.

These principles guide the selection and application of teaching-learning methods in teaching undergraduates **(Fig. 1 and Flowchart 1)**.

TRADITIONAL TEACHING METHODS

Didactic Lectures

Lectures are one of the most commonly used teaching methods. When used effectively, they provide structure, clarity, and foundational knowledge.

A lecture on breastfeeding may include:

- Benefits of breastfeeding for mother and baby
- Physiology of lactation
- WHO and national recommendations
- Common problems such as engorgement, cracked nipples, and mastitis
- Contraindications for breastfeeding

To increase effectiveness, lectures should use images, clinical cases, short videos, and interactive questioning.

Advantages of LGT

Lectures allow coverage of large content efficiently. It is useful for introducing new topics. Teacher can impart his knowledge through his passion and enthusiasm. Students can learn to extract notes in classroom.

Limitations

It is a way of passive learning. The successful lecture delivery depends on oratory skill of lecturer. Teacher acts as information provider rather than being a facilitator. It is not useful method to impart skill training.

It is difficult to assess individual understanding in the class.

Despite limitations, lectures or LGT remain valuable when integrated with active and practical methods.

Interactive Teaching–Learning Methods

Small Group Teaching (Refer Separate Chapter on Small Group Teaching)

Small group teaching is ideal for learning breastfeeding skills because it encourages interaction and personal attention.

Activities may include:

- Discussing breastfeeding case scenarios
- Demonstrating positioning and latch using models
- Peer teaching of counseling

Small groups help students develop communication, empathy, and clinical reasoning.[6]

Problem-Based Learning

Problem-based learning (PBL) involves discussing a real-life problem such as:

- "A mother complains that her 3-day-old baby is not getting enough milk."
- "A mother with inverted nipple"
- "Feeding a newborn with cleft palate and cleft lip"
- "Counseling of breastfeeding to a working mother"

Students analyze the problem, identify learning objectives, and gather information. This method enhances critical thinking, teamwork, and self-directed learning.[7]

Case-based Learning (CBL)

Case-based learning (CBL) uses structured clinical cases aligned with competencies.

For example:

- Poor weight gain
- Sore nipples
- Neonatal jaundice with exclusive breastfeeding
- Breast refusal

The CBL provides context, improves clinical application, and reinforces decision-making.[8]

Demonstration and Re-demonstration (Skill-based Teaching)

Breastfeeding skills require hands-on training. This includes briefing-demonstration and debriefing.

Steps include:

- Faculty demonstrates correct attachment and positioning
- Students observe
- Students redemonstrate using mannequins or volunteer mothers

This "see one, do one, teach one" model is essential for psychomotor learning.[9]

Skill Lab and Simulation-based Learning

Simulation has become a key component of CBME:[10]

- *Breastfeeding mannequins*: Breast models and newborn dolls allow practice of:
    - Positioning (cradle, cross-cradle, football, and side-lying)
    - Proper latch
    - Hand expression of milk
    - Examination of breast and nipple problems

Simulation ensures safe practice without causing discomfort to real patients.

- *Standardized patients*: Trained actors or volunteers (e.g., lactating mothers) simulate real breastfeeding situations. Students practice counseling, diagnosis, and empathy. They are useful for communication-focused competencies.[11]
- *Objective-structured clinical examination (OSCE) stations*: Objective structured clinical examination (OSCE) is an excellent assessment and learning tool.

  Example OSCE stations:
    - Demonstrate breastfeeding positioning
    - Counsel a mother who thinks she has "insufficient milk"
    - Identify incorrect latch
    - Solve a problem of cracked nipples

OSCE provides uniform assessment and structured feedback. This method needs prior planning, checklist for the station. This also needs more human resources and time.

Community and Clinical-based Teaching

- *Bedside clinics in postnatal wards*: Students observe real mothers breastfeeding, identify problems, and practice counseling under supervision. Bedside teaching enhances clinical skills, communication, and real-world understanding.[12]
- *Community visits*: Students visit anganwadis, nutrition rehabilitation centers, and immunization clinics to understand breastfeeding practices at community level. This builds cultural sensitivity and sociobehavioral competence.[13]
- *Breastfeeding week activities (outreach activity learning)*: Participation in events such as World Breastfeeding Week improves knowledge, awareness, advocacy, and leadership skills of the students.

Digital and Technology-enabled Learning

- *E-learning modules*: Videos, animations, and interactive modules help students learn:
  - Physiology of milk production
  - Importance of colostrum
  - Management of breastfeeding challenges
- *Virtual case discussions*: Telemedicine and video-based case discussions allow students to observe real counseling sessions.
- *Mobile Apps*: Apps developed by WHO, UNICEF, and national programs provide guidelines, checklists, and counseling tips for students.[14]

Technology supports flexible, self-directed learning, and revision.

Plenary Session

It helps the students and teachers to interact and discuss the objectives of the session. It also emphasizes what the students learned. During the lesson students review, briefs and reflects on their learning. This helps to find learning gaps and deep learning of the subject.

Roleplay

It recreates practical breastfeeding scenarios, allowing students to develop counseling skills with mothers and their relatives in both one-to-one and group settings. This method also promotes meaningful social engagement and strengthens their insight into cultural beliefs.

Self-directed Learning

Self-directed learning helps medical undergraduates develop confidence and competence in breastfeeding education by prompting them to identify knowledge gaps, seek reliable information, and manage their own learning. By promoting autonomy and aligning with competency-based training, it prepares future doctors to deliver individualized breastfeeding support.

How to plan a SDL:

- Decide topic/subtopic of SDL
- Provide authentic information (textbook, videos, guidelines, and meeting experts) before 2 weeks of scheduled session
- Plan review discussion with students
- Provide feedback

Competency-based Assessment Methods

Assessment is an essential part of learning. CBME recommends multiple, formative, and low-stakes assessments.

Direct Observation of Procedural Skills

Faculty observes and rates students performing skills like breastfeeding counseling.[15] Immediate feedback improves performance.

Mini-CEX (Clinical Evaluation Exercise)

Short assessments during ward postings help evaluate communication, problem-solving, and professionalism.[16]

OSCE and Skills Assessment

Structured stations assess practical competencies.

Viva Voce and Oral Exams

Used to test conceptual clarity and ability to explain breastfeeding issues.

Reflective Writing

Students write reflections on clinical encounters. Helps develop empathy and self-awareness.

Logbooks and Portfolios

Students document their learning experiences, skills performed, and feedback received. This ensures accountability and continuity of learning.

EFFECTIVE COUNSELING TRAINING FOR BREASTFEEDING

Breastfeeding counseling is a core soft skill. Teaching methods must include:

- Roleplay sessions by students
- Communication skill workshops different learning opportunity like clinical posting in pediatrics, OBGY, and community medicine
- Motivational interviewing techniques (PNC clinic, immunization clinic, women forum, and Anganwadi)[17]
- Cultural and emotional sensitivity training (Nukkad natak, Jagran, Jatra, and religious events)

Students should learn how to:

- Encourage exclusive breastfeeding
- Address myths and misconceptions
- Provide solutions for common problems
- Counsel families and caregivers

Good counseling skills help students develop confidence and professionalism.

Every teaching method has its pros and cons along with specific challenges.

Challenges in teaching breastfeeding to undergraduates are as follows.

- Limited faculty time in busy clinical settings
- Large student numbers
- Variations in breastfeeding knowledge among mothers
- Cultural barriers to discussing feeding practices
- Limited simulation resources
- Motivation of teacher and learners

These challenges can be overcome with structured planning, integration of technology, and faculty development programs **(Table 1)**.

CONCLUSION

By using competency-based, student-centered, and interactive teaching–learning strategies, educators can ensure that medical graduates acquire the essential knowledge, skills, and professional attitudes necessary to support breastfeeding mothers and contribute meaningfully to child health.

TABLE 1: Examples of competency and aligned teaching learning method.

	Competency	*Domain*	*Suggested TL methods*
PE 7.4	Describe the composition and types of breast milk and discuss the differences between cow's milk and human milk. Specific learning objectives include: • Describe composition of human milk. • Describe composition of cow's milk. • Enumerate differences between human and cow's milk.	Knows	Lectures, SDL, plenary, SGT, Lectures, SDL, plenary, SGT Videos, plenary, SGD, roleplay
PE 7.7	Perform breast examination and Identify common problems during lactation, such as retracted nipples, cracked nipples, breast engorgement, breast abscess Specific learning objectives include		
	1. Enumerate common problems in the mother during lactation.	Knows	Lecture, SGT, SGD, SDL, bed side clinic, problem-based learning
	2. Examine breast of a lactating mother in an appropriate manner.	Shows how	Skill lab, simulation, case based learning, and DOAP
	3. Identify the common problems after examining the breasting lactating mother viz retracted nipples, cracked nipples, breast engorgement, breast abscess.	Knows, shows how	Skill lab, simulation, case based learning, DOAP, digital/technology-based learning, and problem-based learning
PE 7.9	Educate and counsel mothers for best practices in breastfeeding. Specific learning objectives include:		
	1. Enumerate the best breastfeeding practices.	Knows	Lecture, SGT, SGD, SDL, Bedside clinic, case-based learning, roleplay
	2. Educate mothers for the best breastfeeding practices.	Shows how	Skill lab, simulation, case-based learning, DOAP, roleplay, SGD, plenary discussion, and community-based teaching

The success of teaching lies in selecting appropriate TL method for a specific competency.

REFERENCES

1. Bhutani N, Arora D, Bhutani N. Competency-Based Medical Education in India: A Brief Review. Int J Recent Innov Med Clin Res. 2020;2(2):64-70.
2. National Medical Commission (India). Competency Based Undergraduate Curriculum for the Indian Medical Graduate. New Delhi: NMC; 2018.
3. Prince M. Does active learning work? A review of the research. J Engineer Edu. 2004;93(3):223-31.
4. Hattie J, Timperley H. The power of feedback. Rev Edu Res. 2007;77(1):81-112.
5. Wormald BW, Schoeman S, Somasunderam A, et al. Assessment drives learning: an unavoidable truth? Anat Sci Educ. 2009;2(5):199-204.

6. Steinert Y. Student perceptions of effective small group teaching. Med Educ. 2004;38(3):286-93.
7. Jaganathan S, Bhuminathan S, Ramesh M. Problem-Based Learning - An Overview. J Pharm Bioallied Sci. 2024;16(Suppl 2):S1435-7.
8. Thistlethwaite J, Davies D, Ekeocha S, et al. The effectiveness of case-based learning in health professional education: a BEME systematic review. Med Teach. 2012;34(6):e421-44.
9. McGaghie WC. Mastery learning: it works. Acad Med. 2015;90(1):1-7.
10. Sawyer T, White M, Zaveri P, et al. Learn, see, practice, prove, do, maintain: an evidence-based pedagogical framework for procedural training. Med Teach. 2016;38(1):56-61.
11. Cleland JA, Abe K, Rethans JJ. The use of simulated patients in medical education: AMEE Guide No. 42. Med Edu. 2009;43(9): 1037-44.
12. Ramani S, Leinster S. Clinical teaching: AMEE Guide No. 34. Med Teach. 2008;30(4):347-64.
13. Park K. Park's Textbook of Preventive and Social Medicine. 26th ed. Jabalpur: Banarsidas Bhanot Publishers; 2021.
14. United Nations Children's Fund (UNICEF). UNICEF App Catalogue: Tools for Children, Adolescents, Caregivers, and Frontline Workers. New York: UNICEF; 2024.
15. Ruiz JG, Mintzer MJ, Leipzig RM. The impact of e-learning in medical education. Acad Med. 2006;81(3):207-12.
16. Norcini J. The power of workplace-based assessment. Med Teach. 2007;29:855-71
17. Miller WR, Rose GS. Toward a theory of motivational interviewing. Am Psychol. 2009;64(6):527-37.

CHAPTER 13

Learners Need

Tushar Bharat Jagzape, Arunita Tushar Jagzape

Learning Objectives

- Define the concept of "learners' needs" and explain the purpose of needs assessment.
- Describe the stages of needs assessment in curriculum planning.
- Describe the learner characteristics, styles, environment, and other strategies.
- Differentiate between formal and informal methods of needs assessment suitable for diverse learning environments, including those in LMICs.
- Use of assessment, feedback, and evaluation to refine learner needs.
- Describe the construct of personal learning plans and support of struggling learners.

The needs of the many out-weight the needs of the few.

INTRODUCTION

Need assessment is the first and an integral step during development of curriculum. In order to develop a right training program or curriculum the program developer in case of medical education, the educator must be aware of the deficiencies of the targeted audience.[1] Witkin and Altschuld have defined need as the "discrepancy or gap" between "what is" and "what should be". The gap between the current status and the desired outcome is the need(s).[2] Learners' need assessment is a critical and challenging part of any program related to education. It is a cyclic and dynamic process that occurs throughout the program. This process needs active participation of both the learners and instructors and includes lot of variables. It is not a onetime exercise but a continuous and dynamic process. It starts with the planning and designing phase of the curriculum, setting the objectives, methods of teaching learning to achieve those objectives, assessment, mentoring and finally evaluation of the program and adjusting. Without considering the learning needs, none of the above processes can be carried out.[3]

Let us go through the need assessment during various stages:

- Planning
- Learning
- Assessment

PLANNING

"If you fail to plan, you are planning to fail."

This stage deals with the what, how, and when of the curriculum, i.e., what the learners need to learn, how they will learn and when and how will the assessment be carried out. Well-written learning objectives identified though the need assessment helps faculty and students to achieve these objectives.

- *Need assessment*: The first step is to have clear idea/information about the base line knowledge or skills of the learner. What is the gap to achieve the expected objectives and according to this the intervention to be applied.[4] Too much of dependence on formal need assessment might lead to narrow and instrumental educational process. It should keep in mind educational objectives which are in turn linked with the health needs of the community.[5]

- The process of need assessment can be divided into different stages.[6] In the first stage it is decided from whom the data should be collected (participants), how it should be collected and how it should be analyzed? Actual data collection occurs in the second stage. Both qualitative and quantitative data is gathered. Based on the type of data generated statistical methods are used for the analysis in the third stage. Finally, the result of the data analysis is presented in the appropriate format based on the intended audience.[3]
- *Outcomes of the educational program:* From the information obtained from need assessment the planners can identify the gap and decide on the outcomes of the learning program. Clearly stated learning outcomes are helpful for the students themselves to manage their own learning. Separate outcomes should be specified in relation to the different domains of learning, i.e., knowledge, skills and attitudes.[7]
- *Learning plans for the individual:* Personal learning plans gives the autonomy to the learner over their learning needs and outcomes, i.e., what to learn and how to learn. For this type of planning to be effective clear guidance and timely feedback from the mentors or facilitators is very essential.[7]

LEARNING

- *Depth of learning:* Learning can be surface or deep. Memorization of discrete data without integration with the concepts is the superficial learning. When the learners use the new information to add on to their existing knowledge and understand and develop the concepts, it is called deep learning.[8] A great deal of motivation, efforts and flexibility is required on part of both the student and teacher for developing active, critical and self-regulating learning habits. Transition to active learning needs continuous monitoring from the educators as they have to first assess the students' readiness for active learning. They also have to understand how to encourage active learning and critical thinking skills and keep a vigil to identify students who find it difficult to transit and to active learning and also should have strategies to support these individuals.[3]
- *Styles of learning:* Different individuals have different learning styles. There are various tools to identify the learning style of an individual student like the Myers Brigg Type Indicator, Kolb's learning styles Inventory, the VARK inventory, i.e., visual, audio, read/write, kinetic. Many time it is not possible to categorize into one learning style. The learning style may change over time, context and circumstances or the individual may be multimodal. Students do have different learning preferences and providing resources in different modes gives options to the learner to choose as per their preference. They may benefit from the variety of exposure. Learners also get a sense of autonomy and habit of self-regulated learning.[3,9]

- *Strategies for study:* The learning style has a great influence on the selection of learning strategies. Strategies include discussion, listening, diagramming (physical or mental drawing), mnemonics and other memory devices, hands on rehearsal (developing both mental and physical memory), concept building etc.[10] Learning environment like location, group versus solitary, privacy, noise level, time spent by the student on learning, time of day, time available for study.[10] If the student fails to apply his or her metacognitive skills, then this can lead to choosing an in-appropriate learning strategy. The instructor in such cases may help the student to comprehend and understand the connection between various factors mentioned above by providing timely and effective feedback, motivational support, and a role model.[3]
  - *Environment for learning:* It is well documented that the physical (space, laboratory, campus, library) and intellectual (personal, emotional, and intellectual) learning environment's significantly affects the learning in medical education. Context is essential for situational or experiential learning. The most challenging and authentic environment is the clinical environment. Patient care takes priority over clinical training when in real world there is a conflict between the two. Simulation has a significant role for training in such situation. The transition to clinical training can sometimes be stressful for the students.[11]

ASSESSMENT

Assessment drives learning or in other words, students learn what is assessed. Similarly by communicating the important curricular outcomes, assessment also drives the curriculum. In order to enable students to assess their learning and address any short comings they should be provided with a feedback, against which their progress could be compared. Let us have a look on these assessments or feedbacks in a bit details.

- *Formative assessment/feedback:* The formative feedback is provided to the learner so that they can analyze their own strengths and weaknesses. Medical students often complain that they are not given sufficient feedback. One of the important reason for this complaint is that many times the learners are not able to recognize and understand that they are being given feedback. This is in turn due to failure of the educators to provide an effective feedback.[12] There are few points which should be considered during providing feedback. It can be provided in PNP (Positive Negative positive) format. It should be well timed, based on the direct observation about the specific behaviors. It should not address intentions, but address the decision and actions. It should be in a non-judgmental manner and descriptive. Most importantly it should be a dialog between learner and teacher.
- *Summative feedback or assessment:* It involves certification of student's achievement with respect to the agreed standards. It decides whether the student has passes or failed. Depending on the complexity of learning to be assessed, it is difficult to establish standards of accurately measuring the learning. Hence the grade assigned may not be a true representation of the achievement of the student. It is difficult to have a standardized and coherent scoring system for assessment in clinical settings.[3] Experts have recommended using a mix

of different methods to assess the clinical skills. This will ensure that there are enough observations to make a valid and reliable judgement. Adequate training of the assessors or clinical supervisors will standardize the assessment.[13]

Almost 46 different methods of need assessments are given in the good CPD guide both formal and informal. Various methods or instruments used for assessment in different context are given below. A detailed description of each method is beyond the scope of this chapter and may be found in respective chapters:

1. *Written examination:* This is one of the most common employed method of assessment. The written examination questions can be broadly classified as supply type, which include traditional or modified essay questions, short answers etc. or the selection type which include various types of multiple choice questions(MCQ). Each of the question type has its advantage and disadvantage. MCQs are being used very commonly in assessment. MCQs can be tailor made with respect to the specific learning objectives and can be used for both formative and summative assessment and providing feedback to the learners regarding their strengths and weaknesses.[3]
2. *Assessment in the classroom:* The various techniques of assessment in the classroom can be used to monitor students learning against the objectives of the course. Classroom assessment techniques (CAT) are formative assessment methods more focused on learning. The *one minute paper* (what was the most important learning point from the class), the *muddiest point* (what was the confusing point?) are some specific techniques used for classroom assessment.[14] Information from the CA can be used to modify the teaching during the class itself. The teacher should provide feedback to the students from the information obtained and should be willing to modify the teaching/learning approach based on the assessment. This is one of the most important advantages of CAT as information obtained from the standard testing is acquired after a significant delay.
3. *Workplace assessment:* These methods provide opportunity to assess the students in authentic settings like clinics, wards, or emergency with respect to their skills, critical knowledge, and behaviors. The variety of methods used to do the workplace-based assessment include mini clinical evaluation exercise (mCEX), direct observation of procedural skills (DOPS), mini-peer assessment tool (mPAT) and 360 degree feedback. Since these are observer rating based assessment methods there is a variability due to inherent bias in human judgement. This can affect the reliability and validity of the methods. However the opportunity of observation followed by formative assessment and feedback is critical in identifying learners' needs and the various options of addressing those needs.[3] Paradoxically some studies have observed that even though the scores of multisource feedback indicate that changes were required in the practice many recipients were unlikely to do so.[15]
4. *Objective structured clinical examinations (OSCEs)*: OSCEs are serious of clinical challenges-scenarios-reports, arranged in the form of series of stations. All the three domains knowledge, skills and attitudes of medical students can be assessed by using OSCE stations. These stations may include stations for history taking,

examination and professional behaviors including counseling stations. Though individual station has high objectivity in assessment, the reliability depends on the number of stations and observers. Hence larger number of stations and multiple observers are recommended.[3]

OSCEs can identify gaps in knowledge, skills and behavior of the learners and can be used to provide a feedback to the learners regarding the same. This can be done during both formative and summative assessments. Apart from this OSCEs can provide feedback regarding the identified potential weakness in a curriculum to the instructor.

- *Self-assessment:* This is a skill which enhances the metacognitive development of the learner and also academic progress. The positive effect of self-assessment on teacher-learner relationship can further advance the learning. Students become more responsible for their own learning by doing self-assessment. The students are encouraged to identify and address their own learning needs. When combined with self-reflection learners are able to understand themselves in a better way and motivates them to gain more knowledge. Self-assessment may be done with the help of diaries, log books, journals or weekly reviews. The various positive outcomes of self-assessment incudes improved cognitive and non-cognitive performance, enhancement in the critical thinking, more independent learning approach and improvement in the self-assessment accuracy. The students should be provided with opportunities for active learning and self-assessment should be integrated into formative assessment. The residents are supposed to integrate self-generated feedback with the formative feedback into their daily clinical practice. Peer teaching, collaborative learning, simulation and team based learning are the various approaches which increase the students responsibility towards their own learning and progress.[3]

Assessments should be guided by the learning outcomes **(Table 1)**. The learning could be satisfactory based on the predetermined criteria. Some students may not have mastered the contents to the expected level. This might affect the motivation to learn and efficacy of the student pushing them further at risk of subsequent deficiencies with addition of new content. In order to begin with the remediation process for the struggling learner, it is important to identify

TABLE 1: Formal versus informal needs assessment methods for LMICs.

Method type	*Specific technique*	*Purpose and feasibility*
Formal	Written pre-tests (MCQs)	Measures baseline knowledge and gaps; objective and scalable for large groups
	OSCEs	Assesses baseline skills and attitudes in standardized settings; high objectivity, though resource-intensive initially
Informal	One-minute paper	Rapidly identifies main learning points and confusion ("muddiest point"); high-yield and zero-cost
	Direct observation (WPBA)	Assesses skills and behavior in authentic clinical settings; provides immediate formative feedback
	Focus group discussion	Gathers qualitative data on learner motivation and curriculum expectations; simple to implement

the root cause of the deficiencies. Based on the root cause the problem learners can be categorized into four groups:

Students should be motivated to reflect upon their performance and the shortfall should be discussed with them. Reflection on the causes of unsatisfactory performance and the factors which could be linked with the below par performance are crucial in order to plan and for success of the remediation.[3] Important information on the students progress can be provided by an effective self-assessment. This helps in self-identification of the learning gaps. This is very crucial for identifying learning needs and providing appropriate support and remediation **(Table 2)**.

EVALUATION

One of the essential components of the education spiral is evaluation **(Fig. 1)**. Evaluation helps to ensure that the curriculum is effective in meeting the needs of the learner, institution and the society at large. It is focused on the larger outcomes rather than the individuals specific learning needs.

Few commonly used evaluation methods are:

- **Kirkpatrick's method:** This method describes four levels of evaluation: (1) reaction, (2) learning, (3) behavior and (4) result. This model distinguishes between learning and application of the knowledge and skill and has the advantage of evaluation at multiple levels. But it does not takes into consideration the process and context of learning and assumes that higher the level of evidence gathering better is the evidence.
- **Context-inclusive models:** The 3-P (presage factors, process factors and product factors) model given by Biggs and the Stufflebeam's CIPP (context , inputs, process and products) of evaluation tries to address shortcomings of Kirkpatrick's model by including the context. **Student context** refers to the prior knowledge and skills of the learners, their motivation, learning styles, values and expectations' from the program. **Teacher context** include institutional teaching environment like the class room and other resources available for teaching learning, content and structure of the curriculum and the methods of teaching and learning and evaluation. The interaction between teacher and student context and the actual learning that occurs due to this interaction is the process. The results of interaction between presage and process factors are the learning outcomes. The distinct advantage of CIPP model is the

TABLE 2: Categories of struggling learners and remediation focus.

Category	*Description and root cause*	*Remediation focus*
Affective	External personal issues affecting motivation, attention, and memory	Mentoring; addressing stress/personal issues; reorganization of learning plans
Cognitive	Problems with knowledge acquisition, written/oral communication, or integration of information (often easy to remediate)	Additional tutoring; review of study strategies
Structural	Problems related to study skills, time management, or stress management	Review of study strategies; development of time and stress management skills
Interpersonal	Difficulties in interacting with other people (peers, clinical staff)	Guided practice in communication; team-based learning; mentoring

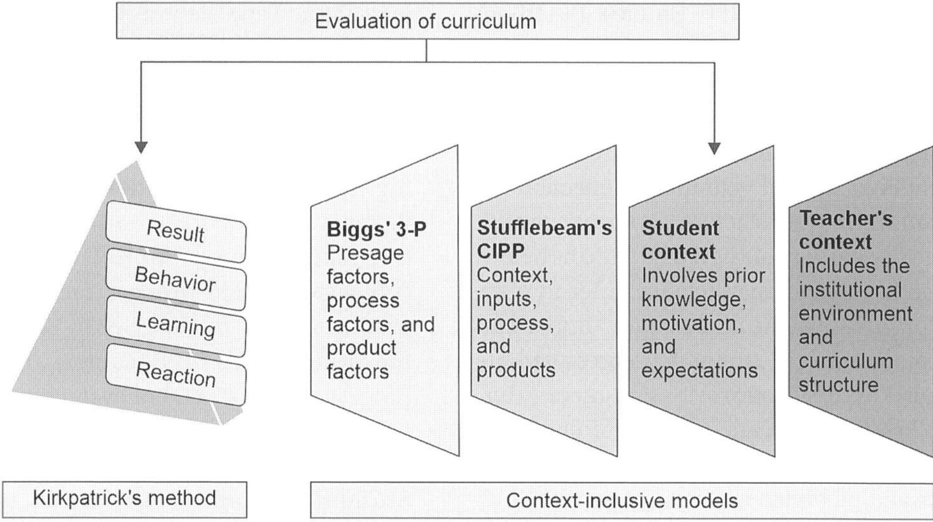

Fig. 1: Curriculum evaluation.

alternating focus among context, inputs, and the process. It helps in program improvement by providing the formative evaluation. Both quantitative and qualitative data should be incorporated in the evaluation method. The evaluation plans should include both formative and summative methods to aid effective decision making.[3]

CONCLUSION/FINAL COMMENTS

Assessing learners' needs is the **foundation and continuous heartbeat** of effective medical education. It is not a rigid protocol but a dynamic, cyclic process that requires the active engagement of both students and educators.

For medical teachers in LMICs, the emphasis should be on adopting resource-appropriate, high-impact strategies: leveraging informal needs assessments, utilizing accessible CATs for rapid feedback, and prioritizing deep learning through contextualized clinical training. Comprehensive and continuous faculty development in needs assessment and feedback skills is thus essential. As Albert Einstein wisely noted, the role of the teacher is not to teach, but to **"provide the conditions in which they can learn"**.

KEY POINTS/TAKE-HOME MESSAGES

1. **Needs assessment is a gap analysis:** It defines the **"discrepancy or gap"** between the learner's current status and the desired competence.
2. **It is cyclical, not static:** Needs assessment is a continuous, dynamic process that runs through the **Planning, Learning, and Assessment** phases.
3. **Assessment drives curriculum:** Students learn what is assessed, making assessment the most powerful tool for shaping curricular outcomes.
4. **Prioritize deep learning:** Instructional strategies must move learners beyond **surface memorization** to **deep learning** involving conceptual integration and critical thinking.
5. **Use PNP for feedback:** Effective feedback is a dialogue. Use the

Positive-Negative-Positive (PNP) format to communicate critical points constructively.
6. **CATs are resource-appropriate: Classroom assessment techniques (CATs)** like the one-minute paper offer immediate, formative feedback that is highly feasible in LMIC settings.
7. **Remediation is categorical:** Deficiencies must be identified and categorized into **affective, cognitive, structural, or interpersonal** groups for targeted and effective remediation.
8. **Ensure multimodal resources:** Provide learning resources in different modes (VARK) to respect varying **learning styles** and encourage **self-regulated learning**.
9. **Evaluation must include context:** Program evaluation models like **CIPP** go beyond results (Kirkpatrick) to include the student and teacher **context** for continuous improvement.

"I never Teach my pupils. I only attempt to provide the conditions in which they can learn" ***Albert Einstein***

REFERENCES

1. Etling A, Maloney T. Needs assessment for Extension agents and other nonformal educators. [Internet]. 1995. Available from: Retrieved from https://files.eric.ed.gov/fulltext/ED388774.pdf
2. Witkin BR, Altschuld JW. Planning and conducting needs assessments: a practical guide. Thousand Oaks, CA: Sage Publications; 1995.
3. Casey B, White, Lou Ann Cooper, Mary Edwards, Jennifer Lyon. Assessing learners' needs. In Oxford Textbook of Medical Education pp. 453-64. Available from: https://doi.org/10.1093/med/9780199652679.003.0039
4. Morrison GR, Ross SM, Kemp JE. Designing effective instruction. Hoboken, NJ: John Wiley & Sons, Inc.; 2006.
5. Bradshaw J. The concept of social need. New Society. 1972;30:640–43.
6. White CB, et al. Assessing learners' needs. In: Walsh K, editor. Oxford Textbook of Medical Education. Oxford: Oxford Textbook; 2013 [cited 2025 Feb 16]. Available from: https://doi.org/10.1093/med/9780199652679.003.0039
7. Challis M. AMEE Medical Education Guide No. 19: personal learning plans. Med Teach. 2000;22:225–36.
8. Papinczak T, Young L, Groves M, Haynes M. Effects of a metacognitive intervention on students' approaches to learning and self-efficacy in a first-year medical course. Adv Health Sci Educ Theory Pract. 2008;13:213–32.
9. Gurpinar E, Bati H, Tetik C. Learning styles of medical students change in relation to time. Adv Physiol Educ. 2011;35:307–11.
10. Genn J. AMEE Medical Education Guide No. 23 (Part 1): curriculum, environment, climate, quality and change in medical education—a unifying perspective. Med Teach. 2001;23:337–44.
11. Cantillon P, Sargeant J. Teaching rounds: giving feedback in clinical settings. BMJ. 2008;337:1292–94.
12. Ende J. Feedback in clinical medical education. JAMA. 1983;250:777–81.
13. Grant J, Chambers G, Jackson G, editors. The good CPD guide. Sutton: Reed Healthcare; 1999.
14. Leahy S, Lyon C, Thompson M, Williams D. Classroom assessment: minute by minute, day by day. Educ Leadership. 2005;63:19–24.
15. Sood R, Singh T. Assessment in medical education: evolving perspectives and contemporary trends. Nat Med J India. 2012;25:357–64.

CHAPTER 14

Microplanning A Teaching Session

Aswathy Rajan, Santosh T Soans

INTRODUCTION

Medical education is rapidly evolving globally, as well as in India, making the need for practical teaching sessions paramount. Microplanning refers to the process of planning small, focused teaching sessions—small group, large group, or clinic sessions—with specific objectives, appropriate teaching methods, and evaluation strategies. Microplanning enables teachers to design individual teaching units tailored to specific competencies and learning outcomes.[1]

PRINCIPLES OF MICROPLANNING A TEACHING SESSION

The principles of planning a session are essential for meeting the specific learning requirements of Indian medical graduates.

- *Learner-centered approach*: Competency-based medical education (CBME) emphasizes the need to shift from a teacher-centered to a student-centered approach.
- *Relevance*: As IMGs practice in diverse healthcare settings, teaching should be contextualized to cases and challenges that they are likely to face.
- *Competency aligned*: A teaching session should cover some competencies as outlined in the curriculum.[2]
- *Integration of theory and practice*: There should be an application of learnt theoretical knowledge with hands-on practice.
- *Active learning and engagement*: Interactive classes are encouraged rather than traditional didactic lectures.
- *Continuous assessment*: Session planning should include opportunities for formative/summative assessment, such as self/peer assessment, to track progress and ensure the achievement of learning objectives.
- *Reflection and feedback*: Reflection helps reinforce the learning process, while constructive and specific feedback provides a motivational drive to the learner.

STRUCTURING A TEACHING SESSION

Domain of Learning

- Based on competency, first determine the principal domain (cognitive/psychomotor/affective) that must be targeted in the instructional session.[3]
- If the competency is related to theory topics, it mainly involves the cognitive domain. Topics in which learners are expected to physically do or demonstrate something (e.g., measuring blood pressure/height, or weight) are mainly psychomotor. Topics where learners are exposed to/must participate in roleplays/

counseling/communication, etc., are primarily affective. Most of the time, other domains are also invoked, regardless of the targeted primary domain. For example, one cannot measure a child's weight or counsel a parent without knowing the theoretical aspects of weight measurement/the condition for which counseling is being offered.

Profile of the Target Audience

- Prior knowledge about a particular topic will depend on the phase in which the students belong. For example, phase II students should have basis foundational understanding about the normal structure and function of an organ or organ system. Therefore, depending on the phase of the student, one must determine the level of the appropriate domain which you may need to target. For example, a topic on short stature being taught to a phase II student might require an initial class targeting the cognitive domain on height measurement. The same topic for a phase III student might involve a higher-level cognitive approach, followed by psychomotor skills learning.
- Identify group behavior of the students so that it can be appropriately utilized for the facilitation of learning.

Setting/Materials

- Most of the time, the setting is quite apparent. Theory classes would be conducted in a lecture hall, while clinics might be bedside. However, in any setting, one must be aware of the resources that may be available for the instructional session, thereby helping narrow the choice of teaching/AV aids to be used for the session.
- Simulation class might require preparation/moulage and rehearsal before the class, and can be taken for a smaller group of students.

Session/Activity Duration

- Lecture classes are typically 60 minutes, while Small-group discussions (SGDs) may vary from 60 to 120 minutes. Bedside clinics and simulation classes may last up to 180 minutes.
- One must determine what duration will be appropriate, given the details from the preceding three steps, and ensure that classes are engaging and hence should not be too lengthy.
- Each activity planned in the session also needs to be time-limited and scheduled in advance.

Rationale

- Depending on the session duration and audience, the competencies to be covered must be identified.
- Objectives framed thereby should be achievable within the time duration of the class.
- It should be kept in mind why the topic or subject is essential as per the community or healthcare need, and this importance should be communicated to students.

Strategy

- Plan how the class will be structured.
- *Building an introduction*: The introduction of the topic should be attractive to the students to grab their attention. Thus, it should initiate with a set induction in the form of a case, evidence or story related to the clinical aspect of the assigned topic. The teacher can also incorporate a personal experience to help students relate to it.

- Checking the prior knowledge of the students and linking it with your session content.
- Decide the subtopics/heading that are going to be covered in the class.
- Case-based learning (CBL) can be initiated.
- Depending on the decided teaching method, prepare materials for the exact needs to be prepared by the teacher/ facilitator, which may be audio-visual aids, black/white-board, online platform like Kahoot, or others.
- The assessment question and approaches for the topic can be specified at the beginning or end of the session.
- Prepare take home points of key concepts
- Do keep a slot for taking attendance?

Forming a Lesson Plan (Fig. 1)

A lesson plan is a written guide for the trainer's activities to achieve the intended learning outcomes. It provides specific definitions and guidance on learning objectives, equipment, instructional media, required materials, and training conduct. It gives you, as a teacher, an opportunity to think through in detail how you will approach your teaching and what the most effective way is to help your students learn.

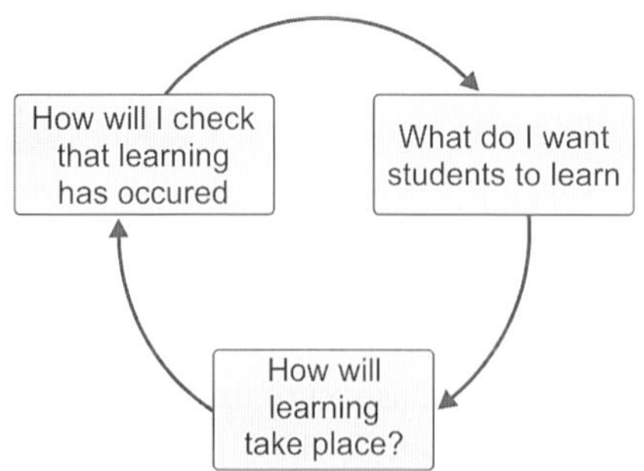

Fig. 1: Forming a lesson plan.

Characteristics of a Good Lesson Plan

- Flexible and should allow some freedom
- Contents should be organized as per attainable objectives
- Neither too brief nor too exhaustive
- Should include student-centered activities
- Relevant, clear, and feasible

Contents of a Lesson Plan

- *Context*: Begin by outlining the session title, the relevant competency area, and what learners are expected to know already or have studied. Consider how this session fits into the broader course structure, including the topics that came before and those that follow.
- *Timing*: Some sessions, like SGDs, may last 60–120 minutes, while clinics may be longer. Be clear about how much time has been allotted for the session, and plan each minute. If the content you're expected to cover doesn't realistically fit within the allotted time, don't try to squeeze everything in. Instead, prioritize key topics and let students know they'll need to explore the rest through self-directed learning (SDL).[4]
- *Participants*: The number of students attending the class should be considered. Typically, if it's a larger group, more time may be needed for discussion and feedback. Reflect on their level of knowledge and experience to tailor your approach accordingly.
- *Equipment*: Take into account the physical environment: what kind of room will you be in? Can students move around or form different groups? Also, note what resources will be available, such as a laptop, projector, internet access, flip charts, and paper.

- *Aims and learning outcomes*: These are often provided as part of the course framework, but if you're developing them yourself, you can refer to the site's learning resource on "making sense of aims and learning outcomes" for guidance.

Lesson Plan Template

LESSON PLAN TEMPLATE

Batch/Class: **Number of Students:**

Subject:

Topic:

Name of the Teacher:

Date:

Duration:

Set Induction/Motivation: Try to assess previous knowledge or trigger learners to create interest in the topic.

Specific Learning Objectives:

-
-
-

Contents:

-
-
-

TL Method: Case or problem-based discussion/interactive lecture/video/roleplay/small group activity/demonstration, etc.

Logistics Needed: AV aids/PPT/charts or models/case report, etc.

Assessment Tool: To assess outcome matching with the objectives.

Follow-up Activity:

DESIGNING A FORMAL TEACHING SESSION

- Identifying required competencies
- Forming specific learning objectives (SLOs)
- Selecting appropriate teaching methods
- Logistics needed
- Assessment tools
- Reflection, feedback and follow-up activity
- Time allocation

Step 1: Identify the Specific Competencies

The goal is to align the session with the competencies of a particular topic defined by the curriculum, which may include patient management, communication, decision-making, or medical knowledge.[5]

Step 2: Forming Specific Learning Objectives

Once the relevant competencies have been identified, one must frame SLOs that enable one to achieve those competencies. These objectives should be *SMART*, targeting specific competencies expected at that stage of learning.

- *S*pecific: Detailed, direct and meaningful, focusing on a particular skill or knowledge area.
- *M*easurable: Quantifiable by assessment to track the learner's progress.
- *A*chievable: Realistic for the learner's current level of competence, time period, and resources available.
- *R*elevant: Relevant to the current real-world scenario.
- *T*ime-bound: Clear time by which the learners are expected to achieve this.

Step 3: Selecting Appropriate Teaching Methods

The teaching methodologies should be selected based on the *learning objectives*. Some competencies may require a combination of teaching methods. For example, for a session on pediatric asthma management, a combination of *CBL* and *hands-on simulation* may be required to complete the learning experience. Some competencies, which involve teaching basic concepts, can be taught through interactive lectures that incorporate presentation slides and live polls to make them more engaging. *SGD or role-playing for specific competencies* that require problem-solving can enable peer-to-peer learning. *Problem-based learning (PBL)* can be used in groups of any size for application practice. It provides hands-on experience and allows learners to practice clinical scenarios. Encouraging the students to explore advances or topics beyond the scope of the competency can be made into *SDL* sessions.

Step 4: Logistics Needed

Once the competency, objectives and teaching learning method have been decided upon, one must plan what the content of the class would be and at the same time consider the learning environment that would be used for the session.

Ensure all materials (e.g., case scenario handouts/slides and assessment tools) are ready before the session.

- *Multimedia/PowerPoint presentations*: Use slides to illustrate key concepts, for example, anatomy, pathophysiology, or algorithms.
- *Visual aids/videos*: Specially for rare clinical cases or findings
- *Clinical guidelines*: To teach the current, evidence-based practices.
- *Case scenarios*: In CBL or SGDs, prepare realistic clinical cases and subquestions which can be solved as a group.
- *Practice tools*: Develop materials such as handouts, growth charts, or diagrams to participate actively

Consider the Learning Environment

- *Space*: If planning a group discussion, ensure there is adequate space for students to arrange themselves in groups. Practical activities and simulations may require setting up a skill lab.
- *Technology*: Utilize appropriate teaching tools such as PowerPoint presentations or pictures and X-rays, digital platforms for online quizzes, or video demonstrations.
- *Materials*: If demonstration of a particular skill is included, have necessary equipment on hand, such as nebulizers, stethoscopes, or mannequins, for hands-on practice.
- *Support*: Some classes, for example, immersive simulations, require teaching assistants or facilitators available to guide learners during interactive activities.[6]

Step 5: Assessment Tools

The aim should be to assess whether learners have achieved the required competencies for the particular class using formative or summative assessments.

- *Formative assessments*: During the session, one can plan continuous assessments in the form of quizzes, questions or, if it was a skill demonstration, then observation of the particular skill. Formative assessment can be followed by immediate feedback to improve students' understanding.
- *Summative assessments*: End-of-session or postsession summative assessments can assess all the objectives taught in that class. This could be in the form of MCQs or short written tests.

For example, formative assessments for a topic such as bronchial asthma could include asking learners to diagnose asthma based on a case scenario or demonstrate inhaler technique. In contrast, summative assessments might consist of a mini-CEX (clinical evaluation exercise) to assess learners' ability to take an effective history, perform a physical examination, and make decisions to manage the case. Clinical sessions may be assessed by objective structured clinical examinations (OSCEs) or by direct observation of procedural skills (DOPS), as applicable. Resource material for assessment must be prepared before the class, such as checklists or digital forms, as deemed appropriate. There are various platforms, such as Kahoot and Socrative, that can be utilized for assessment.

Step 6: Reflection, Feedback, and Follow-up Activity

- *Reflection* helps learners analyze what they have learnt in the session. This can also be done verbally or written into their logbooks. Questions they need to answer can include what they understood well in the class and what they found challenging, or focusing on identifying areas which require practice or improvement.[7]
- *Feedback* can be given by the teacher or peers, either verbally or in writing. Highlight strengths by discussing what went well, while gaps and errors can be pointed out as areas that need improvement. Suggestions can be taken in a written or digital format.
- *Follow-up activity* can be learning reinforcements or further learning beyond the scope of the competency taught that day. Guidance and recommendations for further reading can include videos or articles suggested by the teacher. Assignments or projects can be assigned to the students to reinforce key concepts.

Step 7: Time Allocation

Time must be allocated for various aspects of the class, for example, introduction, content

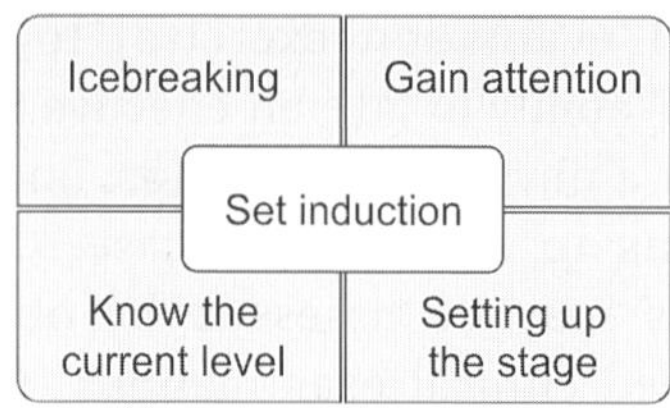

Fig. 2: Set induction.

teaching, discussion, and assessment, which can make the session engaging and crisp. A typical session could be divided as follows:

- *Introduction (5 minutes)*: Set induction **(Fig. 2)** and state the objectives of the class.
- *Teaching (25 minutes)*: Prepared resources can be taught using slides/videos/cases.
- *Interactive learning (15 minutes)*: Roleplay or small group discussions.
- *Assessment (10 minutes)*: Peer or self-assessment.
- *Conclusion (5 minutes)*: Summarize key points, provide feedback, and guidance for follow-up activity.[8]

EXAMPLE OF A TEACHING SESSION PLAN

Topic: Bronchial asthma

Identify competencies as per curriculum

PE 28.19 Describe the etiopathogenesis, diagnosis, clinical features, management, and prevention of asthma in children.

PE 28.20 Counsel the child with asthma on the correct use of inhalers in a simulated environment.

Introduction and Specific Learning Objectives [5 minutes]

Introduction to Bronchial Asthma in Children

- Incidence and prevalence, deaths due to childhood asthma
- Definition of asthma in children as per ATM guidelines

Objectives

By the end of this teaching session, the learners should be able to:

- *Understand* the pathophysiology of asthma and its triggers.
- *Recognize* the clinical signs and symptoms of acute exacerbation of asthma in children.
- *Discuss* the management of a child in acute exacerbation, including initial assessment.
- *List* the drugs used for immediate medical management and devices used for long-term management.
- *Communicate* effectively with parents and caregivers regarding the condition and use of inhaler therapy.

Content [25 minutes]

- *Pathophysiology of asthma in children (2 minutes)*
- *Signs and symptoms (5 minutes):*
  - History taking: Nighttime cough, wheeze, duration, associated symptoms (fever and difficulty in breathing), and potential triggers (viral infection, allergy, etc.).
  - Signs: Tachypnea, grunting, nasal flaring, retractions, cyanosis, and rhonchi
  - Sensorium: Irritability and lethargy
- *Investigations and management of a child with acute exacerbation (8 minutes):*
  - Initial assessment and triage: ABCDE approach and PAT assessment
  - Oxygen therapy: Indications and delivery methods (e.g., nasal cannula and face mask).
  - Medications: Nebulized salbutamol with oxygen, ipratropium bromide, and corticosteroids
  - Monitoring: Pulse oximetry and blood gases

  - Advanced interventions: Intubation and ventilation (when required)
- *Long-term management (5 minutes):*
  - Inhaler therapy
  - Other drug delivery devices—Rotahaler and spacer
- *Parent and caregiver communication (5 minutes):*
  - Explaining the condition and treatment plan
  - Reassuring the family and addressing concerns (e.g., when to seek urgent medical attention)
  - Counsel the child and the caretaker for correct use of MDI and spacer at initiation of therapy and on follow-up

Teaching Methodology (Active Learning Approach)

- *Case-based learning (15 minutes)*:
  - Present a real-life case of a child (e.g., a 12-year-old girl presenting with acute exacerbation of asthma).
  - Ask learners to make a differential diagnosis.
  - Discuss the appropriate management steps, including when to escalate care (e.g., using a nebulizer and starting steroids).
- *Small group discussion (10 minutes)*:
  - Divide the learners into groups of 10 and ask them to discuss:
    - How would they provide long-term management for this child?
    - What treatment would be preferred? What is the dose of medications?
    - Provide feedback on their approaches and discuss best practices.
- *Roleplay (5 minutes)*:
  - Encourage learners to practice communication skills by roleplaying a conversation with a parent/peer.

Assessment Strategies

1. *Formative assessment*: During the *CBL* session, assess if learners can recognize the signs and symptoms. Provide immediate feedback on their clinical reasoning.
2. *Peer feedback*: After the *small group discussion*, allow peers to discuss and debate decision-making and management options.

Resources Required

- *Visual aids*: PowerPoint presentation will include diagrams of the respiratory system and pathophysiology of asthma. It may have clinical photographs/videos showing signs of respiratory distress.
- *Case scenarios*: Prepare realistic case scenarios of children in need of long-term management of asthma for group discussions and roleplaying exercises.
- *MDI*: To demonstrate the correct use of an inhaler in children with and without a spacer/mask.

Reflection, Feedback, and Follow-up Activity

Students should be allowed to reflect on their learning session:

- "What was the most challenging part of managing asthma in children?"
- "How confident do you feel in communicating the treatment plan to parents?"

Feedback can be taken on a digital platform made by the facilitator before the class.

Follow-up activity on newer medications in asthma or GINA guidelines can be shared with the class.

Time Allocation

Time allocation is given in **Table 1**.

TABLE 1: Time allocation.

Session part	*Time*
Introduction	05 minutes
Signs and symptoms, differentials and management	25 minutes
Group discussion	15 minutes
Role-play	05 minutes
Assessment and feedback	10 minutes
Total	*60 minutes*

MICROTEACHING: CONCEPT AND RELEVANCE (FIG. 3)

Microteaching is a scaled-down version of the actual teaching process, aimed at developing specific teaching skills in educators and refining old ones. Allen developed it in the late sixties to improve teachers' skills. It involves teaching microsized lessons of 5–10 minutes, often to a limited number of learners, in a controlled, supportive environment. The key difference between microteaching and traditional teaching is that it focuses on teaching a small portion of the material, allowing for focused feedback and refinement. This Stanford technique involved the steps of *"plan, teach, observe, replan, reteach, and reobserve"*.

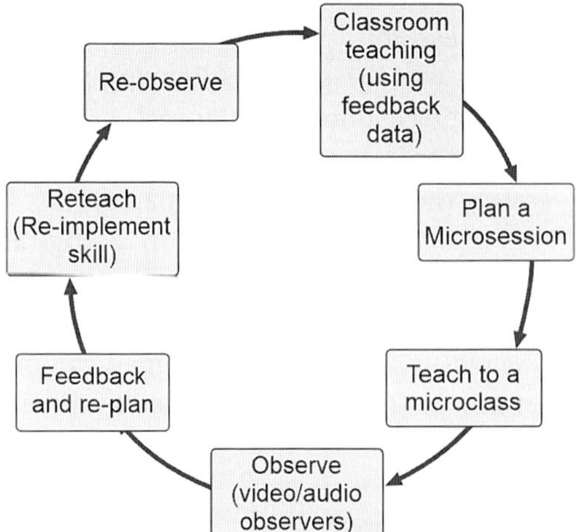

Fig. 3: Concept and relevance of microteaching.

The relevance of microteaching in CBME is that it encourages skill development, is feedback-oriented, allows for simulation of real-life clinical environments, and thereby allows for critical thinking.

Components of Microteaching

- *Lesson planning*: As explained in the previous section, lesson plans must be prepared to target predefined objectives.
- *Set induction*: The initial portion of the class can engage learners by enquiring about previous knowledge.
- *Stimulus variation*: Try to incorporate different teaching techniques so that the students are engaged.
- *Proper audiovisual aids*: Videos/photographs of cases
- *Reinforcement*: Formative assessment or summarizing can be done during the session.
- *Questioning*: Problem/case-based questions to stimulate critical thinking
- *Nonverbal cue*: Effective use of body language as an adjuvant
- *Closure*: Summarize the key points

Advantages of Microteaching

- Microteaching helps in eliminating errors and builds stronger teaching skills for beginners and senior teachers.
- Microteaching increases self-confidence, improves in-class teaching performances, and develops classroom management skills.
- It enables understanding of individual learners.

Limitations of Microteaching

1. Time is the major constraint in the implementation of microteaching sessions.

2. Availability and training of faculty.
3. A lot depends on the motivation of a teacher to improve himself and the ability of the observer to give constructive feedback.

CONCLUSION

Planning a teaching session in accordance with CBME guidelines requires a systematic, thoughtful approach to ensure that all aspects—objectives, content, methods, assessments, and feedback—align with the desired competencies. By focusing on active learning, clinical practice, and continuous feedback, it provides a framework that enables medical learners to develop the skills, knowledge, and ethics needed to become competent and confident healthcare professionals.

REFERENCES

1. Medical Council of India. Competency Based Undergraduate Curriculum for the Indian Medical Graduate, Volume 1-3. New Delhi: Medical Council of India; 2018.
2. van Diggele C, Burgess A, Mellis C. Planning, preparing and structuring a small group teaching session. BMC Med Educ. 2020;20(Suppl 2):462.
3. Ananthakrishnan N. Microteaching as a vehicle of teacher training—its advantages and disadvantages. J Postgrad Med. 1993;39(3):142-3.
4. Hsu T, De Angelis F, Al-Asaaed S, et al. Ten ways to get a grip on designing and implementing a competency-based medical education training program. Can Med Educ J. 2021;12(2):e81-7.
5. Bhatti MA, Ahmed W, Khan RA. Microteaching: A modern technique of teaching. J Ayub Med Coll Abbottabad. 2013;25(1-2):157-60.
6. Kulkarni P. Microteaching-A New Approach to Teaching. J Med Educ Res Pract. 2014;2(1):10-3.
7. Thomas PA, Kern DE, Hughes MT, et al. Curriculum Development for Medical Education: A Six-Step Approach, 3rd edition. Baltimore: Johns Hopkins University Press; 2016.
8. Sood R, Adkoli BV. Medical education in India-problems and prospects. J Indian Acad Clin Med. 2000;1(3):210-2.

CHAPTER 15

Self-directed Learning

Vinod H Ratageri

INTRODUCTION

In recent years, medical education has undergone a significant transformation, shifting from traditional didactic lectures as the primary method of knowledge transmission to a student-centered learning approach. A key component of this transformation is *self-directed learning (SDL)*, which fosters lifelong learning habits essential for medical professionals. SDL encourages students to take ownership of their education, equipping them with the skills needed to navigate the rapidly evolving landscape of medical knowledge and practice. In this chapter, we will cover the principles, benefits, challenges, and strategies of SDL in medical education, with a focus on best practices, evidence-based methodologies, and future implications.[1-4]

DEFINITION AND PRINCIPLES OF SELF-DIRECTED LEARNING[5]

Knowles' (1975) definition of SDL specifies that it is a dynamic, active learning process in which individuals take the initiative, with or without external guidance, to diagnose their learning needs, set goals, identify appropriate resources, implement strategies, and evaluate learning outcomes. It shifts the traditional role of educators from the primary source of knowledge to placing learners at the center, encouraging autonomy and self-regulation. According to Garrison (1997), SDL is an approach where learners assume both personal responsibility and collaborative control over cognitive (self-monitoring) and contextual (self-management) processes to construct meaningful and lasting learning experiences.

In medical education, SDL is particularly crucial as it aligns with the necessity for continuous learning in a rapidly evolving field. It fosters a proactive approach to acquiring knowledge, allowing future healthcare professionals to develop habits that will sustain their lifelong learning journey. Effective SDL involves a cycle of setting learning objectives, seeking relevant information, engaging with the material through various methods, self-assessing progress, and refining strategies based on reflection and feedback.

Key principles of SDL in medical education include:[6-10]

- *Learner autonomy:* Students take active responsibility for setting their learning objectives, designing their study plans, and managing their timelines. They decide what, how, and when to study, enabling a more personalized and efficient learning experience.
- *Self-motivation:* Learning in SDL is driven by both intrinsic and extrinsic motivation. Intrinsic motivation stems from personal interest, intellectual curiosity, and the desire for mastery, while examinations,

career aspirations, and professional expectations may influence extrinsic motivation.

- *Resource utilization:* Effective SDL involves the ability to identify and utilize a diverse range of learning resources, including textbooks, academic journals, online platforms, interactive e-learning modules, peer discussions, mentorship, and hands-on clinical experiences. A successful self-directed learner is adept at filtering and evaluating information for relevance and accuracy.
- *Reflection and evaluation:* Continuous self-assessment is integral to SDL. Learners must engage in reflective practices to analyze their strengths, identify knowledge gaps, and adjust their study strategies accordingly. Tools such as learning logs, portfolios, and feedback mechanisms support this process.
- *Self-pacing and adaptability:* SDL allows students to progress at their own pace, accommodating different learning styles and preferences. Adaptability is essential, as learners must adjust their strategies to evolving academic and clinical demands. This flexibility enhances retention and mastery of medical knowledge.

IMPORTANCE OF SELF-DIRECTED LEARNING IN MEDICAL EDUCATION

Encouraging Lifelong Learning

Medicine is an ever-evolving field that requires continuous learning. SDL cultivates habits that ensure doctors remain up to date on new knowledge and advancements.[11] The ability to seek, critically appraise, and apply new medical knowledge independently is essential for professional growth.

Promoting Critical Thinking and Problem-solving Skills

Medical professionals must analyze complex cases, make evidence-based decisions, and adapt to new information. SDL enhances these capabilities by fostering critical thinking, analytical reasoning, and adaptability in various clinical settings (Schmidt et al., 2013).[12]

Enhancing Motivation and Engagement

When students control their learning process, they engage more deeply with the material and develop intrinsic motivation (Brydges et al., 2010).[13] Medical students who take ownership of their education demonstrate higher levels of academic performance and professional competence.

Aligning with Competency-Based Medical Education

Competency-based medical education (CBME) focuses on developing core competencies rather than time-based training. SDL supports this by allowing learners to progress at their own pace, ensuring competency in essential medical skills.[14] With increasing emphasis on CBME, SDL offers a flexible, individualized approach to achieving the required competencies.

STRATEGIES FOR IMPLEMENTING SELF-DIRECTED LEARNING IN MEDICAL EDUCATION[15-18]

- *Curriculum design to encourage SDL:* A well-structured medical curriculum should incorporate elements that foster SDL. These include:
    - Problem-based learning (PBL): PBL encourages students to seek

information independently by engaging in clinical cases that require critical thinking.
- Flipped classroom approach: Students prepare beforehand by reviewing materials and engage in interactive discussions during class sessions.
- Online and blended learning: It provides access to diverse learning resources, promoting autonomy and flexibility.
- Use of simulation-based training: It encourages active learning through medical simulations and case-based discussions, enhancing clinical reasoning skills.
- Interdisciplinary collaboration: It allows medical students to work with peers from various health disciplines, fostering collaborative SDL.

▪ *Developing self-assessment and reflective skills:* Encouraging students to assess their progress and reflect on their learning experiences enhances SDL effectiveness. Tools such as portfolios, learning logs, self-evaluation surveys, and guided reflection exercises can aid in this process. Reflection-on-action and reflection-in-action are key skills that medical educators should cultivate in students. Additionally, structured reflection sessions in which students discuss their learning experiences with mentors or peers can further reinforce self-awareness and self-improvement.

▪ *Faculty role in facilitating SDL:*
- Mentorship and guidance: Instructors should support students in setting goals and identifying resources, providing timely feedback and encouragement. Faculty should create a supportive learning environment that motivates students to take ownership of their education.
- Providing constructive feedback: Regular formative assessments help students refine their learning strategies and address gaps in knowledge. Feedback should be structured to guide students toward self-improvement while fostering independence.[19]
- Encouraging metacognition: Teaching students to think about their learning processes improves SDL outcomes and fosters deeper understanding (Schmidt & Moust, 1995).[20] Educators should provide tools and frameworks that help students analyze their own learning methods and effectiveness.

▪ *Technology and SDL:* With advancements in technology, various digital resources support SDL, including:
- Massive Open Online Courses (MOOCs): Platforms like Coursera, Khan Academy, and edX offer medical courses that enhance SDL.
- Clinical Decision Support Systems (CDSS): Artificial intelligence (AI)-driven systems provide learners with real-time decision-making assistance.
- Virtual and augmented reality (VR/AR): These technologies simulate medical environments for enhanced learning experiences.
- Mobile learning applications: Apps like Medscape, UpToDate, and Osmosis provide access to a wealth of medical knowledge.
- Adaptive learning platforms: AI-driven tools that personalize content based on individual learning needs, ensuring that students receive targeted and efficient learning resources.

    - Collaborative online learning environments: Discussion forums, virtual study groups, and peer-to-peer learning platforms facilitate knowledge exchange and cooperative SDL.
- *Creating SDL-friendly learning environments:*
    - Encouraging inquiry-based learning: Designing activities that prompt students to explore, question, and research topics independently fosters a habit of lifelong learning.
    - Establishing learning contracts: Agreements between students and faculty outlining learning objectives, resources, timelines, and assessment criteria can help structure SDL while maintaining flexibility.
    - Providing access to diverse learning resources: A well-stocked digital and physical library, access to case studies, and clinical exposure enhance SDL opportunities.

CHALLENGES IN IMPLEMENTING SELF-DIRECTED LEARNING

Despite the numerous advantages of SDL, its implementation in medical education comes with several challenges. These challenges must be addressed to optimize its effectiveness and ensure that students develop the necessary skills for lifelong learning.

Variability in Student Readiness

Not all students enter medical education with the same level of preparedness for SDL. Some may struggle with self-regulation, time management, or goal-setting, making it difficult for them to engage effectively in SDL. Developing SDL skills requires structured guidance, particularly in the early stages of medical training.

Balancing Structured and Self-directed Learning

Medical curricula must strike a balance between SDL and traditional structured learning to ensure that essential competencies are met without overwhelming students with excessive autonomy. While SDL encourages independent learning, some level of guidance is still necessary to provide students with a strong foundational understanding.

Faculty Resistance and Training Needs

Educators may be unfamiliar with SDL methodologies and require training to implement them effectively. Faculty members accustomed to traditional teaching methods might find it challenging to transition to a more facilitative role. Institutional support and professional development programs are essential to equip faculty with the skills needed to foster SDL in students.

Assessment and Evaluation of Self-directed Learning Outcomes

Traditional examinations may not adequately measure SDL competencies. Alternative assessments, such as competency-based evaluations, self-reflective essays, and project-based learning, should be incorporated to provide a more comprehensive evaluation of students' SDL progress.

Resource Availability and Accessibility

Effective SDL relies on diverse, high-quality learning resources, including textbooks, online platforms, medical databases, and clinical experiences. However, disparities in resource availability can hinder SDL implementation, particularly in institutions with limited funding or technological infrastructure.

Student Motivation and Engagement

Self-directed learning requires students to be intrinsically motivated and disciplined in managing their learning. However, maintaining motivation can be challenging, especially amid academic stress, heavy workload, and external pressures. Strategies such as goal-setting, mentorship, and peer collaboration can help sustain motivation and engagement.

Integration of Self-directed Learning with Clinical Training

Integrating SDL into clinical training can be complex, as students must balance SDL with patient care responsibilities, supervised practice, and structured clinical rotations. Providing students with opportunities to engage in SDL while ensuring they receive adequate guidance from clinical mentors is crucial for a well-rounded medical education experience.

FUTURE DIRECTIONS AND RESEARCH OPPORTUNITIES

As the medical education landscape continues to evolve, SDL is expected to undergo significant advancements influenced by technology, pedagogical innovations, and global educational trends. Future directions in SDL implementation may include:

- *Integration of AI and machine learning:* AI-driven learning platforms can provide personalized learning experiences, adapting to students' strengths and weaknesses. AI can facilitate adaptive learning pathways, recommend resources based on individual progress, and provide real-time feedback, making SDL more efficient and targeted.
- *Expansion of VR/AR in SDL:* With advancements in technology, VR and AR can offer immersive learning experiences that enhance SDL. These technologies can simulate real-life clinical scenarios, allowing students to practice medical procedures, improve diagnostic skills, and engage in experiential learning without patient risk.
- *Development of digital learning ecosystems:* Future SDL strategies may involve the creation of interconnected digital learning environments that integrate online courses, interactive simulations, collaborative platforms, and cloud-based resources. These ecosystems will facilitate access to diverse educational materials and foster a more engaging and self-paced learning experience.
- *Innovations in assessment methods:* Traditional assessment models may not fully capture the competencies developed through SDL. Future research should focus on designing competency-based assessments, reflective journals, and AI-powered analytics to effectively evaluate SDL outcomes. Personalized learning dashboards may provide real-time tracking of student progress and areas requiring improvement.
- *Global collaboration and open educational resources (OERs):* The availability of open-access educational resources and global collaborative networks will play a critical role in the future of SDL. Shared medical curricula, cross-institutional collaborations, and virtual mentorship programs can enhance access to

high-quality educational content and broaden learning opportunities.

- *Tailoring SDL to individual learning styles and needs:* Research in cognitive science and learning theories may lead to better customization of SDL approaches based on students' unique learning preferences. Future SDL models could incorporate tailored strategies that accommodate diverse learners, ensuring that education is inclusive and effective for all students.
- *Emphasis on interdisciplinary and collaborative SDL:* Medical education is increasingly recognizing the importance of interdisciplinary learning. Future SDL initiatives may involve collaborations with professionals from other healthcare disciplines, allowing students to develop a holistic understanding of patient care and fostering teamwork skills essential for modern healthcare settings.
- *Longitudinal studies on SDL efficacy:* While SDL is widely promoted, long-term studies examining its impact on medical competency, clinical performance, and patient outcomes are still needed. Future research should focus on evaluating SDL's effectiveness across different contexts to ensure evidence-based improvements in medical education.

By embracing these future directions, SDL can continue to evolve as a powerful educational strategy that prepares medical students for the complexities and challenges of modern healthcare.

CONCLUSION

Self-directed learning is a vital component of medical education, promoting lifelong learning, critical thinking, and self-motivation. While challenges exist, strategic implementation can enhance its effectiveness, preparing medical professionals for the dynamic and evolving nature of healthcare. By fostering a culture of self-directed inquiry and continuous improvement, medical educators can ensure that students are equipped with the necessary skills to adapt and excel in the medical profession.

Summary points

- *SDL fosters lifelong learning* by enabling medical students to continuously update their knowledge and skills, ensuring their competence in an ever-evolving medical landscape.
- *It promotes critical thinking and problem-solving*, essential for clinical decision-making and adapting to new medical advancements.
- *Technology-enhanced SDL*, including AI, VR, and digital learning ecosystems, is expected to play a significant role in the future of medical education.
- *Innovative assessment methods* are required to accurately evaluate SDL competencies, moving beyond traditional examinations to more competency-based evaluations.
- *Global collaboration and open-access resources* will facilitate the sharing of high-quality educational materials, expanding learning opportunities worldwide.
- *SDL requires a balance between autonomy and structure*, as excessive independence without proper guidance may lead to ineffective learning outcomes.
- *Faculty training and institutional support* are crucial for successful SDL implementation, ensuring educators can effectively mentor and guide students.
- *Interdisciplinary and collaborative SDL approaches* are increasingly recognized as vital for developing well-rounded medical professionals prepared for team-based healthcare environments.
- *Future research on SDL effectiveness* should focus on long-term studies examining its impact on clinical practice, patient outcomes, and professional competency.

REFERENCES

1 Aulakh J, Wahab H, Richards C, et al. Self-directed learning versus traditional didactic learning in undergraduate medical education: a systematic review and meta-analysis. BMC Med Educ. 2025;25:70.
2. Lu SY, Ren XP, Xu H, et al. Improving self-directed learning ability using blended teaching. BMC Med Educ. 2023;23:616.
3. Xu X, Li Z, Mackay L, et al. SDL ability during online study. BMC Med Educ. 2024;24:25.
4. Finn A, Fitzgibbon C, Fonda N, et al. SDL and student learning experience. Adv Health Sci Educ. 2025;30:973–1005.
5. Ainoda N, Onishi H, Yasuda Y. Definitions of SDL. Ann Acad Med Singapore. 2005;34:515–9.
6. Anshu, Gupta P, Singh T. SDL in undergraduate curriculum. Indian Pediatr. 2022;59:331–8.
7. Barton J, Rallis KS, Corrigan AE, et al. SDL patterns during COVID-19. J Educ Eval Health Prof. 2021;18:5.
8. Gupta N, Ali K, Jiang D, et al. Learner agency in SDL. BMC Med Educ. 2024;24:1519.
9. Kemp K, Baxa D, Cortes C. Collaborative SDL model. Med Sci Educ. 2022;32:195–207.
10. Buch AC, Rathod H, Naik MD. Scope and challenges of SDL. J Med Edu. 2021;20: e114077.
11. Murad MH, Coto-Yglesias F, Varkey P, et al. SDL in health professions education. Med Educ. 2010;44:1057–68.
12. Schmidt HG, Rotgans JI, Yew EHJ. Process of problem-based learning. Med Educ. 2011;45:792–806.
13. Brydges R, Nair P, Ma I, et al. Directed self-regulated learning. Med Educ. 2012;46:648–56.
14. Frank JR, Snell LS, Sherbino J. Competency-Based Medical Education Framework. Ottawa; 2010.
15. Ginzburg SB, Santen SA, Schwartzstein RM. SDL revisited. Med Sci Educ. 2021;31:229–30.
16. Seraji F, Rahnemo SS. SDL in e-learning environments. Educ Inf Technol. 2025;30: 13331–49.
17. Cook DA, Levinson AJ, Garside S. Internet-based learning. JAMA. 2008;300:1181–96.
18. Driessen E, van Tartwijk J, Vermunt J, et al. Portfolios in medical training. Med Teach. 2007;29:44–9.
19. Prober CG, Heath C. Lecture halls without lectures. N Engl J Med. 2012;366:1657–9.
20. Schmidt HG, Moust JHC. Tutor effectiveness in PBL. Acad Med. 1995;70:708–14.

CHAPTER 16

Learning Domain and Progression of Learning

Swarna Rekha Bhat

"Destroying any nation does not require the use of atomic bombs or the use of long-range missiles. It only requires lowering the quality of education and allowing cheating in the examinations by the students."[1]

INTRODUCTION

A simple definition of learning is the acquisition of knowledge. What we need to understand is that it is not sufficient to acquire knowledge; we should be able to apply it and see it bring about behavior change. As medical professionals, we not only need knowledge but also skills to practice medicine, and we should be able to empathize and communicate with our patients. This holistic learning process lays the foundation for what we call the domains of learning.

DOMAINS OF LEARNING

Domains of learning include cognitive, psychomotor, and affective domains, as described in **Table 1**.

PROGRESSION OF LEARNING[2]

Progression means moving gradually from a basic level to a more advanced level.

TABLE 1: Domains of learning.

Domains of learning	*What do we acquire?*	*What do we use to learn?*
Cognitive	Knowledge	Head
Psychomotor	Skills	Hands
Affective	Attitude	Heart

Learning progression, or the progression of learning, describes how learners progress from basic knowledge, skills, and understanding to more advanced levels in each domain. In medical education, the learner must progress from novice to competent physician. This progression should be defined in the curriculum and assessed longitudinally. The progression of learning in each domain is described further.

Bloom's Taxonomy

Benjamin Bloom, an educational psychologist, described the three domains of learning way back in 1956. These include the cognitive, psychomotor, and affective domains. The cognitive domain relates to knowledge, the psychomotor to skills, and the affective domain to attitude.[3] Simplistically put, these would relate to head, hands, and heart.[1] The concept of the head, hand, heart model is particularly relevant to medical education. The goal of medical education is to produce a competent doctor. For this, a doctor needs knowledge, skills, and a proper attitude to manage patients and their families. Examples for each domain are given in **Table 2**.

TABLE 2: Domains with examples.

Domain	*Example 1*	*Example 2*
Cognitive	Knowing the lifecycle of the malaria parasite	Knowing the causes of birth asphyxia
Psychomotor	Making a blood smear to detect the malaria parasite	Performing bag and mask ventilation on a manikin
Affective	Counseling a patient about the preventive aspects of malaria	Communicating with parents about the condition of their newborn, who has been resuscitated

HIGHER LEVELS OF LEARNING/ PROGRESSION OF LEARNING

Each domain has multiple levels of learning until one masters it. These levels are listed in **Table 3**.

Cognitive Domain[3–5]

In each domain, there are levels of learning, from simpler to more complex. These levels progress from basic knowledge to more sophisticated levels, such as critical thinking.

TABLE 3: Levels of learning.

Cognitive domain	*Psychomotor domain*	*Affective domain*
Knowledge	Perception	Receiving
Comprehension	Set	Responding
Application	Guided response	Valuing
Analysis	Mechanism	Organizing
Synthesis	Complex overt response	Internalizing
Evaluation	Adaptation	
	Organization	

In the cognitive domain:

- *Acquiring knowledge*: In the first level, the learner will learn the facts and will be able to recall what has been previously learnt.
- *Comprehension*: Understanding the facts and making sense of information. It also involves the ability to interpret and explain in your own words.
- *Application*: It involves using knowledge in real-world situations. This stage helps learners in problem-solving.
- *Analysis*: Utilize knowledge to understand the overall structure.
- *Synthesis*: Synthesizing all facts and concluding
- *Evaluate*: To evaluate something based on preset criteria, the ability to back up ideas with evidence.

Anderson and Krathwohl's revised taxonomy classifies these stages into remembering, understanding, applying, analyzing, evaluating, and creating. In the revised version, making is the highest level of cognitive function, in which the learner can make or do something new, using their knowledge and experience.[4]

Simplified classification of cognitive domain:[6]

- Knowledge
- Understanding
- Application

Many other educators have tried to create their own classifications of learning levels. Another example is the SOLO taxonomy by Biggs.[4]

Structure of observed learning outcomes (SOLO taxonomy by Biggs)

- Prestructural
- Unistructural
- Multistructural
- Relational
- Extended abstract

In medical education, these levels of cognitive function help the learner to progress

TABLE 4: Keywords that can be used to assess different levels of cognitive function.

Level	*Keywords*
Knowledge	Write, describe, list, enumerate, arrange, reproduce, and recall
Comprehension	Explain, discuss, identify, interpret, classify, and review
Application	Determine, solve, apply, and illustrate
Analysis	Compare, contrast, analyze, and differentiate
Synthesis	Synthesize, develop, modify, construct, and create
Evaluate	Evaluate, justify, appraise, and assess
Create	Create, design, and reconstruct

from knowing about normal function, what happens when there is a disease/disorder, how to recognize this, how to differentiate this from other similar conditions, what tests are required to confirm diagnosis and treat the condition, and recognize and handle complications or deviations from normal.

Keywords for assessing these levels in the cognitive domain are discussed in **Table 4**, and those for the psychomotor and affective domains are discussed in **Table 5**.[1,3]

Psychomotor Domain[3–5]

Simpson has described levels in the psychomotor domain.

In the psychomotor domain:

- *Perception*: Understand the procedure/skill, for example, providing a bag, mask, and ventilation
- *Set*: Get ready to perform
- *Guided response*: Perform under guidance

TABLE 5: Keywords used to assess different levels in the psychomotor and affective domains.[1,3]

Psychomotor domain	*Words*	*Expectation*	*Affective domain*	*Words*
Perception	Detect and identify	Observes	Receiving	Listen, observe, and recognize
Set	Begin, perform, show, and demonstrate	Learns to perform	Respond	Respond, comply, examine
Guided response	Copy, reproduce, and follow	Performs under guidance	Valuing	Choose, select, differentiate, justify
Mechanism (basic proficiency)	Perform, construct, and demonstrate	Performs independently Basic proficiency	Organization of values	Improve, organize, modify, develop, and integrate
Complex, overt response (expert)	Perform, demonstrate	Performs under difficult situations	Characterization (internalization of values)	Characterize, verify, validate, and practice
Adaptation	Rearrange, revise	Able to adapt in different situations		
Organization	Create, construct, and compose	Able to organize		

- *Mechanism*: Understand the science behind the procedure/ skill, for example, there is a limit to the amount of inflation that needs to be provided.
- *Complex overt response*: Ability to perform under different situations and respond appropriately if there is a problem, and what should be done if chest rise is not occurring.
- *Adaptation*: Adaptation of the skill in other situations, for example, term and preterm neonates. Ability to perform independently.
- *Organization*: Ability to integrate and organize with other skill sets, for example, integrate the skill of providing a bag and mask with different skills required for resuscitation.

To put the levels of the psychomotor domain more simply, they would be: copy/ imitate, practice under supervision, and perform independently.[6] A more detailed but practical description of the levels would be:

- Observe
- Perform under supervision on a mannikin.
- Perform under supervision in a real-life situation.
- Perform independently under uncomplicated situations.
- Perform independently under complex situations.
- Ability to integrate skills.

Other Psychomotor Domains (Dave)[3,5]

- *Imitation*: Observing and imitating someone else.
- *Manipulation*: Performing a skill based on instructions.
- *Precision*: Achieving accuracy and exactness in skill performance without external assistance.
- *Articulation*: Combining and sequencing two or more skills to do them consistently.
- *Naturalization*: Combining and sequencing two or more talents with ease, and carrying them out with little physical or mental effort.

Affective Domain[3–5]

The affective domain refers to counseling, communication skills, ethics, empathy, and values.

In the affective domain:

- *Receiving*: The ability to listen/understand what the parent knows.
- *Responding*: Appropriately after listening/ understanding what the parent knows
- *Valuing*: What does the other person have to say?
- *Organizing*: Organizing and communicating appropriately.
- *Internalizing*: The ability to internalize the process such that the communication/ counseling session becomes a habit and can be performed at any time under any situation.

Simplified classification of the affective domain:[6]

- Receiving
- Responding
- Internalizing

APPLICATION OF LEARNING DOMAINS IN MEDICAL EDUCATION

In the systems approach to medical education, we have input, process, and output. The process consists of:

- Formulating objectives.
- Planning and implementing the learning process.
- Planning and implementing evaluation.

This is also known as the educational spiral.

The three domains of learning we have been discussing should be incorporated into all the processes above to make the educational process more meaningful.

Setting objectives would be different for each domain. Example in the cognitive domain: to enumerate steps in resuscitation; in the psychomotor domain: To demonstrate bag-mask ventilation; and in the affective domain: to counsel parents of an asphyxiated neonate.

While planning teaching and learning methods, focusing on domains is also important. The cognitive domain can be addressed during a lecture, but a higher level of cognition may require something like problem-based learning (PBL). For the psychomotor domain, it must be a demonstration, a video, or observing a procedure, followed by a simulation exercise. For the affective domain, the method could be role-play.

Similarly, for evaluation, the methods will differ based on the domain being tested. Essay questions and MCQs can test cognitive function. The questions must be different to test different levels of the cognitive domain.[7,8] Most often, lower levels of the domain are tested, and we must make a conscious effort to test higher levels of cognition.

Domains are essential in newer teaching and learning methods, such as simulation. All three domains should be incorporated into the planning of a simulation scenario.[9]

APPLICATION OF PROGRESSION OF LEARNING IN MEDICAL EDUCATION

Progression of learning has been described earlier as moving from basic knowledge to more advanced levels, such as critical thinking, moving from basic proficiency to expert level with reference to skills. In medical education, it refers to progressing from a novice student to a competent physician. The progression in each domain has already been described.

It is not easy to maintain continuity in training, and often students learn in parts and then have to integrate all that they have learnt. For example, characteristics of a microorganism are learnt in microbiology and the disease in clinical postings. Assessing this ability to integrate and progress toward becoming a competent doctor is also essential, but it is not often done. So, evaluating progression in each domain and longitudinally throughout the course is essential.[10]

NEWER APPROACHES TO CLASSIFICATION OF THE LEARNING PROCESS: FINK'S TAXONOMY[9,11]

With the widening scope of medical education, newer learning taxonomies have been developed. One of these is Fink's taxonomy of significant learning. The components of Fink's taxonomy are:

- Learning how to learn
- Foundational knowledge
- Application
- Integration
- Human dimension
- Caring

Learning how to learn involves deep learning, self-directed learning, and constructing knowledge. This skill is critical in a clinical setting where the learning environment is unstructured.

Foundational knowledge includes cognitive tasks such as remembering and understanding, like the first levels of Bloom's taxonomy, but it also emphasizes depth of knowledge.

Application includes higher-level thinking, critical thinking, and skill acquisition; integration involves integrating acquired knowledge with existing knowledge, identifying gaps, and resolving any conflicts.

The last two, human dimension and caring, refer to the affective domain of Bloom's taxonomy and include ethics, values, empathy, social skills, and finding job satisfaction.

CONCLUSION

- There are three domains of learning: cognitive, psychomotor and affective.
- Cognitive refers to knowledge, psychomotor to skills and affective to attitude and communication skills.
- Mastery in each of these domains is essential to become a competent doctor
- Each of these domains has different levels, starting from basic to more complex.
- In cognitive, this would be to recall and then move on to critical thinking.
- In psychomotor, this would be from basic to expert level proficiency.
- In addition to assessing progress in the levels of learning in each domain, assessing progression longitudinally through the course is also required.

REFERENCES

1. Islam MA, Said SBHM, Umarlebbe JH, et al. Conceptualization of the head-heart-hands model for developing an effective 21st century teacher. Front Psychol. 2022;13:1-10.
2. Gallacher T, Johnson M. Learning progressions: a historical and theoretical discussion. Research matters, 2019;28:10-6.
3. Singh G, Singh R. Domains of learning: Art of learning in medical education program. Era's J of Med Research. 2020;7(1):79-85.
4. Anand B, Mishra I, Beri G, Chaudhary KL. Types of Learning: Domains of Learning-Cognitive, Affective, and Psychomotor, Learning Theories, Experiential Learning. In extension methods, ICT and education technology. Elite publishing house. 2024;53:82.
5. Hoque EM, Three Domains of Learning: Cognitive, Affective and Psychomotor. J EFL Educ Res. 2016;2:45-52.
6. Shashindran CH. Taxonomy of educational objectives in Medical education principles and practice. In: Nilakantan A, Sethuraman KR, Santosh K, et al. (Eds). Medical Education - Principles And Practice, 2nd edition. Puducherry: NTTC, JIPMER; 2000. pp. 16-23.
7. Perera D, Ramanayake RPJC, de Silva AHW, et al. Domain-specific learning among medical students. J Res Med Educ Ethics. 2012;2(3):264-7.
8. Kim MK, Patel RA, Uchizono JA, Beck L. Incorporation of Bloom's taxonomy into multiple-choice examination questions for a pharmacotherapeutics course. Am J Pharm Educ. 2012;76(6):1-8.
9. Orgill BD, Nolin J. Learning taxonomies in medical simulation. In: Stat Pearls (internet). Treasure Island (FL): StatPearls Publishing; 2025.
10. Vantini I, Benini L. Models of learning, training and progress evaluation of medical students. Clinica Chemica Acta. 2008;393(1):13-6.
11. Branzetti J, Gisondi MA, Hopson LR, et al. Aiming Beyond Competent: The Application of the Taxonomy of Significant Learning to Medical Education. Teach Learn Med. 2019;31(4):466-78.

SECTION 3

Assessment

CHAPTER 17

Principles of Assessment

Somashekhar Nimbalkar

Learning Objectives

- Understand the theoretical foundations and historical evolution of assessment in medical education.
- Apply core assessment frameworks and principles to medical education contexts.
- Select and implement appropriate assessment methods aligned with specific educational purposes.
- Implement modern assessment approaches while ensuring quality assurance and stakeholder engagement.

INTRODUCTION

Assessment is a cornerstone of medical education because it not only judges achievement but also shapes what and how learners study, practice, and improve. Contemporary thinking has shifted from viewing assessment as a single high-stakes event toward designing an integrated assessment programme that supports learning while still enabling trustworthy decisions about progression and competence.

Assessment is multidimensional, balancing various considerations such as validity, reliability, acceptability, educational impact, and feasibility. This allows for assessing students in real educational settings rather than just ensuring testing psychometric strength. Because different levels of competence require different evidence, effective programs combine written tests, simulations, OSCE-style assessments, and workplace-based observations. However, an ideal assessment of a student would be difficult to achieve, as one would need data points over time to align assessment information with coaching, feedback, and fair progression decisions.

PRINCIPLES OF ASSESSMENT IN MEDICAL EDUCATION

Assessment in medical education serves as a cornerstone of the learning process, functioning not merely as an evaluation tool but as a powerful driver of student learning and curriculum development. Assessment practices have evolved from simple measurement-focused approaches to sophisticated, multidimensional systems that emphasize learning, competency development, and preparation for professional practice. This chapter explores the fundamental principles that guide effective assessment in medical education, drawing from contemporary research and best practices in the field.[1,2] The significance of assessment extends beyond grading and certification to encompass formative learning, professional development, and quality assurance in medical education. As medical education evolves toward competency-based models and programmatic approaches, understanding these foundational principles becomes essential for educators, administrators, and policymakers involved in designing and implementing effective assessment systems.[2,3]

THEORETICAL FOUNDATIONS OF ASSESSMENT

Historical Evolution of Assessment

Assessment in medical education has undergone significant transformation through distinct eras, each characterized by different values and approaches. The measurement era focused on objective testing and standardized examinations, emphasizing reliability and standardization. This was followed by the judgment era, which introduced workplace-based assessments and entrustable professional activities (EPAs), recognizing the importance of contextual performance evaluation.[1,3,4] The current systems era represents a paradigm shift toward programmatic assessment, where multiple assessment methods are integrated systematically over time. This approach recognizes that no single assessment can capture the full complexity of medical competence, necessitating a comprehensive system that combines various assessment modalities to provide a holistic view of learner development.[5,6]

Philosophical Underpinnings

Modern assessment philosophy in medical education is grounded in constructivist learning theory, which emphasizes that learning is an active process of knowledge construction rather than passive information absorption. This perspective has profound implications for assessment design, promoting approaches that engage learners in meaningful evaluation activities and provide opportunities for reflection and improvement.[3,7,8] The concept of assessment for learning rather than assessment of learning has gained prominence, emphasizing the formative function of assessment in supporting student development. This shift acknowledges that assessment should serve as a learning tool that provides actionable feedback and promotes continuous improvement throughout the educational journey.[9-11]

CORE PRINCIPLES OF ASSESSMENT

Van der Vleuten's Utility Equation

A foundational framework for understanding assessment quality is *Van der Vleuten's utility equation*, which proposes that the overall utility of an assessment depends on multiple factors working in concert. The equation considers five critical components.[12,13]

Validity represents the degree to which an assessment measures what it intends to measure. In medical education, this encompasses multiple dimensions including content validity (adequate sampling of the curriculum), construct validity (measuring intended competencies), criterion validity (correlation with external performance measures), and consequential validity (positive educational impact).[3,11,13]

Reliability refers to the consistency and reproducibility of assessment results across different occasions, raters, or test forms. While traditionally emphasized in psychometric theory, modern assessment approaches recognize that perfect reliability may not always be necessary if other utility components are strong.[3,6,12,13]

Educational impact focuses on how assessment influences student learning behaviors and curriculum implementation. Effective assessments should promote deep learning, encourage appropriate study behaviors, and align with educational objectives.[3,11,14]

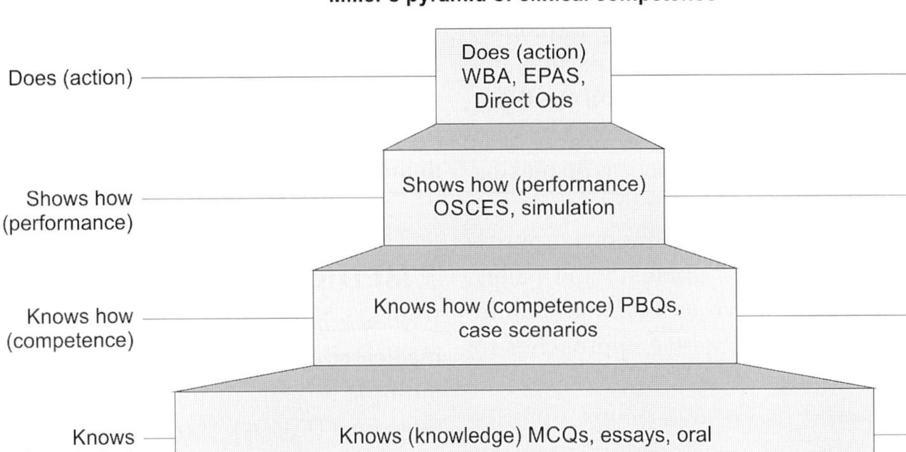

Fig. 1: Miller's pyramid of clinical competence assessment showing the four hierarchical levels and corresponding assessment methods.

Acceptability encompasses stakeholder buy-in, including student satisfaction, faculty engagement, and institutional support. Without acceptability, even well-designed assessments may fail to achieve their intended purposes.[3,15,16]

Cost-effectiveness considers the balance between assessment quality and resource requirements, including time, personnel, and financial costs. Practical implementation constraints must be balanced against assessment goals.[3,13,17]

Miller's Pyramid of Clinical Competence (Fig. 1)

Miller's pyramid provides a hierarchical framework for understanding and assessing clinical competence at different levels. This model has become foundational in medical education assessment design.[4,12,18]

The pyramid progresses from basic factual knowledge (*"Knows"*) through applied knowledge (*"Knows How"*) and demonstrated performance in controlled settings (*"Shows How"*) to authentic performance in clinical practice (*"Does"*). Each level requires different assessment approaches and serves distinct educational purposes.[18,19]

Recent developments have extended Miller's original framework to include additional dimensions such as *entrustment decision-making and professional identity formation*. These extensions recognize that clinical competence encompasses not only technical skills but also professional behaviors, values, and the ability to work independently with appropriate levels of supervision.[4,5,20]

TYPES AND PURPOSES OF ASSESSMENT

Classification by Purpose

Assessment serves multiple purposes in medical education, and understanding these purposes is crucial for selecting appropriate methods and interpreting results.

Formative assessment emphasizes learning and improvement through frequent, low-stakes evaluation activities that provide immediate feedback. Research demonstrates that formative assessment significantly enhances learning outcomes when implemented effectively, particularly when combined with meaningful feedback and opportunities for reflection.[9,10]

Summative assessment focuses on making judgments about achievement levels for grading, promotion, or certification purposes. While necessary for accountability and quality assurance, summative assessment should be balanced with formative approaches to optimize learning.[6,11,13]

Diagnostic assessment helps identify learning gaps and areas needing attention before or during the learning process. This type of assessment is particularly valuable in competency-based medical education, where individualized learning pathways may be necessary.[3,21,22]

Ipsative assessment compares learners' current performance with their own previous performance, emphasizing personal growth and development over time. This approach is particularly relevant in longitudinal assessment programs and portfolio-based evaluation systems.[5,6]

ASSESSMENT FUNCTIONS IN COMPETENCY-BASED MEDICAL EDUCATION

The shift toward competency-based medical education (CBME) has transformed assessment functions and requirements. CBME emphasizes *outcome-based evaluation* focused on demonstrated competencies rather than time-based progression. This approach requires assessment systems that can capture complex, multidimensional competencies and support individualized learning pathways.[5,21,22]

Entrustable professional activities (EPAs) have emerged as a key assessment framework in CBME, linking assessment directly to professional responsibilities and practice requirements. EPAs represent discrete units of professional practice that can be fully entrusted to learners once they have demonstrated sufficient competence.[4,5,23]

TRADITIONAL ASSESSMENT METHODS

Written examinations remain fundamental in medical education assessment, encompassing multiple formats including multiple-choice questions (MCQs), short-answer questions, essay questions, and modified essay questions (MEQs). Recent research emphasizes the importance of aligning question design with appropriate cognitive levels according to *Bloom's Taxonomy*.[13,24]

Analysis of medical education assessments reveals that many examinations focus disproportionately on lower-order cognitive skills (remembering and understanding) rather than higher-order thinking skills (applying, analyzing, evaluating, and creating). Effective assessment design should incorporate questions across all cognitive levels to promote comprehensive learning and clinical reasoning development.[24-27]

Oral examinations provide opportunities for direct interaction between examiners and learners, allowing assessment of communication skills, clinical reasoning, and professional attitudes. While potentially subjective, structured oral examinations can provide valuable insights into learner competence when properly designed and implemented.[3,13]

PERFORMANCE-BASED ASSESSMENT

Objective structured clinical examinations (OSCEs) represent a significant advancement in clinical skills assessment, providing standardized evaluation of clinical competencies in simulated environments. OSCEs allow assessment at the "Shows How" level of Miller's Pyramid, bridging the gap between knowledge and real-world performance.[7,18,19]

Research indicates that OSCEs demonstrate good reliability and validity for assessing clinical skills, though concerns exist about their artificial nature and potential disconnect from authentic clinical practice. Contemporary developments emphasize the need to balance standardization with authenticity in OSCE design.[7,19]

Simulation-based assessment extends performance evaluation to complex clinical scenarios and rare situations that may not be encountered in routine clinical practice. High-fidelity simulation environments allow assessment of technical skills, decision-making, teamwork, and crisis management in controlled, reproducible settings.[12,19,28]

WORKPLACE-BASED ASSESSMENT

Workplace-based assessment (WBA) represents the pinnacle of authentic evaluation, assessing learners in real clinical environments with actual patients. WBA methods include direct observation, case-based discussions, multisource feedback, and clinical supervisor reports.[15,16,29,30]

Recent research highlights both the potential and challenges of WBA implementation. While WBA offers high contextual validity and opportunities for meaningful feedback, issues of variability, standardization, and supervisor training remain significant concerns.

Mini-clinical evaluation exercise (Mini-CEX) provides a structured approach to workplace-based assessment, combining direct observation with immediate feedback. Studies demonstrate that Mini-CEX can be effective for both formative and summative purposes when implemented with adequate frequency and quality feedback.[10]

TECHNOLOGY-ENHANCED ASSESSMENT

The integration of *digital technologies* in assessment has expanded opportunities for innovative evaluation approaches while addressing traditional limitations of time, cost, and standardization. Technology-enhanced assessment includes computer-based testing, adaptive testing, automated scoring, and artificial intelligence applications.[23,31,32]

Artificial intelligence (AI) applications in assessment are rapidly evolving, with potential for automated essay scoring, clinical reasoning evaluation, and personalized feedback generation. However, careful consideration of validity, bias, and ethical implications is essential as these technologies are integrated into medical education assessment systems.

MODERN ASSESSMENT APPROACHES

Programmatic Assessment

Programmatic assessment represents a paradigmatic shift from individual high-stakes examinations to systematic, longitudinal evaluation systems. This approach integrates multiple assessment methods over time, using competency committees to make holistic judgments about learner progress and readiness for advancement.[5,6,22]

Key principles of programmatic assessment include *proportionality* (assessment burden matches importance), *triangulation* (multiple sources of evidence), and *longitudinality* (assessment over time). Research demonstrates that programmatic assessment can provide more robust decision-making while reducing individual assessment stakes and promoting learning.

Implementation of programmatic assessment requires significant organizational change, including faculty development, data management systems, and cultural transformation. Successful programs emphasize stakeholder engagement, clear communication, and gradual implementation strategies.[5,21,22]

Competency-based Assessment Systems

Competency-based assessment systems align evaluation practices with defined competency frameworks such as the *CanMEDS model, ACGME Core Competencies,* or institutional frameworks. These systems emphasize outcome-based evaluation and individualized progression based on demonstrated competence rather than time-based advancement.[21,33]

Milestone-based assessment provides structured frameworks for tracking learner development across competency domains. Milestones offer observable, measurable markers of progression that can guide both formative feedback and summative decision-making.[22,23]

The integration of EPAs *with competency-based assessment* creates powerful frameworks for linking assessment to professional practice requirements. This integration helps ensure that assessment systems prepare learners for the realities of clinical practice while maintaining educational rigor.[4,5,21,23]

QUALITY ASSURANCE IN ASSESSMENT

Validity Framework

Ensuring assessment validity requires systematic attention to multiple dimensions of evidence. Modern validity theory emphasizes *construct validity* as the overarching concept that encompasses all other forms of validity evidence:

Content validity ensures that assessments adequately sample the intended domain of knowledge, skills, and attitudes. This requires systematic curriculum mapping, expert review, and alignment between learning objectives and assessment content.[3,13,17]

Construct validity focuses on whether assessments truly measure the intended competencies or abilities. Evidence for construct validity includes factor analysis, correlation studies, and expert judgment about the relationship between assessment tasks and target constructs.[34]

Criterion validity examines the relationship between assessment results and external measures of performance. This includes concurrent validity (correlation with other measures of the same construct) and predictive validity (ability to predict future performance).[3,13]

Consequential validity considers the broader impacts of assessment on learners, curriculum, and educational systems. This includes intended positive consequences (enhanced learning, improved preparation) and potential negative consequences (teaching to the test, student stress).

Reliability Considerations

While reliability remains important in assessment design, contemporary approaches recognize that *perfect reliability may not always be necessary or achievable.* The appropriate level of reliability depends on the assessment purpose, consequences of decisions, and availability of multiple sources of evidence.[6,13]

Generalizability theory provides a framework for understanding and optimizing reliability across multiple facets of assessment, including content sampling, rater consistency, and occasion effects. This approach allows assessment designers to identify the most important sources of measurement error and develop targeted improvement strategies.[12]

Inter-rater reliability becomes particularly critical in performance-based and workplace-based assessments where subjective judgment plays a significant role. Strategies for enhancing inter-rater reliability include rater training, structured evaluation forms, calibration exercises, and regular feedback on rating patterns.[12,16,23]

Feedback and Improvement Systems

Effective assessment systems incorporate *continuous quality improvement* processes that monitor assessment effectiveness and identify areas for enhancement. This includes regular review of assessment data, stakeholder feedback, and outcome evaluation.[6,9]

Assessment analytics using learning management systems and assessment databases can provide valuable insights into assessment effectiveness, learner performance patterns, and areas needing attention. These data-driven approaches support evidence-based decision-making about assessment design and implementation.[6,23]

CONTEMPORARY CHALLENGES AND FUTURE DIRECTIONS

Trust and Assessment Systems

Recent literature emphasizes *trust as a foundational requirement* for effective assessment systems. The erosion of trust in assessment among learners, faculty, and other stakeholders has significant implications for assessment effectiveness and educational outcomes.[1]

Building trustworthy assessment systems requires attention to *transparency, fairness, consistency, and meaningful stakeholder engagement.* This includes clear communication about assessment purposes and processes, consistent application of standards, and opportunities for learner voice and feedback.

Context and Culture in Assessment

Recognition of the *sociocultural context* of assessment has grown significantly, with increasing attention to how cultural, institutional, and system-level factors influence assessment effectiveness. Assessment systems must be designed and implemented with sensitivity to local contexts while maintaining educational quality and standards.[1,33,35]

Equity and inclusion considerations are increasingly important in assessment design, ensuring that evaluation methods do not inadvertently disadvantage learners from diverse backgrounds. This includes attention to language barriers, cultural differences, and varying educational backgrounds.[16,33,36]

Technology Integration and Innovation

The rapid advancement of *educational technology* creates both opportunities and challenges for assessment in medical education. While technology can enhance efficiency, standardization, and accessibility, it also raises questions about validity, security, and educational impact.[17,32]

Artificial intelligence and machine learning applications in assessment show promise for automated scoring, personalized feedback, and adaptive testing. However, careful validation and ethical consideration are essential as these technologies are integrated into high-stakes assessment systems.[23,31]

Workplace Learning and Assessment Integration

The integration of *learning and assessment in clinical environments* requires sophisticated approaches that balance educational goals with patient care responsibilities. This includes developing assessment methods that capture the complexity of clinical practice while providing meaningful feedback for learner development.[15,29]

Interprofessional assessment is becoming increasingly important as healthcare delivery evolves toward team-based care models. Assessment systems must adapt to evaluate collaboration' communication' and teamwork skills across professional boundaries.[30]

IMPLEMENTATION STRATEGIES AND BEST PRACTICES

Faculty Development

Successful implementation of modern assessment approaches requires *comprehensive faculty development* programs that address both technical skills and conceptual understanding. Faculty development should encompass assessment design principles' implementation strategies' and ongoing quality improvement.[17,37,38]

Assessment literacy among faculty is essential for effective implementation. This includes understanding assessment theory' practical skills in method selection and implementation' and ability to use assessment data for decision-making and improvement.

Institutional Support Systems

Effective assessment systems require *robust institutional support* including administrative leadership, resource allocation, and technological infrastructure. This includes investment in assessment technology, data management systems, and personnel dedicated to assessment coordination.[5,6,21]

Change management strategies are crucial for successful assessment implementation, particularly when transitioning from traditional to innovative approaches. This includes stakeholder engagement, communication strategies, and phased implementation approaches.[5,21,22]

QUALITY MONITORING AND EVALUATION

Assessment systems require *ongoing monitoring and evaluation* to ensure effectiveness and continuous improvement. This includes regular review of assessment data, stakeholder feedback, and outcomes evaluation.[6]

Assessment research and evaluation should be integrated into institutional assessment programs to generate evidence about effectiveness and identify areas for improvement. This includes both internal evaluation and participation in broader research initiatives.[3,6]

CONCLUSION

The principles of assessment in medical education provide a foundational framework for designing, implementing, and evaluating effective assessment systems that serve both learning and accountability functions. As medical education continues to evolve toward competency-based models and programmatic approaches, these principles become increasingly important for ensuring that assessment systems support learner development while maintaining educational quality and public accountability.

The integration of traditional assessment wisdom with contemporary innovations in technology, workplace-based evaluation, and systems thinking creates unprecedented opportunities for enhancing assessment effectiveness. However, successful implementation requires careful attention to validity, reliability, educational impact, and stakeholder engagement within the specific context of each educational program.

Future developments in assessment will likely emphasize greater integration of learning and assessment functions, increased use of technology and artificial intelligence, and enhanced attention to equity, inclusion, and cultural sensitivity. The continued evolution of assessment practices must balance innovation with proven principles, ensuring that new approaches genuinely enhance rather than merely complicate the educational enterprise.

The ultimate goal of assessment in medical education remains the preparation of competent, caring, and professional physicians who can provide excellent patient care in increasingly complex healthcare environments. By adhering to sound assessment principles while embracing appropriate innovations, medical educators can create assessment systems that truly serve this fundamental purpose.

KEY LEARNING POINTS

- Assessment has evolved from a measurement-focused approach to a sophisticated, multidimensional systems approach.
- Van der Vleuten's utility equation identifies five critical, interdependent components of assessment quality.
- Miller's pyramid provides a hierarchical framework for understanding clinical competence and selecting appropriate assessment methods.
- Programmatic assessment represents a paradigm shift toward systematic, longitudinal evaluation that reduces assessment stakes while enhancing decision-making quality.
- Trust, transparency, fairness, and meaningful stakeholder engagement are foundational requirements for effective assessment systems.
- Successful implementation of modern assessment approaches requires comprehensive faculty development, robust institutional support systems, and ongoing quality monitoring.

REFERENCES

1. Caretta-Weyer HA, Smirnova A, Barone MA, et al. The Next Era of Assessment: Building a Trustworthy Assessment System. Perspect Med Educ. 2024;13(1):12-23.
2. Kassam A, de Vries I, Zabar S, et al. The Next Era of Assessment Within Medical Education: Exploring Intersections of Context and Implementation. Perspect Med Educ. 2024;13(1):496-506.
3. Aslam P, Ilyas T, Anwar M, et al. Assessment in Medical Education: Evolving trends. Phys Educ Health Soc Sci. 2025;3(2):257-61.
4. ten Cate O, Carraccio C, Damodaran A, et al. Entrustment Decision Making: Extending Miller's Pyramid. Acad Med. 2021;96(2):199.
5. Cheung WJ, Bhanji F, Gofton W, et al. Design and Implementation of a National Program of Assessment Model - Integrating Entrustable Professional Activity Assessments in Canadian Specialist Postgraduate Medical Education. Perspect Med Educ. 2024;13(1):44-55.
6. Schut S, Maggio LA, Heeneman S, et al. Where the rubber meets the road - An integrative review of programmatic assessment in health care professions education. Perspect Med Educ. 2021;10(1):6-13.

7. Majeed GM, Islam J, Nandakumar G, et al. Progress Testing in UK Medical Education: Evaluating Its Impact and Potential. Cureus. 2024;16(1):e52607.
8. Lakhtakia R, Otaki F, Alsuwaidi L, et al. Assessment as Learning in Medical Education: Feasibility and Perceived Impact of Student-Generated Formative Assessments. JMIR Med Educ. 2022;8(3):e35820.
9. Fuentes-Cimma J, Sluijsmans D, Riquelme A, et al. Designing feedback processes in the workplace-based learning of undergraduate health professions education: a scoping review. BMC Med Educ. 2024;24(1):440.
10. Gupta SK, Srivastava T. Assessment in Undergraduate Competency-Based Medical Education: A Systematic Review. Cureus. 2024;16(4):e58073.
11. Jamieson J, Palermo C, Hay M, et al. Assessment practices for dietetic students: An updated systematic review (2017-2024). Nutr Diet. 2025;82(5):467-86.
12. Ismail OM, Said UN, El-Omar O, et al. Theories and Practices in Learning and Assessment for Postgraduate Medical Education: A Review. Cureus. 2024;16(11):e74160.
13. Al-Wardy NM. Assessment Methods in Undergraduate Medical Education. Sultan Qaboos Univ Med J. 2010;10(2):203-9.
14. Tabish SA. Assessment Methods in Medical Education. Int J Health Sci. 2008;2(2):3-7.
15. Andreou V, Peters S, Eggermont J, et al. A needs assessment for enhancing workplace-based assessment: a grounded theory study. BMC Med Educ. 2024;24(1):659.
16. Siriwardena AN, Phung VH, Emerson K, et al. Perceptions and experiences of trainers and trainees of UK workplace-based assessment for general practice licensing: a mixed methods survey. Educ Prim Care. 2024;35(5):147-59.
17. Shrivastava SR, Hidayah RN. Designing a Faculty Development Program on Electronic Question Banks: Schedule, Evaluation, and Sustainability Plan. J Sci Soc. 2025;52(2):181.
18. Witheridge A, Ferns G, Scott-Smith W. Revisiting Miller's pyramid in medical education: the gap between traditional assessment and diagnostic reasoning. Int J Med Educ. 2019;10:191-2.
19. DeBiasio C, Pageau P, Shefrin A, et al. Point-of-Care-ultrasound in undergraduate medical education: a scoping review of assessment methods. Ultrasound J. 2023;15(1):30.
20. Cruess RL, Cruess SR, Steinert Y. Amending Miller's Pyramid to Include Professional Identity Formation. Acad Med. 2016;91(2):180.
21. Frank JR, Karpinski J, Sherbino J, et al. Competence By Design: a transformational national model of time-variable competency-based postgraduate medical education. Perspect Med Educ. 2024;13(1):201-23.
22. Emke AR, Torre D, Aagaard EM. Competency-Based Education and Programmatic Assessment in Undergraduate Medical Education: Describing the Gateway Experience of Successful Design and Implementation. Acad Med. 2025;100(11):1268.
23. Spadafore M, Yilmaz Y, Rally V, et al. Using Natural Language Processing to Evaluate the Quality of Supervisor Narrative Comments in Competency-Based Medical Education. Acad Med. 2024;99(5):534.
24. Ramavat M, Prajapati T, Akhani PN, et al. Analysis of Physiology Theory Question Papers for Competency-Based Medical Education Implementation in Gujarat: A Pilot Study. Cureus. 2024;16(7):e65642.
25. Javaeed A. Assessment of Higher Ordered Thinking in Medical Education: Multiple Choice Questions and Modified Essay Questions. MedEdPublish. 2018;7:128.
26. Muhayimana T, Kwizera L, Nyirahabimana MR. Using Bloom's taxonomy to evaluate the cognitive levels of Primary Leaving English Exam questions in Rwandan schools. Curric Perspect. 2022;42(1):51-63.
27. Bajpai R, Gavali Y, Rukadikar C. Assessment by modified essay type questions and multiple-choice questions in medical undergraduate students: Which are better in addressing higher cognitive skills? Natl J Physiol Pharm Pharmacol. 2024;14(10):2041.

28. Chebly KO, Hernández E, Cifelli M, et al. Evaluation of an International Point of Care Ultrasound (POCUS) Training Program for Internal Medicine Physicians. POCUS J. 2025;10(01):19-26.
29. Verhees MJM, Landstra AM, Engbers R, et al. Exploring workplace-based learning in distributed healthcare settings: a qualitative study. BMC Med Educ. 2024;24(1):78.
30. Holmboe ES. Work-based Assessment and Co-production in Postgraduate Medical Training. GMS J Med Educ. 2017;34(5):Doc58.
31. Souto MEVC, Fernandes AC, Silva ABS, et al. A multi-model longitudinal assessment of ChatGPT performance on medical residency examinations. Front Artif Intell. 2025;8:1614874.
32. Morjaria L, Burns L, Bracken K, et al. Examining the Threat of ChatGPT to the Validity of Short Answer Assessments in an Undergraduate Medical Program. J Med Educ Curric Dev. 2023;10:23821205231204178.
33. Mukurunge E, Nyoni CN, Hugo L. Assessment approaches in undergraduate health professions education: towards the development of feasible assessment approaches for low-resource settings. BMC Med Educ. 2024;24:318.
34. Guth TA, Wolfe RM, Martinez O, et al. Assessment of Clinical Reasoning in Undergraduate Medical Education: A Pragmatic Approach to Programmatic Assessment. Acad Med. 2024;99(8):912.
35. Ward B, Diug B. Prioritising and reflecting on context in medical education. Med Educ. 2022;56(1):20-2.
36. Binda DD, Kraus A, Gariépy-Assal L, et al. Anti-racism curricula in undergraduate medical education: A scoping review. Med Teach. 2025;47(1):99-109.
37. Abdelkreem E, Abo-Kresha SA, Ahmed EA, et al. Needs assessment for faculty development at an Egyptian medical school: a triangulation approach. Int J Community Med Public Health. 2020;7(5):1669-79.
38. Heydari S, Adibi P, Omid A, et al. Diamond goals not graphite! A triangulation approach to clinical teachers' needs assessment. Med J Islam Repub Iran. 2021;35:96.

CHAPTER 18

Assessment of Knowledge: Methods

Nilofer Mujawar

INTRODUCTION

Having defined competency, we now move on to assessment of the competency achieved. Why do you need to assess it? An assessment of a competency certifies that the learner has the required abilities to perform a job effectively.

Within the framework of competency-based medical education (CBME) framework started by the Medical Council of India in 2019, at the end of the learning period, an Indian Medical Graduate (IMG) has acquired skills to don the role of a health care provider. The attributes of the IMG are five in number—clinician, leader, communicator, lifelong learner, and professional, which in 2023 were increased to seven with the addition of critical thinker and researcher.

For CBME to be successful, assessment of a competency is crucial since CBME is essentially an outcome-based model of education. Competency-based education has been defined as an outcome-based approach to the design, implementation, assessment, and evaluation of a medical education program using an organizing framework of competencies.

One does not acquire competency in one go. In fact, every competency can be broken down into sequential small parts called milestones. To achieve a competency, one acquires the knowledge then the skill and attitude to implement it. Hence, assessing one competency would warrant assessment over a period of time before the learner can be certified as competent. The teacher needs to identify the stage of the learner and modify the further teaching.

The medical education pattern of assessment so far as 2019 was easy to design and implement. Described as a summative pattern of assessment, it did not provide the stage of learning that the student was in. Competency-based assessment is more comprehensive in evaluating the stage of learning. It is reinforced by authentic and instant feedback which improves learning as the deviation in learning is identified early and rectified.

The National Medical Mission in alignment with the regulations of Graduate Medical Education, 2019 Part II document (Assessment Module for Undergraduate Medical Education 2019) has given the following definitions in its document:[1]

- *Summative assessment:* (University examination) an assessment conducted at the end of instruction to check how much the student has learnt.
- *Formative assessment:* An assessment conducted during the instruction with the primary purpose of providing feedback for improving learning.
- *Internal assessment:* Range of assessments conducted by the teachers teaching a particular subject with the express

purpose of knowing what is learnt and how it is learnt. Internal assessment can have both formative and summative functions.

- *Validity:* Degree to which the inferences drawn from assessment are supported by empirical evidence or theoretical rationale.
- *Reliability:* Degree of confidence that can be placed in the results. Depending on the context, it can be in terms of precision, consistency, or reproducibility.
- *Competency:* An observable activity of the health professional with a judicious and consistent mix of knowledge, skills, attitudes, and communication.

For the teacher who has taught the particular competency, assessment provides a gauge to what extent the student is adept and whether he is ready to move to the next level. For the student who has received feedback that he is now capable of doing a particular competency, it not only gives him the confidence but also the eagerness to improve upon his skills in actual situations. Thus, it is obvious that competency-based assessment (CBA) is a longitudinal process with feedback to the learner guiding further achievements.

For understanding the achievement of any competency, it is Miller's pyramid which is always referred to. Another important referral is Bloom's taxonomy of educational objectives. In clinical teaching Miller's Pyramid, proposed by psychologist George Miller in 1990, consists of four levels that represent the progression of clinical competence in medical education[2] **(Fig. 1)**:

1. *Knows:* This level indicates the basic knowledge that a learner possesses. It involves recalling facts and information relevant to clinical practice.
2. *Knows How:* At this level, learners understand how to apply their knowledge in clinical scenarios. They can describe procedures and processes but may not have practiced them yet.
3. *Shows:* This level reflects the ability to demonstrate skills in a controlled environment, such as a simulation or during supervised practice. Learners can show how to perform a procedure or apply their knowledge in practice.
4. *Does:* The highest level of the pyramid, where learners can independently apply their skills and knowledge in real clinical settings. This level indicates competence in performing clinical tasks without supervision.

BLOOM'S TAXONOMY (FIG. 2)

It consists of six hierarchical levels of learning:[3,4]

1. *Remembering*: Recall facts and basic concepts
2. *Understanding*: Explain ideas or concepts
3. *Applying*: Use information in new situations
4. *Analyzing*: Draw connections among ideas
5. *Evaluating*: Justify a decision or course of action
6. *Creating*: Produce new or original work

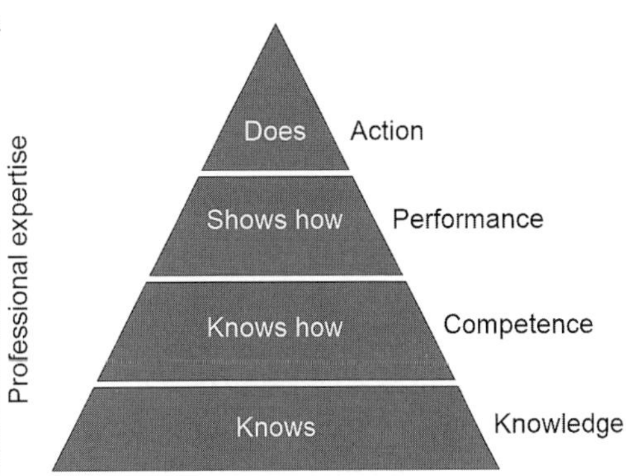

Fig. 1: Miller's pyramid.

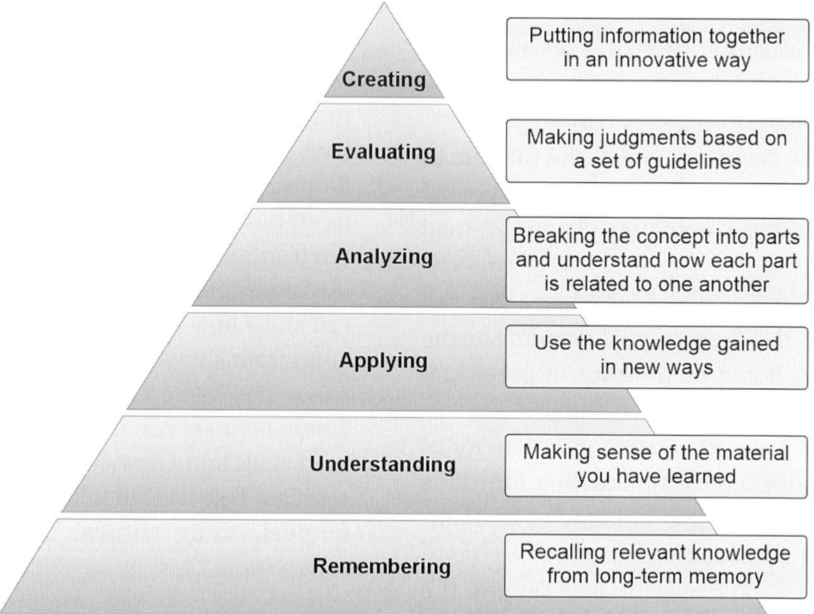

Fig. 2: Bloom's taxonomy.

These levels build upon each other, progressing from basic recall to higher-order thinking skills.

As far as undergraduate medical learning is concerned if one refers to Miller's pyramid, the level expected would be "shows" as "does" would mean ability to perform independently on the patient. According to Bloom's taxonomy, the learner would be on level 5, that is level of evaluation.

Adding to these two referral structures in 1996, Van der Vleuten proposed a conceptual model for defining the utility of an assessment tool.[5] Accordingly, he derived some criteria for judging an assessment tool:

- Validity (does it measure what it is supposed to be measuring?)
- Reliability (does it consistently measure what it is supposed to be measuring?)
- Educational impact (what are the effects on teaching and learning?)
- Acceptability (is it acceptable to staff, students, and other stakeholders?)
- Cost

The Medical Council of India, Assessment Module for Undergraduate Medical Education Training Program, 2019 states that the features of CBA are as follows:

- CBA operates within the framework of competencies. Assessment tools should align with competencies/objectives.
- CBA should help to acquire competencies/objectives (assessment for learning) and their certification (assessment of learning).
- CBA is continuous and ongoing process with opportunities for providing developmental feedback.
- Direct observation of students improves utility of CBA and feedback.
- Multiple assessors, multiple tools, and multiple assessments improve the validity and reliability of CBA.

All competencies have an element of different domain that is knowledge, attitude, and skill. A teacher may have to use more than one method of assessment before declaring the learner competent. In India, the summative examination is used to give the final result of whether the learner has cleared the examination and can be declared as pass or fail. The results would be declared by the University after the examiners convey the results to the University office confidentially. On the other hand, the formative assessments are carried out by the teachers at the college level and are ongoing as the learner starts attending the clinical terms. Thus, the formative assessments are ongoing assessment while the summative are held at the end of the term.

The pattern for the university examination is a set pattern followed by the colleges consisting of a theory examination and a practical examination which has varied little from the traditional examination format.

It is the formative assessment which will be elicited here. Since it is a longitudinal ongoing assessment, it is conducted while the teacher is instructing the learner. The assessment is happening there and then, and the teacher provides the feedback to the learner. Thus, feedback is the backbone of formative assessments and cements the learning process. Internal assessments (IA) recommended by the National Medical Mission are part of the process and are used by the teachers both for formative and summative assessment. It aids in covering a greater number of topics.

As mentioned earlier, a competency needs to be assessed in more than one domain. So, what can be done? Here comes the concept of a toolbox.

A toolbox is a listing of available tools (and rating forms, if required), which are suggested for a particular competency or sub-competency and aims at improving the value of assessment data.[6]

METHODS

Teachers need to research various methods and use their experience and expertise to choose assessment methods. Dividing the competency into its domains of knowledge and performance, they can create their own toolbox to apply to a particular domain.

ASSESSMENT OF KNOWLEDGE AND ITS APPLICATION

It is not very difficult for the teacher in the CBME to test the domain of knowledge as it has been an integral part of the traditional teaching method. Termed as the theory examination, knowledge is assessed by the written method. The following types of questions are framed for knowledge testing. Some of the verbs used for knowledge domain testing as per Bloom's taxonomy are given in **Table 1**.

Some of the ways in which written examinations are conducted are:

- Multiple choice questions
- Key features questions
- Short answer questions (SAQs)
- Essay questions
- Modified essay questions (MEQs)
- Script concordance test (SCT)

True or false questions encourage guessing and should be avoided. Questions asked should be challenging and have no ambiguity so that marking becomes objective.

ASSESSMENT OF PERFORMANCE

The assessment of performance can be regarded as the most important variation from the traditional method of assessment. In our country, there is no dearth of clinical material where performance can be assessed. But many issues arise when using real patients for this purpose. Thus, there has arisen the concept of simulations.

TABLE 1: Verbs in various levels in knowledge domain (Bloom's taxonomy).

Level	*Suggested verbs*
Knowledge	Define, describe, draw, find, enumerate, cite, name, identify, list, label, match, sequence, write, state
Comprehension	Discuss, conclude, articulate, associate, estimate, rearrange, demonstrate understanding, explain, generalize, identify, illustrate, interpret, review, summarize
Application	Apply, choose, compute, modify, solve, prepare, produce, select, show, transfer, use
Analysis	Analyze, characterize, classify, compare, contrast, debate, diagram, differentiate, distinguish, relate, categorize
Synthesis	Compose, construct, create, verify, determine, design, develop, integrate, organize, plan, produce, propose, rewrite
Evaluation	Appraise, assess, conclude, critic, decide, evaluate, judge, justify, predict, prioritize, prove, rank

Simulations can be mannequins or persons who simulate a patient. Before the actual assessment is done, certain principles should be observed. The principles of good medical practice should be observed. Consent of patients and the caretakers should be taken. If the assessment is done on actual patients then one should consider if the patient is "fatigued" due to the exams. Confidentiality should be strictly observed. The place where the assessment is done should be conducive to the conduct of the exams. A very common issue is the problem of communication in the local language as students from all over the country are admitted in the college.

The following tools are used for performance testing. Each has its pros and cons and should be used judiciously.

- Checklists
- Rating scales
- Objective structured clinical examination (OSCE)
- Short cases
- Long cases
- Mini clinical evaluation exercises (mini-cex)
- Portfolios

FEEDBACK

Feedback is the sheet anchor for the success of assessment.

It actually originated in rocket science where the system uses it to make subsequent adjustments to meet the set goals. In CBA, it is utilized to give the student as to what level he has achieved the competency. It helps identify the strength and weaknesses and plan further course of action.

Good feedback supports learning. Learners who have missed the target learn of their mistakes and progress towards improvement and learners who have achieved the target get confidence in performing the skills.[7]

The General Medical Council in its "Assessment in undergraduate medical education" Advice supplementary to Tomorrow's Doctors (2009) states that good feedback:

- Is specific, nonjudgemental, and descriptive, reflecting on observed behaviors and tasks
- Is provided within a supportive educational environment in which feedback is embedded, explicitly and implicitly

- Is delivered in a timely fashion while recognizing the need for quality control arrangements after assessments and that delaying feedback can help to improve the information provided. Expectations about the timescale for feedback should be explicit, honored, and monitored
- Is planned and considered to be ongoing and frequent, part of a sequence rather than a series of isolated episodes
- Avoids complexity and is restricted in length on any one occasion
- Is founded on respect for and the credibility of the feedback giver
- Is built into the assessment strategy and the curriculum
- Gives students consistent messages (or properly reflects inconsistent performance)
- Helps clarify good performance
- Elicits the learner's thoughts and feelings
- Facilitates the development of self-assessment, reflection, and a desire to learn, develop skills, and to seek out further assessment and feedback
- Delivers high-quality information to students about their learning
- Encourages teacher and peer dialog around learning
- Encourages positive motivational beliefs and self-esteem and avoids creation of anxiety
- Delivers difficult messages about progress in a way which is constructive and could not be construed as bullying
- Acknowledges that some students may need more detailed feedback, particularly in relation to interactional skills and self-presentation where they appear less confident or proficient: consideration should be given to the possibility that cultural or social background and norms may influence both their actions and how they are perceived by others
- Relates to the student's personal goals and establishes mutually agreed goals and provides opportunities to close the gap between current and required performance
- Provides information about teachers that can be used to help shape teaching[8]

The types of feedback:

The feedback is commonly classified as follows:

- Formal and informal feedback based on the process and settings
- Constructive, inspiring, and corrective feedback based on purpose
- Formative and summative feedback
- Sandwich and pendelton feedback based on the delivery

The National Medical Mission has designed the revised Basic Course Workshop (rBCW) in medical education technologies for medical teachers which provides training in tools to be used for lower two levels of Miller's pyramid while the Advance Course in Medical Education (ACME) trains in those for higher two levels.

CONCLUSION

An objective and structured assessment is essential to certify the achievement of competence. The frequent assessment at various stages of learning identifies the level of achievement of the learner.

Assessment in CBME is an ongoing process covering all domains—cognitive, psychomotor, attitudinal. Simulation labs help a student to practice a skill until they are confident of applying in real life situations. A good assessment identifies the areas where the learner needs to practice more. It helps the learner to gain confidence and progress to the next level.

REFERENCES

1. Medical Council of India. Assessment Module for Undergraduate Medical Education Training Program. New Delhi: Medical Council of India; 2019. pp. 1-29.
2. Bloom BS. Taxonomy of educational objectives. Handbook I: Cognitive domain. New York: David McKay; 1956.
3. Miller GE. The assessment of clinical skills/competence/performance. Acad Med. 1990;65(9 Suppl):S63-7.
4. Bloom's taxonomy of measurable verbs. [online] Available from https://www.utica.edu/academic/Assessment/new/Blooms%20Taxonomy%20-%20Best.pdf. [Last accessed January, 2025]
5. Van der Vleuten CPM. The assessment of professional competence: developments, research and practical implications. Adv Health Sci Educ. 1996;1:41-67.
6. ACGME. Toolbox of assessment methods ver 1.0. [online] Available from https://www.partners.org/Assets/Documents/Graduate-Medical-Education/ToolTable.pdf. [Last accessed January, 2025]
7. van der Vleuten CPM, Schuwirth LWT, Scheele F, Driessen EW, Hodges B. The assessment of professional competence: building blocks for theory development. Best Pract Res Clin Obst Gynaecol. 2010;24:703-19.
8. General Medical Council. (2009). Assessment in undergraduate medical education. [online] Available from https://www.gmc-uk.org/cdn/documents/assessment-in-undergraduate-medical-education---guidance-0815_pdf-56439668.pdf. [Last accessed January, 2025]

CHAPTER 19

Setting the Question Paper

Suman Singh

OBJECTIVES OF THE CHAPTER

Upon reading this chapter, readers will be able to:

- Explain the purpose and process of setting a question paper
- Identify the attributes of a good quality question paper
- Know the steps to be taken when setting a question paper
- Set a question paper as per the guidelines
- Conduct audits to check the quality of a question paper set.
- Understand the importance of using technology in the process of setting and assessing the quality of a question paper

INTRODUCTION

"If I had an hour to solve a problem, and my life depended on the solution, I would spend the first 55 minutes determining the proper question to ask... for once I know the proper question, I could solve the problem in less than five minutes" a well-known quote by Albert Einstein is a trigger for educators to think, how relevant and appropriate is this for our education and the quality of graduates being produced by the medical institutions. Can the time spent setting a high-quality question paper and the type of questions posed to our students in assessments equip them to solve the problems they are likely to face as healthcare providers more effectively and efficiently?

Most educators would agree "to a large extent" because every student who joins the educational institution is motivated either internally or externally to answer the questions that are being posed to them by examiners, and this makes the whole assessment process the single most important event in the life of a student.[1] The teachers need to capitalize on this event and spend maximum time in the process of making a plan for assessment and choosing to pose the right kind of questions at the right time using the right framework for their students. This makes assessment of the students the most critical component for any educational institution.[2] Without assessment, the institutions will not exist.

Assessments are being undertaken for various purposes.[3] Broadly, teachers need to inform the students if they are progressing as expected and if not, what are changes that need to be made or things what needs to be learnt.[4] Assessment being done for this purpose is known as the formative assessment and are conducted with the main focus on providing feedback to the students about their performance. Teachers also need to inform the students if they qualify for the next phase of their learning or qualify and are eligible for certification. This is commonly known as summative assessment, where the major focus is on decision-making instead of providing feedback to the learner.[5]

A large majority of students are motivated to learn because of the stimulus provided by the assessment process, and thus, assessment is considered the single most influential factor in learning. This driving influence of assessment has the potential to direct what, how and when a student learns.[5] To make use of this, educators must carefully plan the assessment process and set question papers with the right content, format of assessment, as well as the scheduling of examinations to help them make the right decisions.

Assessment being so critical for learners, it expects the teachers to spend time in planning the process of assessment keeping in mind all the attributes that ensure quality in assessment and make the optimum choice of test methods, tools, occasions, and assessors. This Educational impact of assessment must be remembered while setting the paper. We must assess "what we want the students to learn" as content repeatedly asked in exams will be perceived as important by them.

In this chapter, we intend to understand the process of setting a question paper for written assessment.

Concept and Process of Setting a Question Paper

Let us start learning the concept through posing certain questions to ourselves.

WHAT DOES IT MEAN TO SET A QUESTION PAPER?

Broadly dividing, we assess students on theoretical understanding or the cognitive domain and on practical skill performance or the psychomotor domain. Both these opportunities for assessment requires different types of planning and preparations.[2,3] Valid and reliable methods of assessment are necessary to determine students learning. When assessing the cognitive domain, written assessment becomes the most commonly used option with various types of questions being asked, ranging from long answer questions or essay-type questions (with their variations like structured, modified, case-based, etc.), short notes, short answer questions, and multiple choice questions. Each of these question types are well tested and has its own place in students' assessment with advantages and disadvantages.[6,7,8] We have learned the way to frame good quality questions along with the advantages and disadvantages of all of these.[3] When we intend to assess the learning of theory, a set of questions that are fit for the purpose need to be drawn and assembled in the form of a question paper. This is the meaning of setting a question paper.

WHAT IS THE NEED TO SET A QUESTION PAPER OR WHAT IS THE PURPOSE OF SETTING THE QUESTION PAPERS?

The goal of setting a question paper is to help the students express their learning and gain in knowledge with minimum risk of the "chance factor" playing role in students' performance.[9,10]

We need to know, the purpose for setting a specific question paper. Is it summative and we need to evaluate a student's knowledge gained at the end of a course and take some decisions about progression of the learner/certification/selection to some course, or is it formative/diagnostic, and we need to understand a student's level of learning and help them identify their strength and areas for improvement?

Sometimes results of the assessment process are also important in evaluating the program's effectiveness, but this purpose usually does not influence the way you set the question paper, as learners are kept at the center of setting the question paper and not the program. This is an additional use of test results.

WHAT ARE THE PREREQUISITES TO SET A GOOD QUESTION PAPER?

Prerequisites for setting question paper are:

- Know the purpose of the test
- Get the syllabus for the test
- Have the blueprint for the examination ready based on the purpose
- Decide on the objectives/outcomes that are to be tested by written format
- Decide on the level of cognition expected from the level of learners
- Decide which type of questions will best suit the objective and level, i.e., if a constructed response type (LAQ, SAQ) or supply type (MCQ) of question is required

WHAT IS THE CONCEPT, PURPOSE AND STEPS IN MAKING A BLUEPRINT?

A well-designed blueprint is one of the important educational tools that can improve major aspects of curriculum and assessment, which is beneficial to both faculty and students. Validity threats in the form of paper setters being different from teachers who may not be well versed with the expected learning outcomes from students are real. For an assessment to be valid, the paper or practical exercises should match course content, have proportional weightage of content according to clinical importance, consist of questions/exercises which are unambiguous, neither overly difficult nor easy, and use multiple tools to assess various learning outcomes.

A blueprint provides such a template for the question paper setter and the examiner to evaluate all that is expected from a student at the end of the learning sessions.[11] It determines the content of a test, lists the number and type of questions across the course content, learning objectives, and relative weightage given to each topic included in the assessment. It makes the assessment clear, explicit, and transparent for everyone involved in the process of teaching learning and assessment as it deals with the sampling of content, competencies and tools for assessment in a logical and balanced manner, thus reduces two major validity threats, i.e., construct under-representation and construct irrelevance variance by providing a template for the question paper setter and the examiner to assess all that is expected from a student at the end of learning period.[12]

Steps in constructing a blueprint for assessment:[11]

1. Define the purpose (formative/summative), scope (undergraduate/postgraduate), and level of learner (knows/knows how/shows how/does) before making a blueprint.
2. List the content, domain, and methods of assessment to be used
3. Decide the weightage to be given to content, domain, and methods of assessment.
   When deciding the weightage of content, the steps shown in **Table 1** can be followed.
4. Determine the percentage and types of questions to be constructed from various topics and levels of learning
5. Make a table of specifications with details of the type of questions, the domain, and the methods of assessment
6. Prepare a table of specifications

TABLE 1: Points to be considered while calculating the weightage of a topic/competency/disease in the curriculum.

• For basic sciences • Consider clinical relevance/ application of a topic/competency (I)	For clinical sciences, consider urgency/clinical significance and or preventive potential of a disease (I)	Frequency of occurrence/ application of basic science concept (F)	Importance of the topic of disease/ competency in the curriculum	Score to be assigned to both I and F separately
High	Life-threatening/high preventive potential	Very common	Core/must know area	3
Moderate	Serious but not immediately threatening/ moderate preventive potential	Relatively common	Good to know	2
Little/no clinical relevance	Nonurgent/no or little preventive effect	Rare	Noncore/nice to know	1

- Calculate the relative weightage of each area by multiplying the impact and frequency (I*F)
- Convert the total of (I*F) for all content areas to be included in the assessment and convert them into a fraction of one by dividing the I*F of each topic by the total (T) of I*F, i.e., (I*F/T)
- Multiply the fraction with the total number of items/scores included in the test to get the final weightage of that topic in the assessment blueprint

7. Prepare items/individual questions and organize them as per the paper format

Please note that, when it comes to choosing the tools or methods of assessment to be included in the assessment blueprint, there is no formula or objective way to decide. The nature of the subject and the kind of skills required from the student of that particular phase help in deciding the weightage of the test method and tool. We must remember that no single method is best, and it is always advisable to use a combination of test methods for each domain. The combination of these methods must be developed through discussion and consensus-building with expert faculty. If feasible, it is also advisable to take inputs from related clinical departments; this will enhance the reliability and validity of the assessment process.

Once we get clarity on the content, their weightage, and test methods, a two or three-dimensional matrix with the number and type of test questions from each topic, level of learning, and assessment tool can be made. This matrix helps the paper setter to plan the test. This must be done before writing items for the exam and is a necessary part of standard setting and quality assurance. With a blueprint, the whole process of assessment becomes explicit, transparent, fair, and clear, as this deals with the sampling of content, competencies, and tools. Validity, particularly the construct and content validity of assessment, is enhanced.

WHAT ARE THE NEXT STEPS ONCE WE HAVE ALL THE PREREQUISITES AVAILABLE TO SET THE QUESTION PAPER?

The following are the steps to be followed once we have all the required information for setting a question paper:

1. Draft the individual items based on the purpose/requirements/blueprint. Remember, it is not the type/format of question that decides the learning, but the way questions are framed. Thus, the way teachers frame individual items is of paramount importance. Palmer, EJ.
2. Draft the model answers/key points in students' responses to make scoring uniform by different examiners
3. Assemble the items as per the format/ guidelines given by the university/ institute
4. Review and edit the paper before it is given to students

WHAT ARE THE PARAMETERS OR ATTRIBUTES OF A GOOD QUESTION PAPER?

A framework for designing the question paper is usually available from the university for summative assessment. This has information about the date, time, marks, and type of questions to be asked in a particular examination, along with the instructions for the students. A blueprint for summative assessment is also made available by the university. While for formative and/or internal assessments, institutions devise a design with frequency, format, and marks along with instructions for students.

Along with the format or design of the question paper, the availability of a blue blueprint for the question paper helps in ensuring content and, to some extent, construct validity in the assessment. The paper setter must also be provided with the model question paper with the marking scheme, which can help in framing a good-quality question paper. Thus, a good quality question paper is an appropriately assembled, complete set of good questions.

The following are considered attributes or qualities of a good question paper:

- Each question asked in the paper is crisp and concise. It omits any unnecessary information that requires students to spend time understanding it correctly. The language used in drafting questions is simple, unambiguous, and appropriate for the level of the learner. It is such that a student understands what is expected from the question even when they don't know the answer to it. The responses given by the students will help identify problems in learning for the purpose of providing constructive feedback. We need to remember, "Nothing in the content or structure of [a test] item should prevent an informed student from responding correctly" Gronlund (1998).
- The questions are well-organized, have a logical flow, and are linked to the knowledge and/or skills that are being tested.
- The questions are structured in a manner that will improve consistency between marking by team members.
- The expected response or necessary content in the answer is established in the form of a model answer.
- The question paper is free from errors, including spelling/grammar, with an appropriate layout and spacing.
- The question paper has appropriate mark allocation.
- The question paper includes a mix of different types of questions like LAQ, SAQ, MCQ, and of different levels in Bloom's taxonomy, appropriate for the level of learner.
- The time allotted for completion should correlate with the content expected.

Once the paper is drafted, it needs to be reviewed and refined by the paper setter and then moderated for summative assessment before it is offered to the students. This will ensure that the paper drawn is valid, reliable, error-free, and balanced, which would ensure fair assessment of students.

There are no standardized methods to ensure the quality of a question paper. A checklist can be prepared to check the quality of a question paper set and can have items such as:

1. Are their any unclear test instructions?
2. Are the questions aligned with the objectives and outcomes of the course?
3. Are the questions appropriate and relevant for the level or learner?
4. Would the questions measure what they are intended to measure?
5. Is the language used easy to understand without any ambiguity?
6. Is any terminology confusing and ambiguous?
7. Is the paper overly verbose?
8. Is it using complicated vocabulary?
9. Is the sentence structure difficult or poor?
10. Are there any unnecessary and distracting details?
11. Will these questions help or encourage the students to learn better?
12. Is the question paper designed in a versatile manner that has a balance of both simple and complex topics?

A copyrighted checklist to audit the quality of the question paper is also given for reference.

The vetting committee must be set to review and evaluate question items according to specified criteria. This is necessary to detect and correct flaws to improve the quality.

Also, remember that the confidentiality of information matters when handling exam questions, more so in summative or high-stakes exams. The set procedures and protocols for the security of the information must be ensured. For example, protect files with passwords, use properly sealed and marked as confidential when delivering envelopes containing papers, if possible, hand-deliver rather than send in post. Destroy all rough drafts and ensure no document containing such information is accessible to unauthorized persons. Factors that facilitate the assessment process include good item banking and the availability of centralized management and administrative support for the logistics.

Every paper setter must remember and ensure that when they set exam question papers, the overall impact on students' learning experience is kept at the center.

When setting the question paper, ask the following questions before finalizing the paper:

- Is there anything in the paper that might not be clear to students?
- Do the questions framed test what is intended to be tested?
- Will the question test the learning outcome and help students work in a real setting?
- Is the question relevant and realistic?
- If the answer is yes to all of the above, proceed further.

Use of technology in a paper setting: Teachers face a significant challenge in creating varied and effective exam papers that align with learning objectives. AI-powered question paper generation tools offer a solution by automating the process. These systems can quickly produce consistent, fair, and unbiased assessments based on teacher-defined parameters, including difficulty level, question type, and topic. They utilize tagging systems to categorize questions, ranging from basic to advanced.[13] This technology streamlines question paper creation, saving teachers time and improving the overall quality of assessments.

AI-powered tools enable rapid exam creation and customization. A large number of platforms, such as https://questionpaper.ai, https://play.google.com/store/apps/details, tech.hypatia.OpExamsQuestionsGenerator, https://smallpdf.com/question-generator , https://examin8.com/, https://faq-en.exam.net.,https://www.prepai.io,https://www.quillionz.com/, https://www.testportal.net, etc., are available for the purpose with variable options. Some platforms allow teachers to pre-define MCQs, assign scores, and provide instant student feedback with learning resources. Software like Eklavvya offers comprehensive automation for question paper creation, enhancing efficiency, reliability, accuracy, and security.

While many platforms initially focused on MCQs, newer ones support a wider range of question types, including short answer and essay questions. Many offer extensive question banks. These tools enhance teaching by providing AI-powered quizzes, assessments, and exam generation, saving time and increasing student engagement. Some advanced tools, like questionpaper.ai, can even generate course outcomes and create CO-mapped question papers. They can also assist in designing innovative assessments beyond traditional written exams.

Mobile apps like OpExams QuestionsGenerator allow question generation from any text, and online tools like Smallpdf can create quizzes from uploaded PDFs. Platforms like Examin8 provide complete assessment and learning management solutions. Many integrate with LMS systems, such as Exam.net. Other examples include prepai.io, Quillionz, and Testportal.net. While these platforms offer significant benefits, they typically require faculty training, technical support, and institutional purchase.

These systems also facilitate the creation and maintenance of centralized, secure question banks. Security measures like digital encryption, blockchain, multi-factor authentication, watermarking, and DRM, combined with audit trails, protect exam integrity and prevent leaks. All of these platform requires faculty training, good technological support, and are to be purchased by institutions.

CONCLUSION

Question paper drafting is a critical aspect of educational assessment, requiring careful consideration of various factors to ensure quality and effectiveness. Studies have shown that question papers should cover different cognitive levels according to Bloom's taxonomy, assess various difficulty levels, and encompass all syllabus units. To enhance evaluation standards, a scientific approach to question paper construction is recommended, considering objectives, question types, content areas, time allocation, and difficulty levels.

REFERENCES

1. Rashmi K, Cesar O, Sunia S, Anthony AR, Hester D, Linda S, Cees van der V. The Effect of Assessments on Student Motivation for Learning and Its Outcomes in Health Professions Education: A Review and Realist Synthesis. Acad Med. 2023;98(9):1083-92.
2. Singh T. Principles of assessment in medical education. New Delhi: Jaypee Brothers Medical Publishers Pvt. Ltd.; 2012. pp. 205-13.
3. Al-Wardy NM. Assessment methods in undergraduate medical education. Sultan Qaboos University Med J. 2010;10(2):203-9.

4. Tabish SA. Assessment methods in medical education. Int J Health Sci (Qassim). 2008;2:3-7.
5. Wafubwa R. Role of Formative Assessment in Improving Students' Motivation: A Systematic Review of Literature. The International Journal of Assessment and Evaluation. 2020;28(1):17.
6. Hift RJ. Should essays and other "open-ended"-type questions retain a place in written summative assessment in clinical medicine?. BMC Med Educ. 2014;14:1-8.
7. Schuwirth LW, Van Der Vleuten CP. Different written assessment methods: what can be said about their strengths and weaknesses? Medical education. 2004;38(9):974-9.
8. Palmer EJ, Devitt PG. Assessment of higher order cognitive skills in undergraduate education: modified essay or multiple choice questions? Research paper. BMC Med Educ. 2007;7:49.
9. Mehta P, Ingole N. Mechanics of paper setting: Being a paper setter. The Art of Teaching Medical Students. 2015;3:276-87.
10. Godiyal P, Negi P. Construction of Question Paper. Int J Nurs Educ. 2024;16(1):1-7.
11. Coderre S, Woloschuk W, Mclaughlin K. Twelve tips for blueprinting. Medical teacher. 2009;31(4):322-4.
12. Patil SY, Gosavi M, Bannur HB, Ratnakar A. Blueprinting in assessment: A tool to increase the validity of undergraduate written examinations in pathology. Int J Appl Basic Med Res. 2015;5:S76-9.
13. Gauri N, Ramesh R. "Automatic Generation of Question Paper from User Entered Specifications Using a Semantically Tagged Question Repository." 2016 IEEE Eighth International Conference on Technology for Education (T4E). 2016;148-151.

CHAPTER 20

Assessment of Clinical Skills

Puja Dulloo

INTRODUCTION

Clinical skill assessment is an important component of medical education. It is a cornerstone for guaranteeing that healthcare professionals acquire the competencies necessary for providing safe and effective patient care. With the trend toward competency-based medical education (CBME), high-stakes and reliable clinical skill assessment methods are required for evaluating clinical reasoning, communication, procedural skills, and professionalism. The chapter covers the variety of modalities, advantages, and limitations of each and current trends in clinical skill testing.[1-3]

Clinical skills involve collecting, interpreting, communicating, and performing clinical procedures, including history and physical examinations, counseling, and practical methods.[4]

The significant principles that act as a backbone for practical assessment of clinical skills are illustrated in **Figure 1**, highlighting

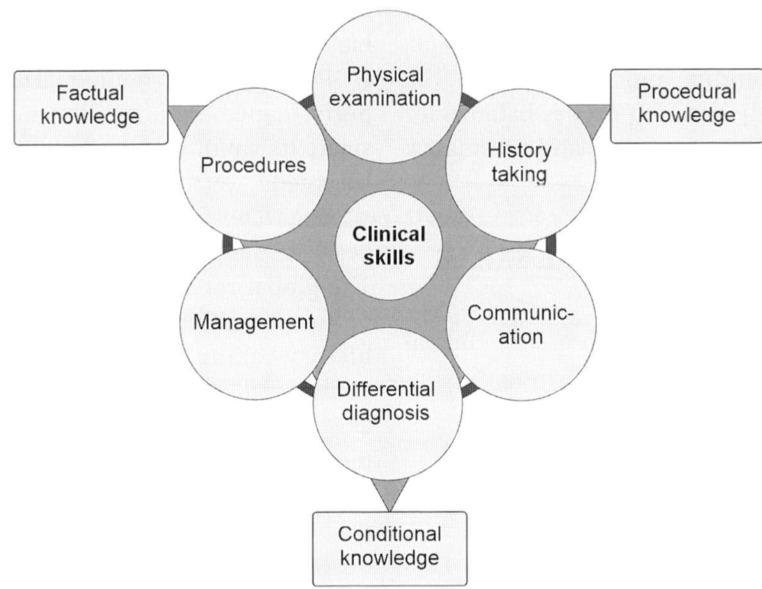

Fig. 1: Components of clinical skills.[5]

Source: Michels ME, Evans DE, Blok GA. What is a clinical skill? Searching for order in chaos through a modified Delphi process. Med Teach. 2012;34(8):e573-81.

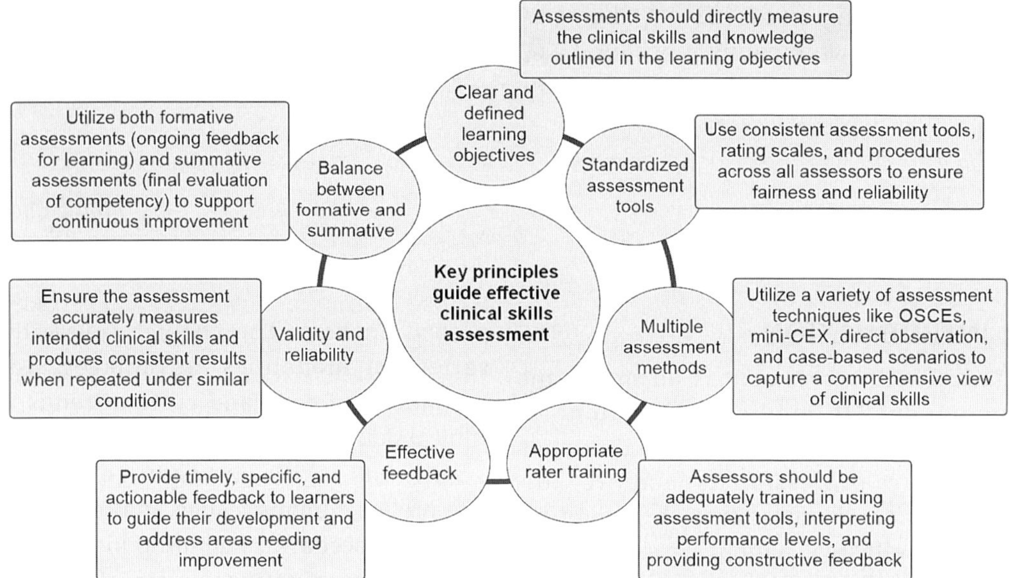

Fig. 2: Principles for practical clinical skills assessment.[6,7]

the process of constructing specific learning objectives, employing standardized assessment tools and employing more than one tool to assess the students, educating assessors on utilizing proper raters and checklists, delivering effective feedback, achieving validity and reliability of the tool and lastly ensuring proper balance for using the tool for formative and summative assessment **(Fig. 2)**.[5]

METHODS OF CLINICAL SKILLS ASSESSMENT

A range of tools is used to assess clinical skills, each with its unique strengths and applications:

Direct Observation of Procedural Skills

The direct observation of procedural skills (DOPS) is a widely used tool for assessing technical and procedural skills in clinical settings. It provides structured feedback on competence and areas for improvement.

The assessment technique, DOPS, has merits in offering feedback and enhancing practical skills, autonomy, relevance, acceptability, and formative nature. Its demerits are stress, time constraints, assessor bias, and coordination. Studies indicate that DOPS is superior to traditional methods, with performance enhancement in the second stage. Its validity and reliability are widely accepted.[8]

The DOPS is a highly structured tool that best assesses procedural mechanistic details. The global ratings scale could be another option for DOPS, this time for assessing history-taking and patient-interaction abilities.[9] Standard, basic procedures such as venipuncture at the foundation level and more complex surgical techniques such as oncologic skin excision and local flap restoration under local anesthesia are among the abilities evaluated. Crucially, actual patients are used for the surgeries as opposed to cadavers, animal models, or simulations.[9]

The surgical trainee chooses an observer, time, and procedure type for

DOPS, reducing stress, preventing rigid deadlines, and eliminating procedural and assessor unfairness. DOPS provides trainees with constructive feedback on procedural competencies for clinical care, reducing observer bias. It allows for rescheduling evaluations and experimentation with optional procedural DOPs. The educational supervisor and final year trainer review the trainee's e-portfolio, including completed DOPS.[9,10]

Direct observation of procedural skills is a cost-effective assessment tool that does not require unique setups or simulated patients. However, its viability can be impacted by patient availability and the short-notice availability of assessors. In busy theaters, finding an assessor with sufficient time can be challenging. The assessment typically lasts 5–15 minutes, followed by feedback. Many physicians prefer a longer timeframe for intimate examinations, informed consent, and patient dignity preservation. Therefore, ensuring adequate time for DOPs is crucial for successful patient care.[9,10]

Objective Structured Clinical Examination

The objective structured clinical examination (OSCE), launched in 1975, measures clinical competence at the bedside using timed stations. It is a versatile assessment tool for measuring healthcare professionals' proficiency in various undergraduate and postgraduate situations.[11] This tool is structured, using direct observational assessments to evaluate clinical competencies, standardized on patients or simulators, guided by checklists and global rating scales.

The OSCE has been applied to test those areas most vital to the performance of health care professionals, such as the ability to get/interpret information, problem-solve, teach, communicate, and manage unexpected patient behaviour.[11]

Components of:[12]

- Multiple stations
- Rotation across stations
- Multiple observations by the examiner
- Uniform time per student, per station
- Strict rotations
- Use of pre-pre-defined marking scheme (checklist)
- Simulated patients/standardized patients

The organization of the stations for OSCE is well explained by Harder RM,[13] highlighting what should be assessed via this tool: components we cannot test by any cognitive assessment tools, such as psychomotor components and affective attributes. The duration of the station ranges from 3 to 15 minutes. However, the time allocated should be adequate to perform the assigned task in every station. There should be at least 10–20 stations with two rest stations for conducting OSCE.[13,14]

Faculty, staff, and students should be sensitized to the tool's use. Before using it, ensure the availability of all resources, human, infrastructure stationary, etc. It is advisable to have a pilot run for the tool.

Modified Type of Objective Structured Clinical Examination

- *Objective structured assessment of technical skills (OSATS):* The tool is designed for objective skills assessment in surgical specialties, and it consists of a global rating scale and procedure-specific checklist for feedback and progress measurement.[15]
- *Team objective structured clinical examination (TOSCE):* The formative assessment tool involves students performing tasks at each station, marking their performance, providing feedback,

improving efficiency, and encouraging peer learning.[15]

Mini-clinical Evaluation Exercise

The mini-clinical evaluation exercise (Mini-CEX) is a workplace-based assessment tool where an assessor observes a trainee conducting a clinical encounter and provides immediate feedback.

Mini-clinical evaluation exercise is a time-efficient method for assessing clinical competence, offering structured feedback to students and faculty, and enhancing decision-making.[16] Mini-CEX is a 10- to 20-minute evaluation of doctor-patient interactions to evaluate students' clinical skills, attitudes, and behaviors crucial for high-quality care.[17]

Norcini et al.'s[17] study found that while mini-CEX measures are similar to performance assessments, their difficulty varies with resident encounters, partially mitigated by examiners overcompensating for patient difficulty and resident interaction with multiple patients. Mini-CEX offers higher fidelity, broader clinical settings, and real-world patient problems, making it an effective evaluation method.[16,18]

Mini-clinical evaluation exercise is most useful when considering the following areas—history, diagnosis, examination, management plan, communication, discharge, and others.[18] The skills assessed strengths—medical interviewing skills, physical examination skills, professional qualities/communication, counseling skills, clinical judgement, organization/efficiency and overall clinical competency in different clinical settings.[18]

Long-case

The long case is a clinical evaluation system used worldwide in undergraduate and graduate medical education.[19] It assesses a candidate's proficiency at Miller's pyramid level,[2] involving a 30–60-minute patient visit, physical examination, oral responses, and submission to examiners. The student spends the first half of the time with a patient, gathers history, performs a physical examination, submits the results to examiners, and then answers the examiner's questions orally.[20]

Specificity of content is crucial for measuring clinical competence, as good performance in one case does not predict good performance in another. A stable assessment requires multiple patient encounters, and traditional long-case assessments are insufficient for reliable assessment.[21] The long case's evaluation relies on an indirect evaluation of competence, with history and examination conducted without examiners.[21] Observations enhance reliability by incorporating competence aspects, as experienced examiners may not accurately assess the same event in conventional long cases, necessitating multiple evaluations.[21]

OBJECTIVE STRUCTURED LONG CASE EXAMINATION RECORDS

The innovative objective structured long case examination records (OSLER) method, or "objective structured long case examination record," improves critical thinking capabilities.[22] According to Gleeson et al.,[23] the method is more organized and includes a 10-point mark scheme (four for history, three for physical examination, and three for management and clinical acumen), which results in better objectivity, validity, and reliability of current practices.[23] All candidates are assessed on identical items. Can be used for both criterion and norm-referenced assessments.[21] OSLER assessment does not require extra time over the ordinary long case. The issues for OSLER and long case remain almost identical. The actual patients in OSLERs can reduce variability in clinical findings. Still, the unstandardized nature of patients and their clinical signs remains a concern, as they cannot be equivalent across candidates.[21]

MULTI-SOURCE FEEDBACK (360-DEGREE ASSESSMENT)

Multisource feedback (MSF) is a formative measure of workplace performance with a four-step procedure where (1) information on a person's observable workplace habits is gathered from questionnaires among the people engaging with the individual; (2) information are consolidated for confidentiality and anonymity; (3) consolidated information, in addition to self-evaluation where applicable, is given to the individual through a report; and (4) the individual receives a meeting with a respected person to reflect on the data and create an action plan.[24]

Multisource feedback is a formative workplace performance measure that gathers observable workplace habits from questionnaires, consolidates them for confidentiality and anonymity, provides a report, and encourages individuals to reflect on the data and create an action plan.[24]

Assessing the attainment level of medical students for communicator, professional, and collaborator roles can be effectively done by MSF. This is due to their visibility to healthcare professionals and patients, and other measures like multiple-choice questions, direct observation of procedures, OSCEs, and performance audits are also used.[25-27]

Multisource feedback gathers feedback from multiple sources, including peers, supervisors, patients, and other healthcare professionals. It provides a holistic view of trainees' competencies, particularly in communication, teamwork, and professionalism.[27]

ENTRUSTABLE PROFESSIONAL ACTIVITIES

Entrustable professional activities (EPAs) are "a unit of professional practice (a task or group of tasks) that can be fully entrusted to a trainee, as soon as he or she has demonstrated the necessary competence to execute this activity unsupervised".[28,29]

The ACGME or CanMEDS competencies form a framework for professionals, providing general descriptions for learners, supervisors, and institutions.[30] However, these frameworks need to be translated into medical practice, and EPAs were created to overcome the fear of being too theoretical for practical application.[30] Cate TO present how the EPAs differ from competencies and the descriptive guidelines for full EPAs to be used by the researcher at their end.[30]

As per Dhaliwal et al.,[31] the EPA tracks real-time performance, which is superior to hoping that the trainee will be capable of doing so. It employs an expert supervisor's subjective, day-to-day views of the trainee against a competency standard. Enhances patient safety by ensuring that a trainee who is requested to carry out an unsupervised activity has already shown a high degree of skill in such an activity. Motivates curriculum developers to consider both the process and outcomes of training. Trainees can measure their learning against expectations, as documented in the EPA and milestone document. A portfolio of EPAs measures medical proficiency. The process is not static; the list can be augmented throughout a lifetime, new EPAs added, or older ones re-learned, as needed.[31]

Bohnen et al.[32] utilized the System for Improving and Measuring Procedural

Learning (SIMPL), a smartphone-based software, to enable real-time intraoperative performance assessment for surgical trainees, hypothesizing its integration into surgical training programs.

TECHNOLOGY IN CLINICAL SKILLS ASSESSMENT

Technological improvements have revolutionized clinical assessment techniques:[31]

- *Simulation-based assessment:* High-fidelity mannequins, task trainers, and virtual reality (VR) offer safe practice and assessment environments. Simulation enhances learning training, particularly during formative assessment, where feedback enhances the learning outcome for the skills. This approach allows the students to perform the technique multiple times without fearing losing or hampering the patient's condition. It is being used increasingly for formative environments, while it is underutilized for summative assessment, specifically in the Indian sub-continent.[33]
- *Artificial intelligence (AI) and virtual patients:* AI-based platforms provide adaptive learning experiences, automated clinical reasoning, and communication skills assessment.

  Virtual patients (VPs) are a hands-on learning tool that allows healthcare and medical students to interact with a computer instead of a patient. Research suggests that these simulations are highly repeatable and can be redeployed to deliver similar experiences to all students. They are also cost-saving for skill development and have favorable to neutral impacts compared to traditional methods like lectures and group discussions.[34-36]
- *Remote and online OSCEs:* Due to the pandemic and the growth of telemedicine, remote OSCEs with videoconferencing technology have become popular. These enable examinations to proceed regardless of logistical impediments. The rapid adoption of virtual OSCE training during the pandemic has shown its effectiveness, with high end-user satisfaction and accessibility. However, challenges such as Internet stability and digital orientation need to be addressed. As the digital age transitions to AI chatbots, there is a growing need for more studies on incorporating learning management systems (LMS) in virtual OSCEs.[37]

CHALLENGES AND FUTURE DIRECTIONS

Clinical skills assessment faces challenges such as resource intensiveness, balancing standardization and variability, requiring skilled assessors for practical evaluation, and the potential integration of AI and automation in future assessments, requiring skilled feedback and training.

CONCLUSION

Clinical skill evaluation is essential to developing skilled, moral, and patient-focused healthcare workers. A well-designed assessment framework should prioritize authenticity across Miller's pyramid, incorporate a variety of techniques, and align with learning objectives. Meaningful evaluation depends on ensuring validity, reliability, feasibility, and educational impact. No single type of assessment is sufficient or valid in isolation; a combination of complementary tools is essential for comprehensive evaluation. In the end, evaluation should serve as a potent catalyst for learning, professional identity development, and ongoing clinical practice improvement rather than merely a gauge of performance.

Summary points

- Clinical skills testing is vital in guaranteeing proficiency in medical practice.
- The main principles are validity, reliability, feasibility, and acceptability.
- There is a range of assessment instruments available, such as OSCEs, Mini-CEX, DOPS, CbD, MSF, and EPAs.
- Technology-aided evaluations like simulation, virtual patients, and AI are designing the future of clinical skill assessment.
- Issues such as resource demands and standardization persist in shaping the assessment approaches.

REFERENCES

1. Norcini JJ, McKinley DW. Assessment methods in medical education. Teach Teach Educ. 2007;23(3):239-50.
2. Miller GE. The assessment of clinical skills/competence/performance. Acad Med. 1990;65(9 Suppl):S63-S67.
3. Epstein RM. Assessment in medical education. N Engl J Med. 2007;356(4):387-96.
4. Andrew Elder. Clinical Skills Assessment in the Twenty-First Century. Med Clin N Am.2018;102:545-58.
5. Michels ME, Evans DE, Blok GA. What is a clinical skill? Searching for order in chaos through a modified Delphi process. Med Teach. 2012;34(8):e573-81.
6. Tabish SA. Assessment methods in medical education. Int J Health Sci (Qassim). 2008;2(2):3-7.
7. Sherali Qizi KM. Five Principles of Assessment: Practicality, Reliability, Validity, Washback, And Authenticity. AJSSHR. 2024;4(06):42-5.
8. Khanghahi ME, Azar FEF. Direct observation of procedural skills (DOPS) evaluation method. Systematic review of evidence. Med J Islamic Rep Iran. 2018;32:45.
9. Khan MAA, Gorman M, Gwozdziewicz L, et al. Direct observation of procedural skills as an assessment tool for surgical trainees. J Pak Med Stud. 2013;3(3):137-40.
10. Denny ML. Pulse Registrar: Taking a look at DOPS (Direct Observation of Procedural Skills). Pulse. 2007.
11. Choudhari S, Maheswari TNU. Objective Structured Clinical Examination (OSCE): A Review. Research J Pharm Tech. 2016;9(8):1-3.
12. Batra B, Norcini J. Developing objective structured clinical examinations (OSCEs). FAIMER-Keele Master's in Health Professions Education: Accreditation and Assessment. Module 1, Unit 3. 4th edition. FAIMER Centre for Distance Learning. CenMEDIC, London; 2016.
13. Harden RM. Twelve tips for organizing an Objective Structured Clinical Examination (OSCE). Med Teach. 1990;12(3-4):259-64.
14. Khan KZ, Ramachandran S, Gaunt K, et al. The Objective Structured Clinical Examination (OSCE): AMEE Guide No. 81. Part I: a historical and theoretical perspective. Med Teach. 2013;35(9):e1437-46.
15. Tejinder S, Piyush G, Daljit S. Assessment of Practical/Clinical Skills in Principles of Medical Education, 4th edition. New Delhi: Jaypee Brothers; 2013. pp. 123-35.
16. Batra P, Batra R, Verma N, et al. Mini clinical evaluation exercise (Mini-CEX): A tool for assessment of residents in the department of surgery. J Educ Health Promo. 2022;11,253.
17. Norcini JJ, Blank LL, Duffy FD, et al. The mini-CEX: A method for assessing clinical skills. Ann Intern Med. 2003;138:476-81.
18. Royal Australasian College of Physicians (RACP). Mini-Clinical Evaluation Exercise (mini-CEX) Rating Form. [online] Available from: https://www.racp.edu.au/docs/default-source/trainees/basic-training/bt-mini-clinical-evaluation-exercise-rating-form.pdf?sfvrsn=acd8341a_10 [Last accessed January 2026].
19. Wass V, van der Vleuten C. The long case. Med Educ. 2004;38(11):1176-80.
20. Ponnamperuma GG, Karunathilake IM, McAleer S, et al. The long case and its modifications: a literature review. Med Educ. 2009;43:936-41.

21. Boursicot K, Fuller R. Clinical and oral examinations. FAIMER-Keele Master's in Health Professions Education: Accreditation and Assessment. Module 1, Unit 6, 4th edition. FAIMER Centre for Distance Learning, CenMEDIC, London; 2016.
22. Wanjari DS, Vagha DS, Mahakalkar DC. Assessment of critical thinking skills of postgraduate students by using the critical self-thinking inventory for clinical examination. Glob J Med Res. 2020;20:33-40.
23. Gleeson F. AMEE Medical Education Guide No. 9. Assessment of clinical competence using the Objective Structured Long Examination Record (OSLER). Med Teach. 1997;19(1):7-14.
24. Lockyer JM, Sargeant J, Introduction to MCC 360: a multi-source feedback initiative. Prepared for Medical Council of Canada, Ottawa, Canada; 2017.
25. Lockyer JM, Violato C, Fidler H. The assessment of emergency physicians by a regulatory authority. Acad Emerg Med. 2006;13(12):1296-303.
26. Lockyer JM, Violato C, Fidler H, et al. The assessment of pathologists/laboratory medicine physicians through a multisource feedback tool. Arch Pathol Lab Med. 2009;133(8):1301-8.
27. Holmboe ES, Durning SJ, Hawkins RE. Practical guide to the evaluation of clinical competence 2nd ed, Philadelphia: Elsevier; 2018.
28. Association of American Medical Colleges. (2014). Core Entrustable Professional Activities for Entering Residency. [online] Available from: https://www.aamc.org [Last accessed January 2026].
29. Gummesson C, Alm S, Cederborg A, et al. Entrustable professional activities (EPAs) for undergraduate medical education – development and exploration of social validity. BMC Med Educ. 2023;23:635.
30. Cate TO. Nuts and bolts of entrustable professional activities. J Grad Med Educ. 2013;5(1):157-8.
31. Dhaliwal U, Gupta P, Singh T. Entrustable Professional Activities: Teaching and Assessing Clinical Competence. Indian Pediatrics. 2015;52:591-7.
32. Bohnen JD, George BC, Williams RG, et al. The Feasibility of Real-Time Intraoperative Performance Assessment with SIMPL (System for Improving and Measuring Procedural Learning): Early Experience From a Multi-institutional Trial. J Surg Educ. 2016;73(6):e118-30.
33. Buléon C, Mattatia L, Minehart RD, et al. Simulation-based summative assessment in healthcare: an overview of key principles for practice. Adv Simul. 2022;7:42.
34. Kononowicz A A, Zary N, Edelbring S, et al. Virtual patients - what are we talking about? A framework to classify the meanings of the term in healthcare education. BMC Med Educ. 2015;15:11.
35. Kononowicz AA, Woodham LA, Edelbring S, et al. Virtual patient simulations in health professions education: Systematic review and meta-analysis by the Digital Health Education Collaboration. J Med Internet Res. 2019;21(7):e14676.
36. Patrick B, Kelley G, Tracii R, et al. Artificial intelligence-driven virtual patients for communication skill development in healthcare students: A scoping review. Australas J Educ Technol. 2024;147427.
37. Saeed E, Hamad MH, Alhuzaimi AN, et al. Virtual Objective Structured Clinical Examination (OSCE) Training in the Pandemic Era: Feasibility, Satisfaction, and the Road Ahead. Cureus. 2024;16(6):e61564.

CHAPTER

21 Professionalism and Ethics: Assessment

Ghanshyam Ahir

Learning Objectives

- Understand medical professionalism and medical ethics.
- State importance of medical professionalism and medical ethics for medical fraternity.
- Conduct assessment of undergraduate and postgraduate medical students regarding professionalism and ethics as per guidelines of regulatory bodies or curriculum of autonomous institutions.

INTRODUCTION

Medical professionalism

Medical professionalism covers a set of duties, competencies, values, virtues, behaviours (professional conduct), outcomes (performance) and relationships that aims to achieve the goals of medicine and promote trust and confidence in the medical profession and the healthcare system."[1]

Professionalism may be defined as "the competence or skill expected of a professional."[2]

"Professionalism is an attitude where individual assumes a particular role."[3]

Medical Ethics

Medical ethics covers as set of the guiding principles for healthcare professionals, ensuring that they prioritize their patients' well-being, treat patients with dignity and respect, and foster trust and confidence in the healthcare system.[4]

Ethics is an inherent and inseparable part of clinical medicine as the physician has an ethical obligation to benefit the patient, to avoid or minimize harm and to respect the values and preferences of the patients and their familes.[5]

IMPORTANCE OF PROFESSIONALISM AND ETHICS IN MEDICAL EDUCATION PROCESS

Healthcare is an environment that requires collaboration built on deeply rooted trust and respect, which are best cultivated through practice of professionalism and ethics.

Studies have shown that medical students who exhibit unprofessional behavior during their training are more likely to repeat in their real-life clinical practice.[6]

Increase in incidences of medical negligence, disputes, and violence against doctors and hospitals indicates the need of training of professional conduct and ethical practice from undergraduate level **(Fig. 1)**.

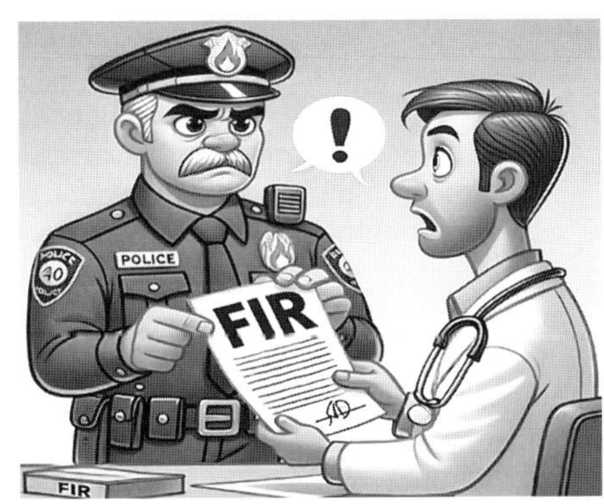

Fig. 1: Consequence of unethical practices.[7]

Any official resource or guidelines were not available on medical education in India until Attitude, Ethics, and Communication (AETCOM) module was rolled out by erstwhile Medical Council of India (now national medical commission India—NMC) in year 2018.

As AETCOM[8] has been enrolled in medical education curriculum, assessment blueprint for both theory and practical component is necessary now **(Tables 1 to 3)**.

TABLE 1: Proposed plan to conduct assessment of professionalism and ethics for MBBS students.

Type of assessment	*Method of assessment*	*Millers pyramid*
Formative and summative	MCQ on Indian Medical Council (Professional Conduct, Etiquette and Ethics) Regulations, consent, patient rights, legal acts of hospital and health staff and public health legislations related to health services, etc.	Knows and knows how
Formative and summative	*Short notes* 1. Differentiate apathy, sympathy and empathy. 2. Enlist ways to improve doctor patient relationship. 3. State the rights of patients.	Knows and knows how
Formative	Attendance in teaching learning assessment session and involvement in learner doctor program as per NMC India Guidelines	Does
Formative	Participation—logbook writing, role play, and portfolio of student	Does
Formative	Participation of student in ICMR short-term studentship (STS) Program and community health research projects	Shows, shows how, does
Formative and summative	Short cases—OSCE—e.g., approach to pediatrics patient with diarrhea using Kalamazoo Essential Elements Communication Checklist[9]	Shows, shows how
Formative and summative	Simulations	Shows, shows how, does

TABLE 2: Proposed plan to conduct assessment of professionalism and ethics for postgraduate students.

Type of assessment	*Method of assessment*	*Millers pyramid*
Formative and summative	MCQ on Indian Medical Council (Professional Conduct, Etiquette and Ethics) Regulations, 2002, good clinical practice, physician code of conduct, consent, patient rights, ethical behavioral skills (obtaining informed consent, assessing decision-making capacity, discussing resuscitation status and use of life-sustaining treatments, advanced care planning, breaking bad news and effective communication)[9] legal acts of hospital and health staff and public health legislations related to health services, etc. Accreditation of organizations, such as NABH, NABL	Knows and knows how
Formative and summative	Short and long cases–OSCE–approach to pediatric patient with diarrhea	Shows, shows how

Contd...

Contd...

Type of assessment	*Method of assessment*	*Millers pyramid*
Formative	Involvement in patient services and teaching learning assessment activities of department	Does
Formative	Participation—E-logbook verification	Does
Formative and summative	Simulations—Kalamazoo Essential Elements Communication checklist[9]	Does
Formative and summative	Patient satisfaction survey	Does
Formative and summative	With the help of standard tools, such as Professionalism Mini-Evaluation Exercise	Does

TABLE 3: Standard tool for assessment of professionalism for postgraduate students.

Professionalism Mini-Evaluation Exercise[10]
Review Committee for Radiation Oncology

Evaluator: ______________ Resident: ______________ Level PGY-1/2/3 Date:____________

	Not Observed	*Not Acceptable*	*Below Expectations*	*Met Expectations*	*Exceeded Expectations*
Listened actively to patient					
Showed interest in patient as a person					
Recognized and met patient needs					
Extended himself/herself to meet patient needs					
Advocated on behalf of a patient					
Demonstrated awareness of limitations					
Admitted errors/omissions					
Solicited feedback					
Accepted feedback					
Maintained appropriate boundaries					
Maintained composure in a difficult situation					
Maintained appropriate appearance					
Was on time					
Completed tasks in a reliable fashion					
Addressed own gaps in knowledge and skills					
Was available to colleagues					
Avoided derogatory language					
Maintained patient confidentiality					
Used health resources appropriately					

Source: ©2015 Accreditation Council for Graduate Medical Education (ACGME).

CONCLUSION

Learning assessment techniques by medical teachers is necessary and continuous structured assessment of professionalism & ethics by multiple assessors will reduce subjectivity and will change professional behaviour of medical students over a period of time.

REFERENCES

1. Low YH, Omar E, Thirumoorthy T. The seven virtues in medical professionalism. Singapore General Hospital Proc. 2009;18:74-9.
2. Ccaps.umn. (2023). 10 ways to show professionalism in the Health Care Field. [online] Available from: https://ccaps.umn.edu/story/10-ways-show-professionalism-health-care-field [Last accessed January 2026].
3. Collier R. Professionalism: what is it?. CMAJ. 2012;184(10):1129-30.
4. Young M, Wagner A. Medical Ethics. In: StatPearls. Treasure Island (FL): StatPearls Publishing; 2025.
5. Singer PA, Pellegrino ED, Siegler M. Clinical ethics revisited. BMC Medical Ethics. 2001;2(1).
6. Modi JN, Anshu Gupta P, Singh T. Teaching and assessing professionalism in the Indian context. Indian Pediatr. 2014;51:881-8.
7. Aiclindia.com. (2024). Protection to doctor in case of FIR (First Information Report). [online] Available from https://aiclindia.com/blog-details.html?ID=39 [Last accessed January 2026].
8. Kulkarni KK, Bhalearo PM, Sarode VS. Communication skills training for medical students: A prospective, Observational, Single Centre Study. J Clin Diagn Res. 2018.
9. Porcerelli JH, Brennan S, Carty J, et al. Resident ratings of communication skills using the Kalamazoo Adapted Checklist. J Grad Med Educ. 2015;7(3):458-61.
10. Acgme.org. (2015). Professionalism Mini-Evaluation Exercise. [online] Available from: https://www.acgme.org/globalassets/430_Professionalism_MiniCEX.pdf [Last accessed January 2026].

CHAPTER

22 Workplace-based Assessment

Shipra Jain

INTRODUCTION

Workplace-based assessment (WPBA) refers to an array of various assessment methods which are conducted to assess subject specific competencies as mandated by regulatory authorities at workplace. This method of assessment is mainly used for postgraduate medical education at present. It aims to link the elements of the golden triangle, viz., learning objectives, teaching-learning methods and assessment techniques in an organized manner. However, WPBAs are not meant to indicate that a learner is competent in a particular process, but it is designed to identify the strengths and weaknesses of the learner so that timely constructive feedback can be provided. Thus, it is frequently used in formative assessment of postgraduate students while currently, its use is restricted for summative assessments **(Fig. 1)**.[1]

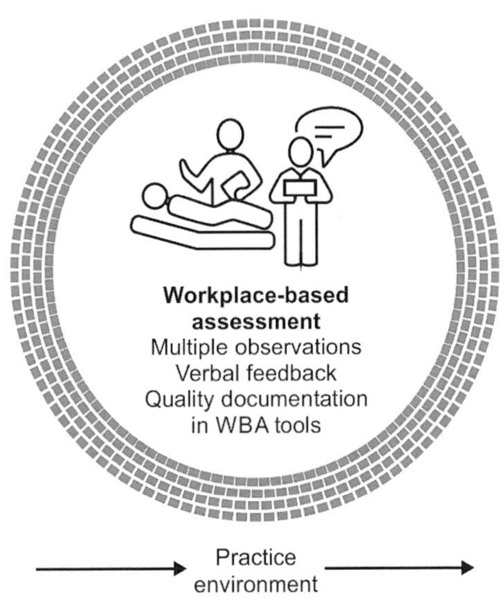

Fig. 1: Workplace-based assessment.

RATIONALE OF WORKPLACE-BASED ASSESSMENT

National Medical Commission has emphasized on the need for competency-based medical education for medical students. The level of competency achieved/not achieved by a student must be periodically assessed and this ideally should occur at his/her workplace. Thus, WPBA would pave the way for competency-based medical education for postgraduate students.

Points in favor of adopting WPBA include:

- Periodic observation at workplace and provision of feedback
- Emphasizes on assessment of clinical skills and soft skills, viz., attitude, ethics, communication, professionalism, and behavior.
- Complies with the higher order in Miller's pyramid.
- Allows to be specific for context and content.
- Overcomes the limitations of conventional methods of assessment.
- Ensures that teaching and learning are aligned with actual practice.
- Promotes reflective thinking.

ADVANTAGES

There are many advantages of workplace-based assessment which include:

- It is a learner-centric method of assessment.
- It ensures that the assessment occurs in actual working environment and removes artificiality.
- It reduces any disruption in work or any extra effort for the assessment.
- It allows assessment to occur in all domains.
- It allows to assess multitude of skills for diverse cases and settings.
- It facilitates assessment of higher order thinking in Miller's pyramid **(Fig. 2)**.
- It emphasizes on assessment of learner's holistic management, viz., documenting, communicating with his/her team, patient, and attendants rather than treating a particular illness.
- It ensures assessment of learner's approach for ethical and legal issues at work.
- It allows assessment to be continuous in nature over a period of learner's training with varying levels of difficulty.
- It provides opportunity of assessment and feedback by multiple assessors.

UTILITY OF WORKPLACE-BASED ASSESSMENT

The utility of an assessment method can be calculated as the product of cost-effectiveness, acceptability, reliability, validity and educational impact. It can be remembered by the mnemonic *CARVE.*

- *Cost-effectiveness:* In terms of manpower, infrastructure, resources, and materials required. Since WPBA actually occurs at workplace where the learner is already overburdened with enormous work, this factor is nullified.
- *Acceptability:* To all stakeholders involved in assessment. Ensuring adequate training of all stakeholders, viz., learners, assessors, and patients would increase the acceptability of WPBA.
- *Reliability:* It should give repeatable results over time. WPBA is reasonably reliable since it requires multiple assessments by multiple assessors. Studies have shown that an average of 6–8 assessment encounters in a year usually give reliable results.
- *Validity:* Ability of a tool to measure what it is expected to. WPBA carries high validity by virtue of it being conducted at real workplace.
- *Educational impact:* The assessment must ensure that the learning has occurred, or the competency has been achieved. WPBA carries high educational impact owing to the number and type of constructive feedback provided to the learner at the end of assessment.

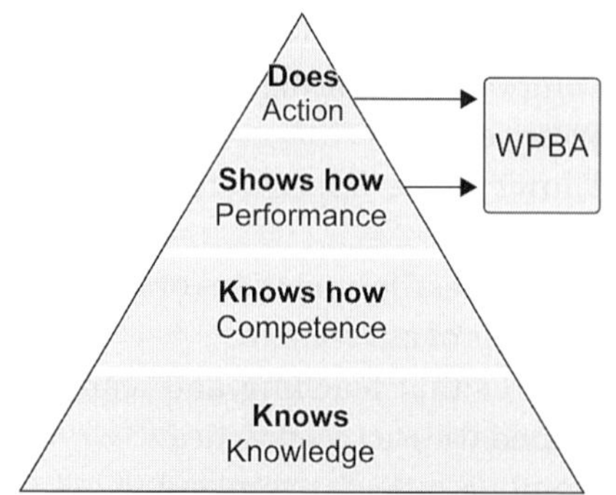

Fig. 2: Miller pyramid.

TYPES OF WORKPLACE-BASED ASSESSMENT TOOLS

A variety of tools are available to facilitate workplace-based assessment as summarized in **Figure 3** here.

Different types of WPBA tools include:

- *Mini clinical evaluation exercise (mini CEX):* It is commonly used in clinical settings and usually takes not >15 minutes. A structured proforma is used for

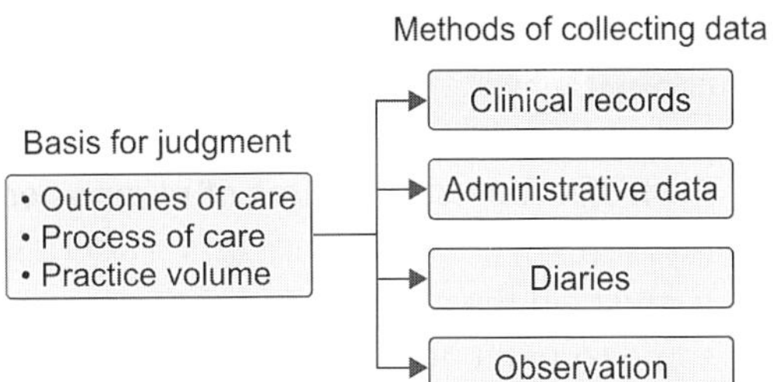

Fig. 3: Workplace-based assessment (WPBA) tools.

assessment of knowledge, skills, attitude, and behavior followed by immediate feedback to the learner by the assessor.

- *Case-based discussion (CBD):* It is an oral workplace-based interview which is done in less than thirty minutes. A case is allotted to the learner by the assessor and the learner sends the clinical information to the assessor before starting CBD. It comprises assessment of clinical judgement for the case which the learner managed on his own.
- *Direct observation of procedural skills (DOPS):* It is designed for assessment of the level of competence of learner in day-to-day practical procedures. It also utilizes a structured proforma for the assessment of skill followed by immediate feedback by the assessor.
- *Clinical work sampling:* It involves direct observation, assessment followed by feedback from assessor on learner's patient management in various domains of patient care (from admission in hospital to discharge of patient).
- *Multisource feedback (MSF):* Also known as 360° feedback, there is structured assessment of learner's performance by people around him/her at workplace, viz., seniors, peers, team members, patients, and attendants in view of his/her professional conduct and behavior. Anonymous feedback is provided to the learner by the assessor.
- *Acute care assessment tool:* It involves structured assessment of learner's ability to period of care at acute ward, night shifts, etc. The assessor observes the learner longitudinally and provides feedback at the end.
- *Consultation observation tool (COT):* It is like mini CEX and involves structured assessment of learner's performance in face-to-face consultation followed by immediate feedback.
- *Audio-COT:* It is COT designed for learner providing telephonic consultation.
- *Clinical examination and procedural skill:* It involves direct observation and assessment of physical examination and procedural skill conducted by the learner.[2] It is commonly used for assessment of examination of breast, rectum, male/female genitalia, prostate, etc.
- *Clinical encounter card:* This method employs cards which are used to record salient points of examination and management of patients seen by the assessor at work for review, assessment, and feedback.

Other workplace-based assessment tools include:

- *Surgeons nontechnical skill:* The learner is rated and assessed on certain intra-operative nontechnical skills which are important for safety of patients, viz., alertness, decision-making, communication with team members, leadership qualities, and ability to work in a team effectively.
- *Nontechnical skills for anesthetist:* It is designed for learners posted in department of anesthesia and includes rating of skills, viz., situational awareness, timely prediction, effective communication, and co-ordination with team members.
- *Objective structured assessment of technical skills:* The learner is assessed based on his/her performance on a station comprising technical skills.

- *Chart stimulated recall:* The assessor uses charts to assess the learner's clinical acumen and decision-making during patient encounters.

FEEDBACK IN WORKPLACE-BASED ASSESSMENT

Workplace-based assessment consists of two prerequisites, viz., assessment which occurs at workplace and provision of feedback to the learner. The importance of giving feedback has been observed in medical education. However, feedback should be based on observation of performance of the learner in the assessment. It should be timely provided to the learner so that he/she may recall his/her errors and appropriate remedial measures can be taken. The process of giving feedback should be such that the learner should not get discouraged after receiving it. It has been observed that *"Sandwich Method"* is widely accepted wherein the errors committed by the learner are sandwiched between the positive points of the learner observed during assessment. It implies that the feedback should be constructive in nature and the result should be improvement in the performance of the learner.

Qualities of feedback:
- Timely
- Constructive
- Objective
- Improvement in performance

POINTS TO REMEMBER BEFORE SUCCESSFUL IMPLEMENTATION OF WORKPLACE-BASED ASSESSMENT IN A MEDICAL INSTITUTION

There are certain key points that need to be kept in mind before implementing WPBA in an institution.[3] These include:

- It needs to address the specific competency.
- It must be able to generate data to facilitate in reflective thinking and remedial measures.
- It must aid the assessor in certification of some competencies.
- It must be able to highlight learner's gaps in knowledge, attitude, and skills for improvement in future.
- Ensure that the practice environment is safe and free from any potential litigation.
- It must be smooth to conduct the assessment.
- The assessment must be acceptable to all stakeholders, viz., learner, patient, and assessor.
- The tool selected for WPBA must be valid and reliable.

DIVERSITY IN WORKPLACE-BASED ASSESSMENT

Since workplace-based assessment occurs at the actual place of work, it can be planned and conducted for diverse range of populations such as:

- Infants and children
- Elderly people
- People with chronic illness such as diabetes, hypertension, etc.
- Vulnerable population
- Patients presenting in emergency care

GRADING IN WORKPLACE-BASED ASSESSMENT

After the assessment is completed, the learner can be graded by the assessor and constructive feedback should be given by the assessor. The grading can be done as:

- Much below the required level of competency[4]
- Below the required level of competency

- Meets the required level of competency
- Exceeds the required level of competency
- Much above the required level of competency

LIMITATIONS OF WORKPLACE-BASED ASSESSMENT

Despite several benefits of WPBA, it should not be considered as a substitute for conventional methods of assessment. WPBA is a valuable additional method for formative assessment of a learner. However, it has been observed that there are chances of students becoming overconfident who perform well in WPBA. On the other hand, slow learners might get discouraged owing to their poor performance and might avoid taking feedback for further improvement. Another limitation of WPBA is that since it is time consuming, learners often prefer junior assessors for their assessment who might not be able to grade their performance accurately. Lastly, most of the tools used for WPBA lack proper standardization which limits the utility of such tools as a reliable method of assessment.

CHALLENGES IN IMPLEMENTATION OF WORKPLACE-BASED ASSESSMENT

Workplace-based assessment seems to be a promising tool for assessment of postgraduates **(Fig. 4)**. However, there are certain challenges which need to be addressed for its successful implementation in curricular framework. These include:

- *Sensitization of learners and faculty:* It is imperative that prior sensitization of students as well as faculty members should be done to ensure that WPBA intends to achieve what is desired.

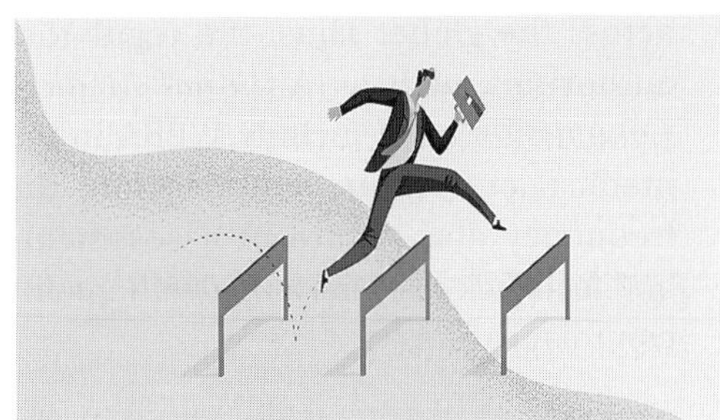

Fig. 4: Challenges in implementation of workplace-based assessment (WPBA).

- *Training of assessors:* This factor is the bottleneck in successful WPBA implementation. The faculties must be trained in two main aspects:
  1. Clarity on what is to be assessed and the standard of assessment.
  2. Provision of valuable feedback which is constructive and timely.
- *Feasibility issues:* Despite having the advantage that WPBA occurs at actual workplace, it has some feasibility issues which include inertia of the assessor. This can be overcome by sensitization of the senior faculties of medical institutions. Additionally, the interested senior assessors may collaborate with their colleagues working in different institutions and design a WPBA model which would motivate others in implementation of WPBA in their respective departments.
- *Mutual respect and trust:* Students usually avoid taking assessments and feedback positively. It is, therefore, imperative for both assessors as well as the student to create an environment of mutual respect and trust such that student does not feel anxious or apprehensive about the entire procedure. This would help in successful implementation of WPBA.
- *Curricular incorporation:* There is consensus on inclusion of WPBA as an assessment method for medical students

across the globe. Thus, the regulatory authorities such as *National Medical Commission* must include WPBA in the medical curriculum emphasizing the frequency and nature of assessments and feedback sessions along with quality control measures.

CONCLUSION

Workplace-based Assessment (WBA) is primarily aimed for postgraduate medical students which evaluates clinical skills, knowledge, and attitude by multiple assessors in real-world settings, moving beyond conventional single examination pattern to provide continuous, constructive feedback for learning and development. It is implemented in the curriculum using various tools like direct observation, Mini-Clinical evaluation exercise (mini-CEX), Case based discussions (CBD), and Portfolios to assess competencies in actual patient care scenarios, crucial for Competency based Medical Education (CBME) as mandated by National Medical commission (NMC).

REFERENCES

1. Prakash J, Chatterjee K, Srivastava K, et al. Workplace based assessment: A review of available tools and their relevance. Ind Psychiatry J. 2020;29(2):200-4.
2. Anderson HL, Kurtz J, West DC. Implementation and Use of Workplace-Based Assessment in Clinical Learning Environments: A Scoping Review. Acad Med. 2021;96(11S):S164-74.
3. Van der Vleuten CP, Schuwirth LW. Assessing professional competence: From methods to programmes. Med Educ. 2005;39:309-17.
4. Singh T, Modi JN. Workplace-based Assessment: A Step to Promote Competency Based Postgraduate Training. Indian Pediatr. 2013;50:553-9.

CHAPTER 23

Objective Structured Clinical Examination for Skills Assessment

Praveen Singh

Learning Objectives

After studying this chapter, readers will be able to:
- Understand the concept and need for OSCE in modern medical education
- Apply principles of blueprinting to design OSCE stations
- Assess clinical competence across multiple domains using OSCE
- Develop standardized checklists and rating scales
- Conduct OSCEs in a fair, objective, and reliable manner
- Implement appropriate standard-setting and feedback strategies
- Evaluate the role of OSCE within a comprehensive assessment framework

"Purpose of this chapter is to provide health care professionals with a comprehensive understanding of OSCE principles, design, implementation, and evaluation for assessing clinical skills effectively."[1,2]

INTRODUCTION

Effective assessment lies at the heart of medical education, ensuring that graduating students possess the necessary competencies for safe and effective patient care. However, traditional methods of clinical and practical examination, while familiar, often fall short of this crucial goal. Consider a typical final practical exam scenario: One student examines blood pressure (BP), another estimates hemoglobin using Sahli's method, a third maps a visual field defect, and a fourth assesses the facial nerve. While each task has clinical relevance, they differ vastly in complexity and the skills tested. This inherent lack of standardization introduces a significant "luck factor," making fair comparison between students difficult and compromising the examination's validity.[1-3]

Beyond the variability in tasks, conventional clinical exams suffer from significant subjectivity. Examiner bias, whether lenient or strict, conscious or unconscious, can heavily influence student scores. Inter-examiner variability (different examiners scoring the same performance differently) and even intra-examiner variability (the same examiner scoring inconsistently over time or across students) undermine the reliability of the assessment. Furthermore, patient variability—differing pathologies, patient temperaments, and willingness to cooperate—adds another layer of inconsistency. Often, these traditional formats, particularly the long case, focus heavily on the student's final synthesis and theoretical discussion, neglecting direct observation of the *process*. We assess the end result—the diagnosis or management plan—but rarely witness *how* the student gathered the history, performed the physical examination, or executed a procedural skill, missing vital opportunities to evaluate fundamental clinical techniques and communication abilities.[4-6]

An ideal assessment system, conversely, should possess several key characteristics. It must be *valid*, accurately measuring the clinical skills and competencies it purports to assess. It needs to be *reliable*, yielding consistent results regardless of the examiner, the specific patient encountered (within standardized limits), or the occasion. *Objectivity* is paramount, minimizing subjective judgment and bias through clear, predefined criteria. An assessment should also be *relevant*, aligning closely with the curriculum's learning objectives and the competencies required for actual clinical practice, and *feasible* within the available resources of time, personnel, and finances.[1,2]

It is precisely to address the shortcomings of traditional methods and strive towards these ideals that the objective structured clinical examination (OSCE) was developed by Harden and colleagues in the 1970s. The OSCE provides a framework to systematically overcome many conventional limitations. By rotating all students through a series of standardized stations, each presenting an identical task (be it history taking from a standardized patient, performing a focused physical examination, interpreting data like an ECG, or executing a procedure on a simulator), it drastically reduces case variability and the "luck factor." The use of detailed, preagreed checklists and trained examiners minimizes subjectivity and enhances objectivity and reliability. Crucially, OSCE allows for the direct observation and assessment of the *process* of care—the "Shows How" level of competence—ensuring that fundamental skills are evaluated alongside knowledge application.[8] While not without its own challenges, the OSCE represents a significant advancement, offering a more structured, objective, and comprehensive approach to evaluating the multifaceted skills essential for medical practice.

THE NEED FOR OBJECTIVE STRUCTURED CLINICAL EXAMINATION IN PRESENT DAY MEDICAL EDUCATION

The shift towards more robust assessment methods like the OSCE is not merely procedural; it stems from fundamental requirements of modern medical training and the recognized limitations of traditional approaches. Several key factors that underscore this necessity are discussed further.

Assessment Drives Learning

It is a well-established principle in education that students strategically focus their learning efforts on what they expect to be assessed. If examinations predominantly test factual recall through written papers or theoretical vivas, students will prioritize memorization. Conversely, when assessments require the demonstration of practical skills—performing a physical examination correctly, communicating effectively with a patient, or executing a procedure safely—students are intrinsically motivated to seek out and engage in hands-on practice. OSCE, by its very nature, signals to learners that demonstrable clinical competence is not just desirable but essential, thereby driving learning towards the acquisition and refinement of these crucial practical abilities.[9,10]

Moving-up on Miller's Pyramid

Competence in medicine exists on a spectrum, often conceptualized by

Miller's Pyramid with four levels: "Knows" (knowledge), "Knows How" (can apply knowledge), "Shows How" (demonstrates skills in a simulated setting), and "Does" (performs independently in practice). Traditional assessments frequently operate at the lower two levels. Written exams test "Knows,"' while case discussions might probe "Knows How." However, ensuring a doctor can actually *perform* requires assessment at the higher levels. OSCE is specifically designed to evaluate the "Shows How" level—observing students as they demonstrate their skills in a controlled, standardized environment. This provides crucial evidence of practical ability, bridging the gap between theoretical knowledge and competent real-world practice.[8,11]

Assessing the Process, Not Just the Outcome

Conventional clinical exams often evaluate the end product—the student's summarized findings, diagnosis, or management plan—without witnessing the steps taken to reach it. Was the patient's history gathered empathetically and systematically? Was the physical examination performed using the correct technique? Were safety protocols like hand hygiene observed during a procedure? OSCE allows examiners to directly observe and evaluate these critical process elements using structured checklists. This focus ensures that proper technique, effective communication, and safe practices are assessed and reinforced; aspects often missed when only the final outcome is considered.[1,7]

Addressing Variability

A major weakness of traditional clinical exams is their susceptibility to variability. Different students face cases of varying difficulty, and examiners may apply different standards or exhibit biases. OSCE directly tackles this by standardizing the assessment experience. All students rotate through the exact same set of tasks or stations. Standardized patients ensure consistent presentations and interactions. Predefined checklists and trained examiners minimize subjective judgment, leading to significantly improved objectivity and reliability, ensuring fairer and more dependable evaluation of competence.[4,5,12]

Relevance to Competency-based Medical Education

The global shift towards competency-based medical education (CBME), including its implementation in India, fundamentally reorients medical training around the achievement of specific, demonstrable competencies. This framework demands assessment methods that can validly determine if these competencies have been acquired. OSCE aligns perfectly with CBME's philosophy by providing a structured means to directly assess a wide range of predetermined clinical skills—procedural, communication, examination, and interpretation—ensuring that assessment methods directly reflect and support the competency-focused goals of the curriculum.[12,13]

UNDERSTANDING OBJECTIVE STRUCTURED CLINICAL EXAMINATION: DEFINITION, PRINCIPLES, AND DOMAINS ASSESSED

The OSCE is fundamentally *an assessment method where components of clinical competence are evaluated in a planned, structured manner, with candidates rotating through stations, each presenting a specific task, often assessed using predetermined checklists.*[1,7] To fully understand its utility, it is helpful to deconstruct the acronym OSCE. *Objective* refers to the minimization of subjectivity through standardized tasks, standardized patients (where applicable), and the use of detailed checklists or rating scales applied consistently by trained examiners. *Structured* highlights the planned nature of the exam—the specific sequence of timed stations, the defined tasks at each station, and the organized assessment format. *Clinical* (or *Practical* in OSPE) signifies its focus on assessing performance in scenarios relevant to clinical practice or laboratory procedures. *Examination* underscores its function as a formal method of evaluating competence.

Several core principles underpin the OSCE methodology. *Standardization* is key, ensuring all candidates face the same challenges under the same conditions. *Objectivity* in scoring is obtained through checklists and trained observers. It fundamentally assesses competence (capability)—(what the candidate *does?*)—rather than just what they know. It allows for *broad sampling* of skills and knowledge across multiple stations, providing a more comprehensive picture of competence than a single long case might. Finally, it emphasizes assessment of the *process* of care, not just the final outcome.

The versatility of the OSCE allows for the assessment of a wide array of competency domains crucial for medical professionals. These include:

- *History taking skills:* Evaluating the ability to gather relevant information systematically, build rapport, and demonstrate empathy.
- *Physical examination skills:* Assessing the correct technique, sequence, and interpretation of physical findings for various body systems.
- *Procedural skills:* Observing the performance of practical tasks ranging from basic procedures such as measuring BP and giving an injection, to more complex ones like inserting an IV line or performing basic life support, often using mannequins or task trainers.
- *Communication skills:* Evaluating interactions with standardized patients or colleagues, such as explaining diagnoses or procedures, breaking bad news, obtaining informed consent, counseling on lifestyle changes, etc.
- *Interpretation skills:* Assessing the ability to analyze data such as electrocardiograms (ECGs), radiographs, laboratory reports, and spirometry results presented at a station.
- *Clinical reasoning and decision making:* Often evaluated through linked stations where initial data gathering leads to subsequent analysis or management planning.
- *Professionalism and ethics:* Observing behaviors like respect for patients, maintaining confidentiality, and demonstrating ethical conduct during interactions.[1,6]

It is crucial to distinguish OSCE from simpler assessment formats like 'spotting'. While spotting tests typically recall of knowledge (e.g., identifying anatomical structures or instruments) targeting the cognitive domain, OSCE focuses on the application of knowledge and the demonstration of skills—the psychomotor and affective domains—evaluating how candidates integrate knowledge, skills, and attitudes in simulated practical scenarios.[8,11]

DESIGNING AND PLANNING AN EFFECTIVE OSCE (THE CORE "HOW-TO")

The success of an OSCE hinges less on the day of the exam and more on the weeks and months of meticulous planning preceding it. It demands a systematic approach, significant resource allocation, and collaborative effort. As Harden noted, "The key to a successful OSCE is careful planning."

Meticulous Planning—the Foundation

- *Team approach:* Implementing an OSCE is rarely a solo endeavor. It requires a dedicated team comprising faculty members (for content expertise, station design, and examining), educationalists (for assessment expertise), administrative staff (for logistics, scheduling, and communication), technical support (for equipment and simulators), and potentially standardized patient coordinators. Clear roles, responsibilities, and timelines are all essential from the outset. Sensitization and orientation of all involved personnel, including nonteaching staff and students, are crucial first steps. Hands-on training for faculty in OSCE principles and checklist development is vital.
- *Resource assessment:* A realistic appraisal of available resources is necessary. This includes:
    - *Space:* Sufficient rooms or areas for the required number of stations, waiting areas, and briefing rooms.
- *Time:* Adequate time for planning, station development, pilot testing, training (examiners and simulated patients), conducting the exam, scoring, and feedback. Faculty time is a major resource consideration.
- *Personnel:* Availability of sufficient trained examiners, simulated patients (if used), and administrative and technical support staff.
- *Equipment:* Mannequins, task trainers, medical instruments, diagnostic images (X-rays and ECGs), laboratory reports, consumables, and other equipment if needed.
- *Budget:* Costs associated with simulated patients' fees, consumables, printing, potential software, and faculty/staff time.[1,14]

Determining Content: Blueprinting the Objective Structured Clinical Examination

- *What is blueprinting?* Blueprinting is the process of creating a map that explicitly links the content and skills assessed in the OSCE stations to the course's learning objectives, curriculum topics, and the competency domains being targeted (e.g., history taking, physical exam, communication, and procedures).
- *Why blueprint?* It serves multiple critical functions:
    - *Ensures content validity:* Guarantees that the OSCE assesses what it is intended to assess, reflecting the taught curriculum and expected competencies.
    - *Ensures balanced coverage:* Prevents overassessment of certain topics/skills and underassessment of others.
    - *Guides station development:* Provides a clear framework for deciding the number and type of stations needed for each area.
    - *Enhances defensibility*: Makes the assessment process transparent and justifiable.

  - *Aligns with student level*: Helps tailor the complexity of stations appropriately for undergraduate or postgraduate levels.[1,14]
- *How to blueprint:* A common approach involves creating a table. One axis lists the key subject areas, clinical presentations, or body systems covered in the curriculum (e.g., Cardiovascular System, Respiratory Emergencies, and Diabetes Management). The other axis lists the core skills or competency domains to be assessed (e.g., History Taking, Physical Examination, Communication, Procedural Skill, Data Interpretation, and Professionalism). The cells within the grid are then populated to indicate which stations will assess which combination of content and skill, ensuring comprehensive coverage according to predefined weightings based on importance and teaching time.

Designing the Stations

- *Number and duration:* Reliability generally increases with the number of stations. A common range is 10–15 stations for summative exams, though fewer may be used for formative assessments. Station duration typically ranges from 5 to 10 minutes, depending on task complexity, allowing time for reading instructions, performing the task, and examiner scoring (plus rotation time between stations).
- *Types of stations:*
  - *Procedure stations (observed):* Candidates perform a specific clinical or practical skill (e.g., examining a joint, demonstrating inhaler technique, performing urinary catheterization on a model, hand hygiene). An examiner observes and scores using a checklist.
  - *Communication stations (observed):* Candidates interact with a standardized patient (SP) or occasionally a real patient (with consent and careful planning). Tasks include taking a focused history, counseling, breaking bad news, explaining a procedure, or obtaining consent. Assessment uses checklists and/or global rating scales (GRS).
  - *Interpretation stations (observed or unobserved):* Candidates interpret clinical data (e.g., ECG strips, radiographs, blood gas reports, and growth charts). This can be an observed station where they explain their findings or an unobserved "question station" where they write down their interpretation and answers to related questions.
  - *Question/response stations (unobserved):* Candidates answer written questions based on a short scenario, image, specimen, instruments, or data provided at the station. These should ideally test higher-order thinking (application and analysis) rather than simple recall, perhaps asking for differential diagnoses, investigation plans, or management steps based on the provided information. They are often used to balance the need for observers.
  - *Linked/couplet stations:* Consist of two or more sequential stations where the task in a later station depends on information gathered or actions taken in an earlier one (e.g., Station 1: Interpret an ECG; Station 2: Answer questions on management based on the ECG diagnosis). This allows assessment of integrated clinical reasoning.

- *Rest stations:* Strategically placed short breaks within the OSCE can help reduce candidate fatigue and anxiety.
- *Writing station instructions (stems):* Instructions provided to the candidate must be crystal clear, concise, and unambiguous. They should set the context (e.g., "You are a junior consultant in the OPD"), state the required task clearly using action verbs (e.g., "Examine the patient's thyroid gland," "Explain the risks and benefits of this procedure to the patient," "Interpret the provided chest radiograph"), and indicate the time available. Instructions should be piloted to ensure they are easily understood.[1,7]

- *Materials and setup:* Each station requires a detailed list of all necessary items: specific equipment (stethoscopes, BP cuffs, and models), props (patient charts, X-ray films, and laboratory reports), consumables (gloves and swabs), instructions sheets for candidates and examiners, checklists/rating scales, and specific setup requirements for the room. Everything must be checked for functionality and availability, including their specific numbers, before the exam.

Developing Checklists and Rating Scales

- *Purpose:* These are the cornerstones of OSCE objectivity. They standardize the observation process, guide scoring, ensure key elements of performance are assessed, minimize examiner bias, and can form the basis for specific feedback.
- *Checklist construction principles:*
  - *Objective-driven:* Directly reflect the specific learning objectives of the task being assessed.
  - *Action-oriented:* List essential, observable actions or behaviors required to perform the task competently. Use clear, unambiguous verbs (e.g., "Palpates apex beat," "Asks about history of allergy," "Washes hands before procedure").
  - *Sequenced logically:* Steps should generally follow a logical flow where applicable.
  - *Focus on key steps:* Include critical actions essential for effectiveness or patient safety. Avoid trivial steps unless crucial to the process. Items may be weighted based on importance.
  - *Binary format:* Typically, uses a simple dichotomous scale (e.g., Done/Not Done, Yes/No, Present/Absent).
  - *Manageable length:* Keep the checklist concise enough for an examiner to use accurately in real-time while observing the candidate during OSCE.
  - *Validation and piloting:* Absolutely essential. Checklists must be reviewed by content experts (internal validation) and ideally piloted with students or junior staff to check for clarity, feasibility, time adequacy, and accuracy. Revisions based on feedback are critical. External validation can enhance acceptability.[1,12]
- *Global Rating Scales (GRS):*
  - *What are they?* Holistic scales are used to assess the overall quality of performance on a specific dimension (e.g., communication effectiveness, procedural fluency, organization, professionalism). They use descriptive anchors for different performance levels (e.g., unsatisfactory, borderline, satisfactory, good, and excellent).

- *When to use?* Particularly useful for assessing qualities that are difficult to break down into discrete checklist items, such as empathy, rapport, confidence, and the overall integration of skills. Often used alongside checklists in communication or complex procedure stations.
- *Combined approach:* Often, the most robust assessment uses a combination: a checklist captures the completion of specific, critical actions, while a GRS captures the overall quality and integration of the performance.

Standardized Patients

- *Role:* SPs are individuals trained to portray a specific patient case consistently and realistically. They can simulate history, emotional responses, and sometimes physical signs. They are invaluable for assessing communication, history taking, and interpersonal skills. Some SPs are also trained to provide feedback or complete assessment checklists from the patient's perspective.
- *Selection and training:* Careful selection is needed to find reliable individuals comfortable with the role. Rigorous training is paramount and must cover: the specific case details (history, affect, and responses), consistent portrayal across all candidates, how to interact naturally, avoiding leading the candidate, accurate use of any checklists/scales they are assigned, and maintaining confidentiality.[4,6,12]

Examiners/Observers

- *Selection:* Should be faculty members or senior residents thoroughly familiar with the content area and ideally with assessment principles. Consistency is aided by using the same examiners for a specific station throughout a cohort if possible.
- *Training:* This is non-negotiable for ensuring reliability and objectivity. Training must cover: OSCE principles, detailed understanding of their assigned station(s) and tasks, accurate and consistent use of the checklist/GRS, avoiding common rating errors (e.g., halo effect—letting overall impression influence specific ratings; horn effect—letting one mistake negatively bias all ratings), maintaining neutrality (observe objectively, do not teach, prompt, or interact unless required by the station design), adhering to timings, and administrative procedures. Practice sessions with mock candidates are highly recommended. Inter-rater reliability checks (having two examiners score independently and comparing results) during training or piloting are valuable.
- *Role clarity:* Examiners must understand their role is solely assessment during the OSCE. They should observe discreetly and score based only on the predefined criteria, resisting the urge to intervene or provide feedback during the station unless specifically designed for interaction.

CONDUCTING THE OBJECTIVE STRUCTURED CLINICAL EXAMINATION

The smooth execution of the OSCE on exam day is the culmination of meticulous planning. Careful attention to logistics and clear communication are vital.

- *Logistics and environment:* The chosen venue must accommodate the number of stations and candidates comfortably.

Clear signage is essential to guide students efficiently through the circuit, usually in a unidirectional flow. Measures should be taken to minimize noise and distractions. Strict procedures must be in place to maintain the confidentiality of station content, preventing candidates who have finished from communicating with those yet to start. Ensure all equipment is functional and backup plans exist for potential failures (e.g., faulty mannequin and absent SP).

- *Briefing:* Comprehensive briefings are essential for all participants:
  - *Students:* Before starting, provide clear, concise instructions covering the format of the exam, the number of stations, the time allocated per station, the signals indicating the start and end of each station and rotation time, rules of conduct (e.g., no interaction with examiners unless part of the task, displaying identification), and emergency procedures. Address any immediate questions to alleviate their anxiety.
  - *Examiners/SPs:* Conduct a final pre-exam briefing to review station specifics, reinforce checklist/GRS usage guidelines, reiterate the importance of timing and neutrality, confirm logistical arrangements, and address any last-minute queries. Distribute necessary materials (checklists and instructions).
- *Execution:* The examination circuit should start promptly. Accurate timekeeping is critical, using bells, buzzers, or visual timers to signal station start, warnings (if used), end, and rotation periods. Coordinators must manage the flow of students between stations smoothly. Completed checklists and answer sheets need to be collected systematically and securely after each candidate finishes the circuit or at designated points. Contingency plans should be activated swiftly if any unforeseen issues arise (e.g., a student feeling unwell, an equipment malfunction).
- *Quality assurance:* Appointing a chief coordinator or lead invigilator is highly recommended. This individual oversees the entire process, monitors timings, ensures adherence to procedures, troubleshoots problems, maintains exam integrity, and acts as a point of contact for examiners and students. Having floating invigilators can also help monitor the process and address minor issues quickly.[1]

SCORING, SETTING STANDARDS, AND PROVIDING FEEDBACK

Once the OSCE is conducted, the focus shifts to scoring the performance, determining pass/fail boundaries, and, crucially for learning, providing meaningful feedback.

- *Scoring:* The objective nature of OSCE facilitates relatively straightforward scoring, primarily based on the predesigned instruments:
  - *Checklist scoring:* Points assigned to each item on the checklist are summed. Items deemed critical for safety or competence may be given higher weightings. A total score per station is calculated.
  - *GRS scoring:* Scores are assigned based on the descriptive anchors for each quality being assessed. These provide a holistic judgment complementing the checklist's specific actions.
  - *Combined Scores:* If both checklists and GRS are used, methods for combining these into a single station

score (e.g., weighted averages) need to be predetermined.
  - *Handling omissions/errors:* Clear rules should exist on how to score missed steps or actions performed incorrectly, particularly regarding critical errors that might warrant failing a station regardless of the total score.
- *Standard setting:* Simply summing scores is insufficient; a defensible passing standard (cut-score) must be established to determine competence. This is especially critical for high-stakes summative exams.
  - *Why Needed:* Ensures the pass/fail decision is not arbitrary but reflects a defined level of minimally acceptable performance. It enhances fairness and the credibility of the assessment.
  - *Methods (Criterion-Referenced Preferred):* While various methods exist, criterion-referenced approaches are generally preferred for competency decisions as they judge performance against a predefined standard, not just relative to peers (norm-referencing).
- *Providing feedback:* OSCE offers excellent opportunities for formative feedback, transforming assessment *of* learning into assessment *for* learning.[9,10]
- *Importance:* Feedback helps students understand their strengths and identify specific areas needing improvement, guiding future learning efforts.
- *Methods:* Feedback should be timely and specific. Options include:
  - *Individual score reports:* Providing students with their scores per station, potentially broken down by checklist item or competency domain. Comparing their score to the pass mark or average performance can be informative.
  - *Narrative comments:* Collating brief written comments from examiners or SPs (if feasible and structured) can provide qualitative insights.
  - *Group debriefing:* Discussing common errors and successful strategies observed across the cohort (while maintaining anonymity) can be highly educational.
  - *Video review:* If stations are video recorded, reviewing performance with a tutor offers powerful feedback opportunities.

ADVANTAGES AND DISADVANTAGES OF OBJECTIVE STRUCTURED CLINICAL EXAMINATION

Objective structured clinical examination offers significant advantages over traditional clinical assessment methods, but it also presents challenges that must be acknowledged and managed.

Advantages

- *Objectivity and reliability:* Through standardized tasks, checklists, and trained examiners, OSCE significantly reduces examiner bias and case variability, leading to more reliable and consistent scores.
- *Validity:* When properly blueprinted against the curriculum, OSCE demonstrates strong content validity. It also has good potential for construct validity by directly assessing the performance of clinical skills.
- *Assessment of performance:* It directly observes what candidates *do* (Shows How), focusing on essential clinical skills, procedures, and communication behaviors—assessing the process, not just the outcome.

- *Wide sampling and comprehensive assessment:* Multiple stations allow for assessment across a broader range of topics, skills, and competency domains compared to a single long case, providing a more holistic view of the candidate's abilities.
- *Standardization and fairness:* All candidates face the same tasks under the same conditions, ensuring a level playing field.
- *Feedback potential:* The structured nature, particularly with detailed checklists, facilitates the provision of specific, targeted feedback to learners, guiding improvement.
- *Positive educational impact (assessment drives learning):* Emphasizing practical skills in assessment motivates students to actively practice and develop these competencies. Student feedback often indicates OSCE is perceived as fairer and more relevant (e.g., studies by Watson, Singh, and Smith).[1,12,15]

Disadvantages and Challenges (with Mitigation Strategies)

- *Resource-intensive:* Requires substantial investment in faculty time (planning, training, examining), administrative support, space, equipment, and potentially SP costs. *(Mitigation: Phased implementation, faculty development programs, resource sharing between departments, utilizing existing simulation center resources).*
- *Compartmentalization (checklist mentality):* Assesses skills in discrete units, potentially failing to capture the candidate's ability to integrate skills and manage a patient holistically. *(Mitigation: Include integrated stations, use GRS alongside checklists, combine OSCE with other assessments like long cases or workplace-based assessments).*
- *Authenticity concerns:* The simulated environment may lack the complexity, uncertainty, and emotional pressure of real clinical encounters. *(Mitigation: Use well-trained SPs to enhance realism, design challenging scenarios, high-fidelity simulation where appropriate, acknowledge limitations).*
- *Examiner/SP fatigue:* Long OSCE circuits can be tiring for examiners and SPs, potentially affecting scoring consistency. *(Mitigation: Schedule adequate breaks, limit the number of candidates per session, and rotate examiners/SPs if possible).*
- *Student anxiety:* The timed, structured nature can be highly stressful for candidates, potentially impacting performance (e.g., studies by Russell and Van der Vleuten). *(Mitigation: Thorough student briefing, practice/mock OSCE sessions, familiarization with the format, creating a supportive exam environment).*
- *Potential for cueing:* Poorly designed stations or checklists might inadvertently cue candidates to the expected actions. *(Mitigation: Careful station design, rigorous checklist piloting, and refinement).*[12]

OBJECTIVE STRUCTURED CLINICAL EXAMINATION VARIATIONS AND FUTURE DIRECTIONS

The fundamental principles of OSCE have been adapted into various formats tailored to specific needs. *Objective Structured Practical Examination (OSPE)* focuses specifically on laboratory or practical skills often found in basic sciences. Other variations include *Objective Structured Long Examination*

Record (OSLER), combining OSCE principles with aspects of the long case; *Objective Structured Video Examination (OSVE)*, using video scenarios; *OSTE (Objective Structured Teaching Evaluation)*, assessing teaching skills; and even *Objective Structured Selection Exam (OSSE)* for admission processes. Looking ahead, technology offers exciting possibilities, including the use of video recording of OSCE stations for remote assessment, quality assurance, examiner calibration, and enhanced student feedback. Virtual reality (VR) and augmented reality (AR) simulations hold potential for creating even more immersive and complex OSCE scenarios, potentially reducing the reliance on physical resources in the long term.[12]

CONCLUSION

The OSCE represents a significant methodological advancement in the assessment of clinical competence. By prioritizing objectivity, structure, and the direct observation of performance, OSCE addresses many inherent weaknesses of traditional clinical examinations, particularly their subjectivity and limited scope. Its ability to assess a wide range of skills—procedural, communicative, interpretive, and clinical reasoning—across multiple standardized encounters makes it an invaluable tool, especially within the framework of CBME.

While acknowledging the considerable resources required for its effective planning and implementation and recognizing that it assesses skills in a somewhat compartmentalized manner, the benefits of OSCE in driving learning towards practical skills and providing reliable, valid data on student performance are substantial. It is not necessarily a replacement for all other forms of clinical assessment but serves best as a cornerstone within a comprehensive assessment strategy, often complemented by methods evaluating integration (like long cases) or performance in the real workplace ("Does" level). When meticulously planned, rigorously executed, and used appropriately—as Harden emphasized, "When used correctly, the OSCE can be highly successful as an instrument to assess competence in medicine"—it significantly enhances our ability to ensure future physicians are equipped with the essential skills for high-quality patient care.[7]

KEY POINTS TO REMEMBER

- *Addresses flaws:* OSCE directly tackles the subjectivity, lack of standardization, and limited scope often seen in traditional clinical exams.
- *Drives relevant learning:* By assessing practical skills directly, OSCE motivates students to learn and practice what truly matters for clinical competence ("Shows How" on Miller's Pyramid).
- *Assesses the process:* Unlike methods focusing only on the outcome, OSCE allows direct observation and evaluation of *how* students perform procedures, communicate, and conduct examinations.
- *Objectivity through structure:* Standardization is key—achieved via identical stations, timed rotations, clear tasks, detailed checklists, and trained examiners/standardized patients (SPs).
- *Meticulous planning is crucial:* Successful OSCE implementation requires significant upfront planning, including team coordination, resource assessment, and faculty/staff training. *Do not underestimate the planning phase.*
- *Blueprint for validity:* Always map your OSCE stations to curriculum objectives and competency domains (blueprinting)

to ensure you are assessing the right things fairly and comprehensively.

- *Checklists and rating scales are core tools:* Develop clear, objective, and validated checklists for specific actions and consider GRS for overall qualities (like communication). These are essential for standardized scoring.
- *Training is non-negotiable:* Examiners and SPs *must* be rigorously trained on their roles, the specific stations, and the use of assessment tools to ensure reliability and consistency.
- *Standard setting is essential:* For summative OSCEs, establish a defensible pass/fail standard (cut-score) using recognized methods (e.g., Angoff and borderline) rather than relying on arbitrary percentages.
- *Feedback maximizes learning:* Use the detailed information gathered during OSCE to provide specific, constructive feedback to students, turning assessment *of* learning into assessment *for* learning.
- *Resource intensive:* Be prepared for the significant investment required in terms of faculty/staff time, space, equipment, and potentially SP costs.
- *Part of a system:* OSCE is powerful but has limitations (e.g., compartmentalization). It is most effective as part of a broader assessment strategy that may include workplace-based assessments or traditional long cases to evaluate skill integration and performance in real settings (Does).
- Remembering these points will help ensure that OSCE is used effectively as a valid, reliable, and educationally beneficial assessment tool.

REFERENCES

1. Harden RM, Gleeson FA. Assessment of clinical competence using an objective structured clinical examination (OSCE). Med Educ. 1979;13:41-54.
2. Harden RM, Lilley P, Patricio M. The Definitive Guide to the OSCE. Edinburgh: Elsevier; 2016.
3. Newble D. Techniques for measuring clinical competence. Br J Anaesth. 1984;56:221-229.
4. van der Vleuten CPM. The assessment of professional competence. Adv Health Sci Educ. 1996;1:41-67.
5. Wass V, van der Vleuten C, Shatzer J, Jones R. Assessment of clinical competence. Lancet. 2001;357:945-949.
6. Barrows HS. Uses of standardized patients. Acad Med. 1993;68:443-451.
7. Harden RM, Stevenson M, Downie WW, Wilson GM. Assessment using OSCE. Br Med J. 1975;1:447-451.
8. Miller GE. The assessment of clinical skills/competence/performance. Acad Med. 1990;65:S63-S67.
9. Schuwirth LWT, van der Vleuten CPM. Assessment of medical competence. Med Educ. 2006;40:309-317.
10. Nicol DJ, Macfarlane-Dick D. Formative assessment and self-regulated learning. Stud High Educ. 2006;31:199-218.
11. Downing SM, Yudkowsky R. Assessment in Health Professions Education. New York: Routledge; 2009.
12. Hodges B. OSCE! Variations on a theme by Harden. Med Educ. 2003;37:1134-1140.
13. Frank JR, Snell LS, Ten Cate O, et al. Competency-based medical education. Med Teach. 2010;32:638-645.
14. Dent JA, Harden RM, Hunt D. A Practical Guide for Medical Teachers. 5th ed. Elsevier; 2021.
15. Singh T, Gupta P, Singh D. Principles of Medical Education. 4th ed. New Delhi: Jaypee Brothers; 2013

CHAPTER 24

Assessment for and of Learning

Sara Dhanawade

INTRODUCTION

Assessment is a powerful tool in education. It is generally acknowledged that assessment drives learning. In the broad sense, assessment refers to the processes employed to make judgements about the achievements of students over a course of study.[1] It directs learning by signaling what is important and ensures that learning has occurred. Nevertheless, learning is dependent on the type of assessment used and whether or not timely feedback is given. Elton and Laurillard (1979)[2] stated that "the quickest way to change student learning is to change the assessment system." Assessment should be linked to the learning outcomes and teaching methods.

The Medical Council of India (2019) has proposed five different roles of the Indian Medical Graduate (IMG), namely clinician, leader, professional, life-long learner, and communicator. To ensure that the desired outcome is achieved, these attributes, at least the core competencies, must be assessed before they are allowed to practice in society. It is evident that while some of these qualities are easy to define and measure, others are not easily measurable.

Clinical competence or professional competence is a multidimensional construct and therefore needs a multidimensional assessment.[3]

Miller (1990)[4] proposed a hierarchical model of assessment of clinical competence. It starts with the assessment of cognition and ends with the assessment of behavior **(Fig. 1)**.

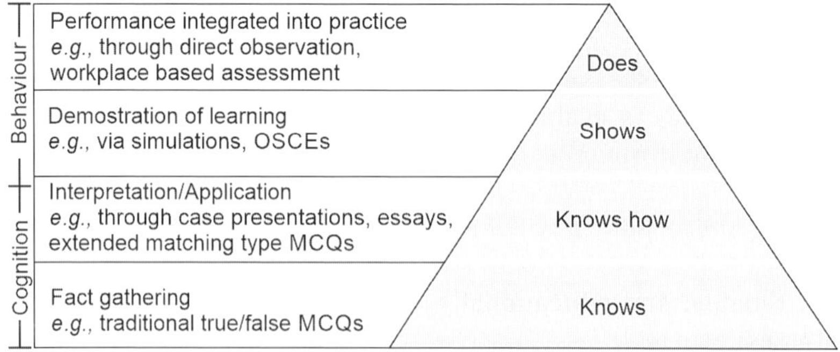

Fig. 1: Miller's hierarchical model of assessment of clinical competence.

As we move up the model, the task resembles real practice. The cognitive assessment deals with knowledge and its application (knows, knows how). The assessment of behavior deals with the assessment of competence under a controlled environment (shows how) and competence in practice (does). This spans over the levels of Bloom's taxonomy of educational objectives from the level of comprehension to the level of evaluation.

Traditionally, in medical education, the focus is on summative assessment, which occurs at the end of the year. However, Competency-Based Medical Education (CBME) requires a robust, multifaceted assessment system that places more emphasis on formative assessment. We will now look at the six key features of effective assessment in CBME.

- *Assessment needs to be more frequent and continuous*: Frequent assessment with effective feedback helps learners progress and reach where they are expected to reach. However, feedback in medical education is a complex process demanding specific skills on the part of the assessor. Feedback is only as good as the assessment that informs it.[5] Inaccurate assessment leads to ineffective feedback. The faculty needs to develop good observation skills, as one cannot give feedback on something that one has not observed. Feedback needs to be constructive and nonjudgmental, which should guide trainees towards meaningful "assessment seeking behavior."
- *Assessment must be criterion-based*: A norm-referenced assessment based on comparison of trainees within an institute generally results in setting the standard below appropriate expectations. Hence, criterion referencing is important, especially for core and certifiable competencies. However, the major challenge remains in training the faculty to be accurate observers and better assessors of performance. Criteria should be developmental, defined as milestones or benchmarks marked, and this allows the program to identify whether the trainee is progressing in the right direction. Milestones become the blueprint for assessment and help to select appropriate assessment methods.
- *Assessment should be contextual*: Assessment in an authentic setting (work-based assessment) is an essential component of CBME. Although faculty who work along with trainees are in an excellent position to directly observe their skills and give real-time feedback, studies have shown that faculty frequently fail to identify deficiencies in trainees' clinical skills.[6]
- *Assessment tools must meet the minimum standard of quality*: Vleuten (1996) proposed a conceptual model for deciding the validity of an assessment tool. The criteria were: (1) Validity (does it measure what it is supposed to measure?), (2) reliability (does it consistently measure what it is supposed to measure?), (3) acceptability (Is it acceptable to stakeholders?), (4) educational impact, and (5) cost effectiveness. The weighting of the criteria depended on the purpose for which the assessment tool was used. For summative purposes, such as certification, more weightage was given to reliability, whereas for formative purposes, such as improvement, more weightage was given to educational impact.[7]

One of the best-studied assessment tools for direct observation is mini-CEX.

Having said that, one must remember that any work-based assessment tool is only as good as the person using it.[8,9] So, finally, it boils down to developing skilled faculty who are keen and accurate observers.

- *Assessment should incorporate more qualitative approaches*: This includes narratives and reflection writing. Studies have shown that valuable information can be obtained through this in certain difficult-to-assess competencies like professionalism.[10]
- *Assessment should be done by multiple assessors*: Ideally, assessments should be done by multiple methods, in multiple settings, by multiple assessors to make it more valid.

TYPES OF ASSESSMENTS

Depending on the primary purpose for which it is conducted, it can be classified as formative and summative. Formative is for enhancing learning, and summative is for the purpose of certification. Before we choose the type of assessment, we need to consider certain key questions. (1) Why do we assess, or the purpose of the assessment?, (2) What are we trying to assess?, and (3) Who should assess?

Assessment in medical education is crucial as certification gives the candidate a license to practice as an autonomous doctor dealing with human lives. Hence, it is important that appropriate methods should be used to assess their learning, which includes many critical skills **(Table 1)**.

ASSESSMENT FOR LEARNING

Assessment for learning (AFL), also known as formative assessment, uses feedback to improve student learning. Although both terms are often used interchangeably, it must be remembered that traditional formative assessment, where only the teacher is informed about the students' performance, does not qualify as AFL. Similarly, traditional formative assessment does not focus on the progress of the learner along the learning trajectory. Students are important stakeholders in AFL.

AFL is defined as "the process of seeking and interpreting evidence for use by learners and their teachers to decide where the learners are in their learning, where they need to go, and how best to get there" (The Assessment Reform Group 2002) **(Fig. 2)**.

Klenowski (2009)[11] defined AFL as "part of everyday practice by students, teachers and peers that seeks, reflects upon and responds to information from dialogue, demonstration and observation in ways that enhance learning."

Benefits of Assessment for Learning

- AFL helps students understand their progress and identify areas for improvement.

TABLE 1: Summative versus formative assessment.

Summative	*Formative*
Assess the performance of students at the end of an instructional period	Assess the performance of students throughout the course
Focuses on the product to ensure that the minimum standard has been attained	Focuses on the process
For certification as pass/fail	To improve learning through feedback
High stakes	Low stakes

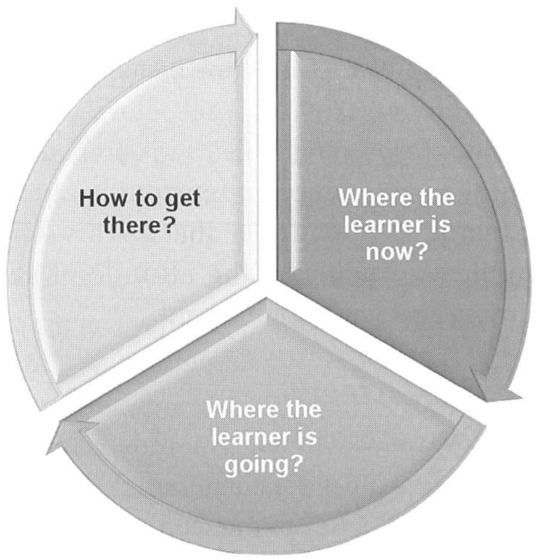

Fig. 2: Assessment for learning.

- It helps students learn better, rather than just achieve a better mark.
- AFL helps students develop the skills to be independent learners (self-regulated learners).

Assessment for learning is usually used throughout the teaching and learning process and can include formal and informal assessment activities.

Among the different roles of IMG, it is the role of "clinician" that is most commonly assessed. We need to ensure that all competencies are assessed in some way or other, as it is pertinent for patient safety, accountability, and the ability to work in a team. It is impossible to assess each and every competency at summative assessment.

Hence, formative assessment gives a wider opportunity to assess most of the competencies. A competency-based assessment that links learning outcomes with specific learning objectives requires continuous and frequent assessment. Formative assessment is the best example of the interdependence of input, processes, and output in the educational system.

Cycle of Learning

Assessment for learning should be a planned activity. The overall strategy and methods to gather information about student learning should be incorporated into the curriculum. In AFL, we identify what we want the students to learn, provide learning opportunities, evaluate whether they have learned what we want them to, and give constructive, actionable feedback to help students learn better. It is an ongoing cycle that helps us monitor our teaching and continually improve student learning **(Fig. 3)**.

Components of Assessment for Learning

Learners and teachers are the most important stakeholders of AFL. Only motivated and willing students open to feedback and ready to act upon feedback will benefit. In the same way, a teacher who is ready to dedicate time for providing feedback, suggesting remedial measures, and monitoring the progress of the student is equally important in the process.

The fundamental elements of AFL are:

- Formulating statements of intended learning outcomes.[12] This should be explicitly communicated to the students.

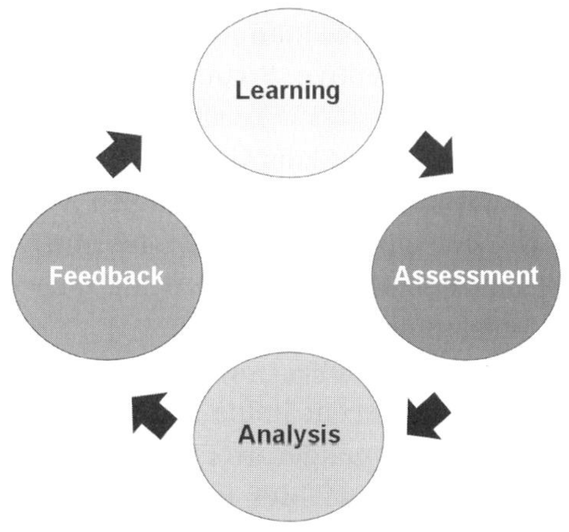

Fig. 3: Cycle of learning.

- Creating an educational environment and learning experiences for students to achieve the intended outcome.
- Selecting appropriate assessment methods.
- Feedback—characteristics of effective feedback hold true for feedback in AFL too. Feedback should be clear, specific, based on direct observation, and should be delivered in a non-judgmental manner.
- Monitoring learning progression. This helps teachers to identify learning gaps and plan instructions.

Methods of Assessment for Learning

Assessment for learning must be introduced in a continuous fashion longitudinally throughout the course using routine teaching and learning activities.

- *Written tests*: Written assessment criteria and how marks are computed can be provided beforehand and used subsequently for correcting. Written comments can be given, but they should be specific and not vague.
- *Classroom teachings*:[13] Seminars and tutorials provide opportunities to learn from assessment.
- *Clinical teaching*: Case presentations, miniclinical evaluation exercise (Mini-CEX), Objective Structured Clinical Examination (OSCE), Direct Observation of Procedural Skills (DOPS), and other Workplace-Based Assessment (WPBA) provide opportunities for learning in clinical settings. This is particularly useful for learning clinical skills.
- *Reflections*: Reflecting on a particular session or event helps recapture their experience, ponder over it, and evaluate it. Thus, it provides opportunities for identifying learning gaps and promoting self-directed learning.[14]

Portfolios

A portfolio is a collection of assignments and professional work that showcases an individual's learning, skills, and competence. Portfolios give ample opportunities to the evaluator to provide feedback. This helps students to inculcate the attitude of self-learning and self-improvement.[15,16]

Peer Assessment

This is the process by which a student assesses their peers against a set benchmark. Students may respond better to the feedback received from their peers than from the tutor. It must be remembered that anonymity should be maintained in peer assessment.

Reflections, portfolios, and peer assessment improve the metacognitive skills of the student. However, it is not the method, but its use to improve learning that makes it an AFL.

Strengths of Assessment for Learning

Assessment for learning allows teachers to identify areas where students struggle, thus enabling targeted interventions and individualized learning plans. By offering immediate feedback on performance, students can improve their understanding before moving on to more complex concepts. It promotes self-regulated learning (SRL), and students can take ownership of their learning and monitor their progress. Regular AFL can keep students actively engaged in the learning process and boost their confidence, and motivate them to learn. It promotes lifelong learning skills in students. Another important positive point to keep in mind is that frequent low-stakes assessments reduce the stress and anxiety associated with high-stakes summative exams.

Weaknesses of Assessment for Learning

Designing, administering, and providing feedback can be time-intensive for faculty, especially in large classes. Effective use of AFL demands well-trained and motivated faculty who can provide constructive, actionable, and timely feedback to students. There is always an element of inconsistency depending on the assessment method and faculty involved. A single assessment will not provide enough information about students' knowledge and skills. Hence, needs to be done frequently using different methods and by multiple assessors.

Overall, AFL are considered a valuable tool in medical education when implemented effectively. However, purely formative assessments are not taken seriously by students as well as teachers, and ideally, both formative and summative assessments should be merged.

ASSESSMENT OF LEARNING

This is the traditional and most commonly used method, also called summative assessment. Assessment of learning judges the overall progression of students in a systematic fashion. It has decision-making power and is hence considered a high-stakes examination. As students cannot escape the impact of summative assessment, it is important to design the assessment methods appropriately.[16] It is well accepted that what is not assessed is not learnt by the students. However, it is pertinent to note that summative assessment has limited learning value.[17] All assessments essentially become assessments of learning unless they are conducted with the purpose of improving students' learning. Assessments where the results are going to be used to make educational decisions essentially become summative or an assessment of learning, whether it is a university examination or an internal assessment examination (**Flowchart 1**).

Flowchart 1: Assessment of learning.

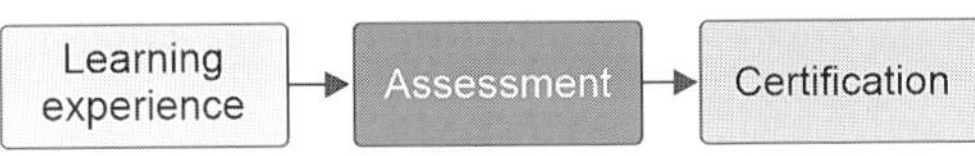

Strengths of Summative Assessment

- Provide a summary of a student's performance.
- Effectively measures learning outcomes.
- Promotes accountability both for students and teachers.
- Inculcates a sense of accomplishment in students.
- Encourages to maintenance of consistent educational quality and standards.
- Serves as a basis for licensing and accreditation.
- Provides data to the institution to assess the effectiveness of curriculum implementation.

Drawbacks of Summative Assessment

Summative assessments in medical education can have many drawbacks.

- Being a high-stakes examination, it can create a high-pressure environment and induce anxiety and stress.
- Summative assessments focus on a single performance, rather than gradual growth over time.
- Students tend to focus on what is likely to be asked in the exam rather than learning in depth with the goal of knowledge acquisition. This encourages rote learning.
- Summative assessments can negatively impact a student's motivation to learn.

- Summative assessments can be expensive to develop and administer, requiring a lot of resources.
- As students learn just with the intention to pass, generally shortly before the assessment, it can lead to inefficient learning.

To overcome these drawbacks, teachers should use assessment blueprints based on models, such as Miller's pyramid (1990), Bloom's taxonomy (1956), and Dreyfus' model (1980) of skill acquisition.

METHODS OF ASSESSMENT

A good summative assessment should adequately reflect the evaluation of necessary clinical competencies. How students perform in SA influences their educational progress. Hence, ensuring robustness of assessment is so important.

Current methods of summative assessment, such as written and oral exams, need to be improved to have a better impact on the learners. Multiple choice questions (MCQs) are very popular in medical education at both undergraduate and postgraduate levels. However, educators need to be aware that poorly constructed MCQs facilitate success based on savviness or test-wiseness of students rather than their knowledge. Educators must strive to create the fairest MCQs possible for students, particularly keeping in mind their prominent use in high-stakes examinations

Methods of Assessment in Medicine

See **Table 2.**

SIMULATION-BASED ASSESSMENT

There is growing evidence of the utility of simulation-based assessment in formative contexts, as relevant and representative clinical scenarios can be used to train learners in a safe environment. Simulation adds value to the educational training process with feedback. Students can make mistakes and learn from them without risking harm to patients, thus improving clinical competence. It offers a platform to assess soft and complex skills, such as communication, teamwork, professionalism, and decision-making. The challenges include its expensive nature and limited evidence about the effectiveness of simulation-based assessment in evaluating competence and performance. Hence, advancing to the next step of using simulation for summative assessment needs a rigorous and evidence-based approach, looking at the feasibility and validity. There are currently limited experiences, like the OSCE, and no guidelines for further advancements.

Future of Simulation-based Training

Artificial intelligence (AI) is expected to play a significant role in simulation-based training. Virtual Reality (VR) and augmented reality (AR) applications can enhance personalized learning experiences.

Strategies to Improve Summative Assessments

Integration of Multiple Assessment Methods (A combination of MCQs, OSCE, DOPS, and Mini-CEX, etc.), Enhancing Objectivity and Standardization (conducting examinations with trained faculty, standard rubrics, blue printing, using standardized patients), Incorporation of Technology and reducing biases (Computer assisted assessment, using virtual reality, AI driven assessment tools), Regular Faculty Training (OSCE, OSPE, Osler's method).

TABLE 2: Methods of assessment in medicine.

Method	Domain	Type of use	Limitation	Strength
MCQ	Knowledge	Summative	• Difficult to write • Cues	• High reliability • Computer graded • Efficient
SAQs	Knowledge	Summative Some formative	• Reliability dependent • on the training of graders	• No cueing • Assess problem-solving
Essays	Knowledge	Summative Some formatives	• Time-consuming • Interrater reliability	• No cueing • Higher order thinking required
DOPs/ MINI-CEX Oral	Skills Attitude Knowledge Attitudes	Formative Some summative Summative Some formatives	• Time-consuming • Selective behaviors • Subjective • Time-consuming • Training of examiners	• Feedback by • experts • Feedback by • experts
Simulator	Skills Attitudes	Formative Some summative	• Expensive • Can be artificial	• Tailored to • educational goals • Often reliable • and credible
Peer	Attitudes	Formative	• Confidentiality • Anonymity • Student buy-in	• Correlation with future clinical performance
Self	Knowledge Skills Attitudes	Formative	• Training required	• Fosters reflection and learning
Portfolio	Knowledge Skills Attitudes	Formative	• Time-consuming • Students select the best material	• Fosters reflection and learning

Source: Adapted from Epstein RM. Assessment in medical education. N Engl J Med. 2007;356(4):387-96.

Assessment as Learning

In this type, students are themselves accessors of their own learning. Students monitor their own learning, ask questions, and use a range of strategies to decide what they know and can do. It encourages students to take responsibility for their learning. Herein, students are trained to make effective use of formal and informal feedback to improve learning along with self-assessment. Assessment as Learning can be used to inculcate SRL by promoting active learning habits.

Challenges of Assessment and Way Forward

The task of assessment in medical education is highly challenging and likely to become more demanding in times to come. There is a lack of evidence linking assessment with safe practice.[18] Certain aspects of competence, like knowledge, can be reliably assessed using MCQs, extended matching, and essay questions. Similarly, OSCEs, DOPS, Mini-CEX, and OSLER are effective frameworks to assess clinical skills.[19] In contrast, attitude, communication, and professionalism are more difficult to assess. Hence, multimodal assessment from a number of assessors should be used to overcome these challenges and provide broader insights into a trainee's competence.

Incorporating Assessment for Learning in Curriculum

Despite the clear advantages of AFL, it is not widely incorporated in the true sense in medical colleges across India. The difficulties faced include:

- *Faculty development*: This is the most crucial intervention but often neglected. Medical colleges should have an adequate number of faculty and should have strong faculty development programs (FDPs). Hands-on training workshops on various aspects of assessment should be made part of FDPs.
- *Educational environment*: The Educational environment must be conducive and supportive for AFL to thrive. Institutions must try to promote the culture of self-regulated or self-directed learning in the students rather than just focusing on passing exams.
- *Programmatic assessment*: Institutions must implement processes to assess how AOL and AFL are conducted. Institutional instructional goals[20] and assessment criteria should be well-designed.
- *Mentorship*: Strong mentorship programs can create a conducive environment and boost AFL.

CONCLUSION

Assessments should be directly aligned to expected outcomes (competency achievement). Overall assessment should be planned to keep in mind the balance of formative and summative methods. The best practices should be adopted to make assessments more robust and effective. Following strategies can be adopted—triangulation of assessment, effective provision of feedback, opportunities for improvement by maintaining clear transparency and standards, use of programmatic assessment, training of accessors in competency framework and improving inter-rater reliability, establishing monitoring committees at institutional level, developing policies for remediations and improvement, ensuring content validity by blueprinting, building assessment literacy among learners (orientation to assessment system and expectations), addressing biases and use of technology, systematic alignment of assessment methods to ensure both progression and certification.[21,22]

REFERENCES

1. Harlen W. (2005). Teachers' summative practices and assessment for learning: Tensions and synergies. [Online] Available from https://doi.org/10.1080/09585170500136093 [Last accessed January, 2025].
2. Elton LRB, Laurillard DM. Trends in research on student learning. Studies in Higher Education. 1979;4(1):87-102.
3. Sood R, Singh T. Assessment in medical education: evolving perspectives and contemporary trends. Natl Med J India. 2012;25(6):357-64.
4. Miller GE. The assessment of clinical skills/competence/performance. Acad Med. 1990;65(9 Suppl):S63-7.
5. Holmboe ES, Sherbino J, Long DM, et al. The role of assessment in competency-based medical education. Med Teach. 2010;32(8):676-82.
6. Holmboe ES, Yepes M, Williams F, et al. Feedback and the mini clinical evaluation exercise. J Gen Intern Med. 2004;19(5 Pt 2):558-61.

7. van der Vleuten CP, Schuwirth LW. Assessing professional competence: from methods to programmes. Med Educ. 2005;39(3):309-17.
8. Landy FJ, Farr JL. Performance rating. Psychological Bulletin. 1980;87(1):72-107.
9. In: Murphy K, Cleveland JN (Eds). Understanding Performance Appraisal. Social, Organizational and Goal Setting. Gurugram: Sage Publications, Thousand Oaks; 1952. pp. 442-83.
10. Hemmer PA, Hawkins R, Jackson JL, et al. Assessing how well three evaluation methods detect deficiencies in medical students' professionalism in two settings of an internal medicine clerkship. Acad Med. 2000;75(2):167-73.
11. Klenowski V. Assessment for Learning revisited: an Asia-Pacific perspective. Assessment in Education: Principles, Policy Pract. 2009;16(3):263-8.
12. McManus S. (2008). Attributes of effective formative assessment. Washington DC: Council of chief State School Officers. [Online] Available from https://schoolturnaroundsupport.org/resources/attributes-effective-formative [Last accessed January, 2025].
13. Black P, William D. Assessment and classroom learning. Assessment in Education. 1998;5(1):7-74.
14. Mahajan R, Badyal DK, Gupta P, Singh T. Cultivating Lifelong Learning Skills During Graduate Medical Training. Indian Pediatr. 2016;53(9):797-804.
15. Joshi MK, Gupta P, Singh T. Portfolio-based learning and assessment. Indian Pediatr. 2015;52(3):231-5.
16. Boud D, Keogh R, Walker D (Eds). Reflection: Turning Experience into Learning, 1st edition. London: Routledge; 1985.
17. Linn RL. Assessments and Accountability. Sage J. 2000;29(2):4-16.
18. Epstein RM. Assessment in medical education. N Engl J Med. 2007;356(4):387-96.
19. Palmer EJ, Devitt PG. Limitations of student-driven formative assessment in a clinical clerkship. A randomised controlled trial. BMC Med Educ. 2008;8:29.
20. Sadler R. Formative assessment and the design of instructional systems. Instructional Science. 1989;18:119-44.
21. Airasian PW. Measurement driven instruction: A closer look. Educational Measurement: Issues and Practice. 1988;7:6-11.
22. Alderson JC, Banerjee J. Language testing and assessment (Part 1) Language Teaching. 2001;34:213-36.

FURTHER READINGS

1. Buléon C, Mattatia L, Minehart RD, et al. Simulation-based summative assessment in healthcare: an overview of key principles for practice. Adv Simul (Lond). 2022;7(1):42.
2. Kassam A, de Vries I, Zabar S, et al. The Next Era of Assessment Within Medical Education: Exploring Intersections of Context and Implementation. Perspect Med Educ. 2024;13(1):496-506.
3. Schuwirth L, van der Vleuten C, Durning SJ. What can programmatic assessment in medical education can learn from healthcare? Perspect Med Educ. 2017;6(4):211-5.
4. Schuwirth LWT, van der Vleuten CPM. A history of assessment in medical education. Adv Health Sci Educ. 2020;25(5):1045-56.

CHAPTER 25

Assessment for Selection

Ajay Gaur

Learning Objectives

- Describe the fundamentals of evaluation for selection and their significance in guaranteeing validity and reliability in critical decision-making.
- Evaluate the suitability of different written and selection-type assessment methods for use in selection by comparing and contrasting them.
- Explain the function of computer-based and online evaluation tools in large-scale selection and examine their benefits, drawbacks, and security issues.
- Describe programmatic approaches to selection and talk about how using a variety of evaluation modalities improves decision-making and lessens bias.

INTRODUCTION

One of the most potent factors influencing student behavior is assessment, which is essential to the teaching-learning process. In medical education, where lifelong learning, competency, and safety are critical, evaluation needs to be carefully planned, executed, and utilized. Knowledge acquisition, skill practice, attitude formation, and internalization of professional behaviors are all ensured by effective assessment. It is a method for, as, and of learning rather than just an instrument for measuring it.[1]

Clinical competency is based on knowledge, which should be evaluated with purpose, structure, and intent. Four levels are highlighted in Miller's Pyramid (1990), which is frequently used in medical education: knows, knows how, shows how, and does. Knowledge (knows) and comprehension (knows how) constitute the base of the pyramid. Testing performance in controlled environments (shows how) and in real-world scenarios (does) becomes more important as we climb the pyramid. Over the past ten years, more advanced techniques have supplanted conventional methods of assessment in medical education. Assessment of clinical competence is becoming more popular than assessment of knowledge. Therefore, a systematic evaluation of foundational knowledge must still be part of the assessment of clinical competence.

Newble's paradigm for clinical competence is another excellent example of this idea (Newble, 1992). Clinical competency necessitates the development of appropriate attitudes, mastery of pertinent knowledge, and proficiency in interpersonal, technical, clinical, and communication skills, all of which are interconnected. Each of these influences' clinical performance and the standard of patient care.

Finding students who have the knowledge, abilities, and attitudes necessary for success in medical school depends heavily on assessment for selection. Selection-oriented assessment must prioritize fairness, objectivity, dependability, and predictive validity in contrast to standard classroom assessment. It decides who gets competitive opportunities, advances to more advanced levels, or enrolls in a training program.

As a result, selection tests need to be technically solid, strategically planned, and in line with the skills that future healthcare professionals are anticipated to possess.[2] The principles, forms, and techniques of assessment that are particularly appropriate for selection procedures are described in this chapter, with a focus on written exams, objective formats, online techniques, and contemporary developments that improve decision-making.

FOUNDATIONS OF SELECTION ASSESSMENT

Understanding the competencies needed for admission into or advancement within medical training is the first step in conducting an effective selection of evaluation. Decisions about selection must follow:

- *Validity*: Assessing what really counts 2.
- *Reliability*: Administering and rating consistently.
- *Objectivity*: Little influence from the examiner.
- *Transparency*: Precise guidelines and evaluation standards.
- *Feasibility*: Controllable logistics and resources.
- *Equity*: Accessibility for every applicant.
- *Predictive value*: The capacity to project future results.

We are reminded by models like Miller's Pyramid that the foundation of competency is basic knowledge. The objective of selection is to find applicants who possess the fundamental information and cognitive abilities required to develop into skilled practitioners rather than to evaluate complete clinical performance.

Strong knowledge is a predictor of future clinical performance, according to numerous studies. Declarative and procedural knowledge assessment is therefore still essential to the selection process.

PROGRAMMATIC APPROACHES FOR SELECTION

Instead of depending just on one test, modern systems are increasingly using a combination of methodologies. Programmatic evaluation incorporates:

- Standardized tests, interviews, portfolios, and several low-stakes exams.
- Tests of situational judgment (SJTs).
- Decision accuracy is increased, and bias is decreased using a mixed, multimodal selection procedure.

WRITTEN ASSESSMENT METHODS FOR SELECTION

Because they provide large topic sampling, consistency, and effective scoring, written exams are still often utilized in selection processes. When a large number of students need to be assessed, written assessment methods are popular since they are inexpensive and simple to administer.

Essay questions, structured essay questions, and modified essay questions are among the different written evaluation tools.

- Questions with brief answers.
- Multiple-choice questions (MCQs) and their variations.

Written evaluation methods can be either closed-ended or open-ended, depending on the desired response type. Closed-ended inquiries are typically of the selection of kind and offer a list of possible replies. Multiple-choice, or closed-ended, questions.

Examinees must respond to open-ended questions in their own terms. This chapter will concentrate on open-ended written assessment styles. Questions may be context-rich or context-free, depending on the format of the stimuli.[3] Factual knowledge is typically assessed in a context-free question with straightforward (yes/no) considerations. Context-free queries do not elicit the same mental processes as questions that are directly tied to a situation and request decisions. Candidates mostly use propositional reasoning in context-rich questions, weighing various information units against one another to reach a choice.[4] These include the following methods:

Essays

Essays are subjective and have poor reliability, but they do allow for evaluation of the depth of thought and language. Students are encouraged to produce extended responses to broad issues in essays, and they are permitted to examine different aspects of the subject. The essay question type can be used to evaluate a student's depth of comprehension, breadth of knowledge, organizational skills, and capacity for critical analysis. Their application in high-stakes selection is restricted unless they are used in conjunction with many qualified evaluators and unambiguous rubrics.

Short Answer Questions

Short answer questions (SAQs) assess fundamental knowledge and memory of facts. When organized around clinical scenarios, they can evaluate reasoning and offer greater objectivity. Instead of being discursive, the required responses are succinct and sequential. SAQs are employed when objectivity and score dependability are desired. They are adept at evaluating particular subject areas. They are typically used to test "must-know" topics. They are particular and ought to have one-of-a-kind responses. When the spontaneous creation of the response is a crucial component of the stimulus, SAQs should be employed.

There are various kinds of short response questions:

- *Completion type*: The keyword is blocked in order to test an important fact.
- *Ideal response format*: Specific answers in the form of multiple facts or a labelled diagram are preferred.
- *Open SAQs*: These provide respondents with some leeway in their responses. All potential responses to these kinds of inquiries should be included in the key.

Compared to essay questions, quick response questions take significantly less testing time. The cost of writing and editing them is lower. Additionally, a larger percentage of the syllabus and multiple subject areas can be covered in a short amount of time by using numerous relevant SAQS.

Modified Essay Questions

Modified essay questions (MEQs) use a series of case-based questions to examine clinical reasoning. They must, however, be expertly constructed and consistently scored—conditions that are frequently challenging in large-scale selection of tests. Testing problem-solving skills is not only the most challenging but also the most overlooked of the three domains of cognitive ability (recall and recognition, data interpretation, and problem solving). All of Bloom's levels may be tested by modified essay questions, which can also be used to evaluate knowledge of recall, understanding, analysis, synthesis, and evaluation. A problem or case scenario is given to the learner together with a context in a modified essay topic. The contexts are then connected to the questions. The questions are presented in a step-by-step manner using a real-world approach to problem-solving. The objective is to assess information of practical significance and the capacity to logically analyze and resolve an issue using common clinical scenarios. In MEQs, a consensus over the marking pattern must be reached before deciding on the paper's structure and content distribution. The intended responses will be more succinct, the more precise and factual the questions. These questions might not necessarily assess the higher levels of intellect, even though this makes grading more objective and consistent. The more one wanders into developing an interpretation of facts and problem-solving issues, the more "softer" becomes the marking pattern, and it is more difficult to assess papers objectively.[5]

SELECTION-TYPE QUESTIONS IN HIGH-STAKES ASSESSMENT

Objective questions can be classified as either supply-type, in which the student must provide the right response, or selection-type, in which the student must choose the right response from a list of possibilities. Objective formats are perfect for selection of decisions since they promote dependability and decrease examiner bias.

The following is a list of the most popular selection methods used in written assessments:

- *True-false questions*: This kind of question consists of a statement that the learner must mark as true (T) or untrue (F). In its most basic form, the statement (or stem) consists of a single concept that the student assigns a true or false rating. It is also possible to nest these questions into a scenario. Despite their simplicity, they are prone to guesswork and lack discrimination. They have limited value in rigorous selection settings.
- *MCQs*: Because of its vast content sample and high dependability, MCQs are the most used selection instrument. Case-based MCQs improve validity by evaluating thinking and application rather than just memorization.

  The learner is required to "choose one answer from a list" of potential responses for these questions. They are frequently called "one-best" or "single best" response types. The "stem" of these questions is a problem, question, or statement with three to four possible replies. The alternative choices are referred to as "distractors," while the right response is known as the "key." MCQs may be "context dependent," necessitating careful interpretation and analysis. Case studies, scenarios, graphical data, and tabular data are examples of contexts (Collins, 2006). Effective MCQs include:
    - Focused, clear stems
    - One right response
    - Distractions that are plausible
    - Context-based scenarios
- *Multiple response questions*: These are similar to MCQs but involve the selection of more than one answer from a list. They reduce guessing and test comprehensive understanding.
- *Ranking questions*: These require the student to relate items in a column to one another and can be used to test the knowledge of sequences, order of events, or level of gradation.
- *Assertion-reason questions*: True-false questions and MCQs are combined in these questions. Cause and effect can be investigated, and links can be found using assertion-reason testing. This category's items enable testing of more complex problems that call for a

higher degree of expertise.[6] It is possible to think of assertion-reason questions as variations on the true-false question format. Every item has a claim that is connected to a justification. The student must determine whether both the claim and the reason are true on their own, and if they are, whether the reason provides a convincing justification for the assertion. Each item, A, B, C, D, or E, is marked with a predefined code to signify the solution. To put it another way, each item in an assertion-reason question is made up of two connected items: an assertion and a reason. This approach is helpful for determining causality and conceptual links. They assist in distinguishing strong candidates and call for higher-order thinking.

- *Matching questions*: Two lists of statements, words, or symbols that must be matched with one another make up matching items. The amount of items in the two lists varies, and those in the longer list that don't match those in the shorter list operate as distractions.[7] Evaluate associations, sequencing, and categorization well, particularly when extensive content coverage is required.
- *Extended matching questions (EMQs)*: A list of possibilities, a theme, a "lead-in" question, and a few case studies or vignettes are the main components of EMQs. This is a type of MCQ in which the student is asked to provide a diagnosis based on a brief problem or vignette with specifics. The goal is to reduce the recognition effect that arises from the numerous ways that vignettes and options can be combined in ordinary MCQs. The items can be used to assess knowledge applications or problem-solving skills by substituting cases for facts. These kinds of questions are common in the medical field for similar reasons, and they can assess advanced abilities if they are written effectively.[7] EMQs are very good at evaluating diagnostic reasoning and reducing cueing. For advanced-level selection testing, they are perfect.
- *Key-feature questions (KFQs)*: At each step of the consultation process, KFQs are created to evaluate reasoning and decision-making abilities. This format aids in evaluating a student's capacity to make key judgments, such as selecting necessary and economical investigations, making a diagnosis, or offering suitable short-term and long-term patient care based on the information supplied. The purpose of these questions is to accurately assess problem-solving skills while maintaining a high degree of reliability. KFQs concentrate on crucial phases in the clinical decision-making process. They are useful in evaluating candidates' ability to solve problems.[8,9]

In general, the best evidence for selection decisions comes from a combination of MCQs, EMQs, and KFQs.

COMPUTER-ASSISTED ASSESSMENTS

Computer-based objective forms of evaluation are developing technologies with enormous potential for enhancing assessment in medical education. In addition to several practical advantages, computer-based testing can allow the construction of more valid evaluations.[10,11] The expenses and skills required to use this technology should not be undervalued, despite its popularity among candidates, because of its effective marking and delivery. Large-scale administration, automated scoring, instant feedback, improved security controls, and multimedia (pictures, videos, and simulations) integration are some benefits of these approaches. Other difficulties include restricted psychomotor assessment capabilities, cybersecurity threats, identity verification and integrity, and network problems. These techniques make it possible to assess intricate cognitive processes in a scalable, standardized fashion, which is perfect for high-stakes selection.

A few computer-assisted assessment methods are:

- In graphical hotspot questions, a marker pointer is moved to the desired location in order to pick one or more areas of the screen. Labeling and constructing questions are examples of advanced hotspot question kinds. In medical school labs, these kinds of inquiries are probably going to supplement, if not completely replaced, cadavers, microscopes, and tissue sections.
- Text/numerical questions require typing text or numbers into the keyboard.
- One word, code, or phrase that has no bearing on the remainder of a piece is used in sore finger queries. It might be offered as a text input or "hot spot" question. For formative purposes, similar ones are already used in medical education.
- Students must arrange the text or graphic elements in each preset order when answering sequencing questions. These are especially useful for assessing fundamental science and clinical curriculum knowledge of pathways and techniques.
- The assessment of virtual medicine would greatly benefit from field simulation questions, which provide simulations of actual situations or tasks.

The benefit of selection-type questions is that they are objective, but they demand more from the pupils than just memorization. They can be a very helpful tool for evaluating even higher levels of knowledge when properly structured and combined with other forms of evaluation.

ASSESSMENT AS LEARNING IN THE SELECTION CONTEXT

Assessment as learning (AaL) principles improve transparency and readiness, even though selection assessment is mainly summative:

- Students comprehend the selection criteria.
- Candidates learn self-regulation through mock exams and feedback and reflection improves exam preparation and lessens bias associated with unfamiliarity.
- Although AaL does not directly select candidates, it improves fairness and reduces anxiety.

CONCLUSION

Selection evaluation must strike a balance between objectivity, fairness, rigor, and practicality. Because they provide dependability and extensive subject coverage, objective written formats—particularly MCQs, EMQs, and KFQ—form the foundation of high-stakes selection. Large-scale, safe, and varied testing techniques are made possible by digital developments, which further improve assessment quality.

In the end, selection tests need to be evidence-based, learner-centered, and in line with the skills needed by aspiring medical professionals. A well-thought-out selection process guarantees that the most competent and dedicated students enroll in medical school, improving the standard of healthcare provision.

REFERENCES

1. Anshu S. Assessment of knowledge: Free response type questions. In: Anshu S (Ed). Principles of Assessment in Medical Education, 2nd edition. New Delhi: Jaypee Brothers Medical Publishers Pvt. Ltd; 2022. pp. 30-8.
2. Mahajan R, Virk A, Saiyad S. Assessment as learning. In: Mahajan R, Singh T (Eds). Perspectives in Medical Education, 1st edition. 2025. New Delhi: CBS Publishers and Distributors; 2025. pp. 137-44.
3. Schuwirth LW, Van der Vleuten, CPM. Different written assessment methods; what can be said about their strengths and weaknesses? Medical Education. 2004;38(9):974-9.
4. Schuwirth LW, Verheggen M, Van der Vleuten, et al. Validation of short case-based testing using a cognitive psychological methodology. Medical Education. 2000;35:348-56.
5. Irwin WG, Bamber JH. The cognitive structure of the modified essay questions. Medical Education. 1982;16(6):326-31.
6. National Forum for the enhancement of Teaching and Learning in Higher education. Assessment of/ For/ AS learning. [Online] Available from https://www.teachingandlearning.ie/our-priorities/student-success/assesment-of-for-as-learning/ [Last accessed January, 2026].
7. Nitko AJ. Educational assessment of students. Upper Saddle River. 2004. NJ: Merrill Prentice Hall.
8. Case SM, Swanson DB, Extended matching items: A practical alternative to free-response questions. Teaching and learning in Medicine. 1993;5(2):107-15.
9. Page G, Bordage G, Allen T. Developing key-feature problems and examinations to assess clinical decision-making skills. Academic Medicine. 1995;70(3):194-201.
10. Scalise K, Gifford B. Computer-based assessment in e-learning: a framework for constructing "intermediate constraint" questions and tasks for technology platforms. J Technol Learn Assess. 2006;4(6). Available from: http://www.jtla.org. Accessed January 4, 2026.
11. Collins C, Duncan A. Re-designing computer-based assessment tests for use as a learning tool: Profiling tacit learning processes instead of measuring learning outcomes. Assessment design for learner responsibility. [Online] Available from https://www.oecd.org/content/dam/oecd/en/publications/reports/2010/08/the-nature-of-learning_g1ghfff3/9789264086487-en.pdf [Last accessed January, 2026].

CHAPTER 26

Internal Assessment

Sandeep Shrivastava, Archana Dhok

HISTORY OF INTERNAL ASSESSMENT IN MEDICAL EDUCATION

INTRODUCTION

Internal assessment (IA) in medical education has evolved significantly over time, transitioning from a narrow focus on final examinations to a dynamic, continuous process embedded within the learning experience. This evolution reflects broader shifts in medical education, including the increasing emphasis on competency-based education (CBE) and the growing recognition of the need for a more holistic approach to student evaluation. This section outlines the historical development of internal assessments in medical education, highlighting the key changes and milestones.[1]

EARLY MEDICAL EDUCATION AND TRADITIONAL ASSESSMENT MODELS

In the 19th and early 20th centuries, medical education was primarily apprenticeship-based, with students learning directly under the supervision of experienced physicians. Assessment during this period was largely informal and sporadic, if it existed at all. Physicians-to-be observed and assisted their mentors in clinical settings, with little standardization in educational practices or assessment methods. Examinations, when they did occur, were minimal and often confined to oral examinations or tests that measured theoretical knowledge rather than practical skills.

As medical education began to formalize in the late 19th century, the curriculum became more structured. With this shift, formal assessments, particularly final examinations, began to take shape. However, these assessments were largely summative, designed to evaluate students at the end of their course or degree program. Students were expected to demonstrate their knowledge and competence through written examinations, oral examinations, and practical tests, but there was little ongoing or internal assessment. This approach limited opportunities for continuous feedback and progression tracking during the educational process.

MID-20TH CENTURY: EMERGENCE OF FORMALIZED INTERNAL ASSESSMENT

The mid-20th century saw a significant shift toward the formalization of internal assessment systems within medical schools. The Flexner Report of 1910, led by Abraham Flexner, was instrumental in this transformation. Flexner's work advocated for a more standardized, structured, and scientifically grounded approach to medical education, emphasizing the importance of rigorous curricula and objective, and formal assessment methods.

In line with Flexner's recommendations, medical schools began to develop more structured courses and curricula, and internal assessment systems started to reflect this new emphasis on comprehensive medical knowledge.[2] However, despite these changes, internal assessment remained largely focused on written examinations that tested theoretical knowledge. Practical assessments, such as clinical examinations, were still rare, and the feedback process during training was often limited. Many medical schools also relied heavily on external examinations or board examinations to certify the competence of their students, relegating internal assessments to secondary importance.

1970S-1990S: SHIFT TOWARD CONTINUOUS ASSESSMENT AND COMPETENCY MODELS

By the 1970s, the medical education community began to recognize the limitations of traditional assessment methods. These approaches were often criticized for focusing too heavily on theoretical knowledge while neglecting essential clinical skills, communication abilities, and professional behaviors. As a result, the focus gradually shifted toward competency-based assessment models,[3-5] which were seen as a more holistic means of evaluating students across a broad range of skills and competencies.

During this period, the concept of continuous assessment gained traction.[6] The new approach emphasized ongoing evaluation rather than relying solely on final examinations. Key developments included:

- *Practical examinations:* The use of clinical skills assessments and objective structured clinical examinations (OSCEs) became more common. These practical assessments allowed educators to observe students' clinical competencies firsthand, ensuring that students could apply their theoretical knowledge in real-world clinical settings.
- *Formative assessments:* Ongoing feedback through formative assessments became an integral part of the medical education process. These assessments provided students with continuous feedback on their performance, enabling educators to identify areas of weakness and offer timely remedial support. This shift marked a move away from traditional summative-only assessments to a model that fostered learning and improvement over time.

As medical schools around the world adopted these new approaches, internal assessment systems were restructured to incorporate clinical skills evaluations, performance assessments, and formative feedback. This helped bridge the gap between theoretical knowledge and practical application, ensuring that students were not only knowledgeable but also competent in the critical aspects of patient care.

EARLY 21ST CENTURY: COMPETENCY-BASED MEDICAL EDUCATION AND INTERNAL ASSESSMENT

The early 21st century marked a turning point in medical education with the global adoption of competency-based medical education (CBME). CBME focuses on achieving specific competencies across multiple domains, including medical knowledge, clinical skills, communication, and professionalism. This shift necessitated a more comprehensive and continuous system of internal assessment, one that could track students' progress across the various competencies and provide continuous feedback.[7]

With CBME's introduction, internal assessment became more structured and formalized. The assessment framework evolved to include:

- *Competency tracking:* Internal assessment now focused not only on measuring theoretical knowledge and practical skills but also on tracking students' development across a broader range of competencies. This required a more granular approach to assessment, with evaluations being integrated throughout the course to reflect continuous learning and improvement.
- *Feedback loops:* Continuous feedback mechanisms became a central feature of the internal assessment process. Students received regular evaluations that allowed them to reflect on their progress, identify areas for improvement, and take corrective action before the final examinations.
- *Certification of competencies:* As part of CBME, students were required to demonstrate mastery in specific competencies, with these achievements being documented in logbooks or portfolios. This ensured that graduates were competent in all aspects of medical practice, including clinical skills, communication, professionalism, and teamwork.

RECENT DEVELOPMENTS AND THE ROLE OF TECHNOLOGY

In recent years, internal assessment in medical education has increasingly embraced technological innovations.[8] Digital tools and platforms have streamlined and enhanced the assessment process, making it more efficient and accessible. Some key developments include:

- *E-portfolios and digital logbooks:* E-portfolios and digital logbooks have become common tools for documenting competencies and achievements. These digital platforms provide students and instructors with an organized and transparent system for tracking progress, making it easier to monitor learning outcomes and areas that require further development.
- *Online formative assessments:* Many medical schools now incorporate online formative assessments, such as quizzes, case-based discussions, and simulation exercises. These tools provide opportunities for students to test their knowledge and skills in a low-stakes environment, while instructors can offer immediate feedback and identify gaps in learning.
- *Simulation-based assessments:* Simulation-based assessments, including virtual patient encounters and mannequin-based simulations, have gained prominence in medical education. These simulations allow students to practice and demonstrate their skills in a controlled environment, reducing the risk to patient safety while offering valuable assessment opportunities.
- *Data analytics:* The use of data analytics in internal assessment is also on the rise. By analyzing trends in student performance, educators can identify patterns, predict challenges, and tailor remediation efforts to support struggling students more effectively.

These technological advancements have not only increased the efficiency of internal assessment but also enabled a more accurate and comprehensive tracking of student performance across multiple competencies. With the use of digital tools, feedback is faster, more detailed, and easily accessible to both students and instructors, enhancing the overall learning experience.

In summary, internal assessment in medical education has come a long way from its humble beginnings as an informal, final-examination-based process to a dynamic and continuous evaluation system that tracks students' progress across multiple domains. The integration of CBE, formative assessments, and technological tools has significantly shaped how medical students are evaluated. These changes have made the assessment process more holistic, efficient, and effective, ultimately ensuring that medical graduates are well-prepared for the complexities of modern medical practice.

CURRENT SCENARIO OF INTERNAL ASSESSMENT IN COMPETENCY-BASED MEDICAL EDUCATION

INTRODUCTION

Assessment is an integral part of any educational framework, particularly in the realm of medical education, where it plays a crucial role in shaping the learner's professional development and ensuring that they are adequately equipped to handle the demands of their profession. Assessment serves not only as a tool for evaluating student performance but also as a means to guide learning, provide feedback, and create opportunities for improvement. In the context of the *CBME* model, internal assessment is an ongoing process that supports the holistic development of medical students.

The *competency-based curriculum (CBC)* is designed to emphasize the acquisition of specific competencies that are required for medical practice, focusing on skills, knowledge, attitudes, and behaviors that contribute to a competent healthcare professional. The shift to this curriculum in India, starting in 2019, marked a significant change in how medical education is structured and assessed. Internal assessment under the *CBME* framework has been designed to ensure that students acquire the requisite competencies and are prepared for the professional challenges they will face.

This chapter explores the role of internal assessment within the *CBME* framework, focusing on its structure, implementation, components, and feedback mechanisms. The primary objective of this chapter is to provide a comprehensive understanding of internal assessment, its importance, the methods used to evaluate student performance, and its impact on students' learning outcomes.

COMPETENCY-BASED MEDICAL EDUCATION: AN OVERVIEW

Competency-based medical education represents a paradigm shift in medical training, emphasizing outcomes over time-based learning. In a CBC, the focus is on the acquisition and demonstration of specific competencies—whether cognitive, technical, or interpersonal—rather than on completing a fixed number of hours or courses. The primary goal of CBME is to prepare students to be competent professionals by ensuring that they possess the necessary skills and knowledge to perform in real-world settings.

The transition to *CBME in India* began in 2019 and is mandated for all phases of the *MBBS* course. This shift has necessitated significant changes not only in the curriculum content but also in the methods of assessment.

Traditional assessments that primarily relied on summative examinations have now been supplemented or replaced by a more dynamic and continuous system of evaluation, which includes *internal assessments* that track students' progress over time.

As per the revised *CBME guidelines 2024* by the *Undergraduate Medical Education Board (UGMEB),*[9-11] internal assessments are designed to be *continuous and formative,* providing feedback that helps learners to develop necessary competencies across all phases of their education. The guidelines ensure that internal assessment marks are separate from summative assessments and must be communicated regularly to students for transparency and accountability.

CONCEPT AND PURPOSE OF INTERNAL ASSESSMENT

Internal assessment in the context of *CBME* is a continuous evaluation process that tracks a student's performance across various domains, such as *knowledge, skills,* and *attitudes.* Unlike traditional assessments, which may focus on final examinations, internal assessments are longitudinal in nature, allowing instructors to monitor student progress over time and provide ongoing feedback.

The primary purpose of internal assessment is to serve as a *feedback mechanism* that helps students to understand their strengths and areas for improvement. In this context, assessment is not just a tool for assigning grades but an integral part of the *learning process.* It provides *formative feedback* that supports *learning* and *competency development.* Through continuous assessment, educators can identify students' needs and take *remedial action,* ensuring that students acquire the competencies required to succeed in their professional roles.

In a *CBC,* internal assessment is designed to be comprehensive and *multidimensional.* It aims to evaluate not only academic performance but also the development of key professional competencies, such as *clinical skills, communication abilities, ethical behavior,* and *professionalism.* By evaluating students across multiple competencies, internal assessment helps to ensure that learners are well-rounded and capable of meeting the demands of the medical profession.

PROCESS OF INTERNAL ASSESSMENT

The internal assessment process in *CBME* is a *longitudinal and continuous* one, designed to evaluate students throughout the academic year rather than at the end of the course. This process is intended to track a learner's development across all *competency domains* and provide an opportunity for teachers to offer constructive feedback. Internal assessment in this context is meant to be *formative*—i.e., to inform and guide learning—rather than merely summative.

Internal assessment is typically carried out by *faculty members* who are teaching specific subjects within the institution. Since each faculty is closely involved in the teaching and learning process, they are best positioned to assess student progress on a regular basis and identify areas for improvement. In this way, internal assessment helps to ensure that teaching is responsive to student needs and students receive personalized guidance to foster their growth.

The assessment of competencies in a *CBC* often involves evaluating a student's *clinical skills, procedural skills,* and *soft skills,* such as *communication, professionalism,* and *ethics.* The range of competencies assessed will depend on the specific phase of training, but overall, the process ensures that students are developing holistically as medical professionals.

Internal assessments can take a variety of forms, including:

- *Written examinations* (theory assessments)
- *Practical examinations* (clinical assessments)
- *Objective structured clinical examinations (OSCEs)*
- *Objective structured practical examinations (OSPEs)*
- *Directly observed procedural skills (DOPS)*
- *Mini clinical evaluation exercises (Mini-CEX)*
- *Clinical case studies and presentations*
- *Peer assessments*
- *Feedback from patients, peers, and faculty*
- *Logbook evaluations*

These assessments are integrated into the overall process of learning, helping both students and faculty to identify areas of strength and areas requiring attention.

COMPONENTS OF INTERNAL ASSESSMENT

The internal assessment process in *CBME* comprises several key components that allow for a thorough and well-rounded evaluation of students. These components help to ensure that all relevant competencies are evaluated and that feedback is provided in a timely manner.

- *Theory assessment:* Theory assessments in the form of *periodic examinations* (usually three or more per year) are used to evaluate students' understanding of theoretical knowledge. These assessments ensure that students are acquiring and applying foundational medical knowledge. Theory examinations are typically conducted in both *formative and summative formats,* with feedback provided on performance.
- *Practical/clinical assessment:* In the clinical or practical component of internal assessment, students are evaluated on their *hands-on skills,* such as conducting physical examinations, performing diagnostic tests, and applying clinical knowledge in real-world scenarios. *OSCEs* and *OSPEs* are designed to assess specific competencies in a structured and standardized manner.
- *Certification of competencies:* Each phase of the curriculum includes a set of *certifiable competencies* that students must demonstrate. These competencies are documented in a *logbook,* which serves as a record of the student's learning and progress. The logbook is regularly reviewed by faculty to ensure that the student is meeting the required milestones.
- *Other learning activities:* Various academic and extracurricular activities are also evaluated as part of internal assessment. These may include *seminars, problem-solving exercises, home assignments,* and participation in *healthcare projects.* Such activities allow for the development of critical thinking, research skills, and *professionalism.*
- *Logbook evaluation:* The *logbook* is an essential component of the internal assessment process. It serves as a detailed record of all learning activities, competencies achieved, and assessments completed. Regular review of the logbook ensures that students are progressing through the curriculum and meeting all required milestones.

FEEDBACK AND REMEDIAL MEASURES

A central feature of *competency-based internal assessment* is the *provision of feedback*. Feedback is not only essential for helping students to identify their strengths and weaknesses but also for guiding them toward remediation if necessary.

- *Timely feedback:* Students should receive feedback on their performance at regular intervals—at least once every 3 months. Feedback should be constructive, highlighting areas for improvement and offering suggestions for how to address deficiencies.
- *Structured feedback:* Feedback should be structured and specific, addressing the particular competencies evaluated. Both faculty and students must be sensitized to giving and receiving feedback effectively, ensuring that it leads to positive learning outcomes.
- *Remedial measures:* Students who fall behind or fail to meet the required competencies must be provided with *remedial action*. Remediation can take the form of additional teaching sessions, assessments, or clinical practice. Faculty must ensure that these interventions are documented and students complete them in a timely manner.

In cases where students fail to meet internal assessment requirements, such as insufficient internal assessment marks or low attendance, *remedial classes* and *supplementary examinations* are offered to allow students to catch up and improve their standing before the final university examinations.

CONCLUSION

The history of internal assessment in medical education reflects broader changes in the philosophy of medical training. From early apprenticeship models with minimal assessment to the adoption of CBE with continuous, multidimensional evaluations, internal assessment has evolved into a sophisticated and formative process. Today, internal assessment serves not only as a tool for grading but as a critical mechanism for promoting *learning* and ensuring that medical students acquire the full range of competencies required to be effective healthcare providers.

The shift toward *CBE* and the integration of *continuous assessment* represent significant steps forward in ensuring that future physicians are not only knowledgeable but also proficient in their clinical skills, communication, professionalism, and ethics. The future of internal assessment in medical education will likely continue to evolve, with ongoing advancements in assessment technology and methodology ensuring that medical education keeps pace with the demands of the profession and the healthcare system.

REFERENCES

1. Shah N, Desai C, Jorwekar G, et al. Competency-based medical education: An overview and application in pharmacology. Indian J Pharmacol. 2016;48(Suppl 1):S5-9.
2. Badyal DK, Singh T. Internal assessment for medical graduates in India: Concept and application. CHRISMED J Health Res. 2018;5(4):253-8.
3. Frank JR, Snell LS, Cate OT, et al. Competency-based medical education: Theory to practice. Med Teach. 2010;32(8):638-45.
4. Medical Council of India. (2019). Competency Based Assessment Module for Undergraduate Medical Education. [online] Available from https://www.nmc.org.in/wp-content/uploads/2019/10/

Module_Competence_based_02.09.2019.pdf [Last accessed January, 2025].
5. Gonçalves Cristóvão HL, Gonçalves Cristóvão NB, de Moraes Castellari LM, et al. Continuous assessment in medical education: Exploring students' views on the progress test. PLoS One. 2024;19(12):e0314848.
6. Aftab MT, Tariq MH. Continuous Assessment as a Good Motivational Tool in Medical Education. Acta Med Acad. 2018;47(1):76-81.
7. Starting Point, Teaching Entry Level Geoscience. (2025). Short Glossary of Assessment Terms. [online] Available from https://serc.carleton.edu/introgeo/assessment/glossary.html [Last accessed January, 2026].
8. Flexner A. Medical Education in the United States and Canada. From the Carnegie Foundation for the Advancement of Teaching, Bulletin Number Four, 1910. Bull World Health Organ. 2002;80(7):594-602.
9. Hammoud MM, Barclay ML. Development of a Web-based question database for students' self-assessment. Acad Med. 2002;77(9):925.
10. Salam A, Yousuf R, Allhiani RF, et al. Continuous Assessment in Undergraduate Medical EducationTowards Objectivity and Standardization. Int J Hum Health Sci. 2022;6(3):233-6.
11. Shrivastava S, Shrivastava T, Samal N, et al. A Study on Academic Appraisal Program: An Innovation towards Quality Assurance in Undergraduate Medical Education. Am J Educ Res. 2016;4(11):798-805.

SECTION

4 Miscellaneous

CHAPTER

27

Online Teaching–Learning Assessment

Meenal Batta, Shashi Kant Dhir

INTRODUCTION

In the era of the increasingly digital world, the medical education sector is also witnessing a profound transformation in the way assessments are conducted. Online assessment, defined as the "use of digital platforms to evaluate knowledge, skills, or competencies", has emerged as a cornerstone of this evolution. What started as a niche solution few years ago, has grown into a mainstream method of evaluation across medical educational institutions, training programs, as well as certification processes. The COVID-19 pandemic in 2020 accelerated the adoption of online assessment. With lockdowns forcing educational institutions and workplaces to pivot to remote operations, online assessments became the norm and the necessity. This period also spurred significant advancements in proctoring technology and accessibility features, ensuring that online assessments could cater to a broader demographic profile.[1]

The significance of online assessment lies in its ability to adapt to the needs of a global and diverse audience. By offering unparalleled flexibility, scalability, and efficiency, online assessments have not only addressed logistical challenges associated with traditional methods but have also paved the way for innovative approaches to testing. However, they are not without challenges, including concerns around security, equity, and technical reliability.[2] This chapter delves into the various tools, advantages, challenges, implementation strategy, technological advancements, and future prospects of online assessments, highlighting their transformative impact in the medical education.

EVOLUTION OF ONLINE ASSESSMENT

The journey of online assessment began with the advent of computer-based testing in the late 20th century. During this period, assessments were conducted offline, typically on dedicated computer terminals. Subsequently, the rise of the internet, enabling online platforms to host assessments and eliminating the need for physical presence in a specific location led to the development of much more comprehensive assessment tools. After the COVID-19 pandemic, the usage of the online tools has risen exponentially in the medical field.

The initial online assessment constituted only of the MCQs and focused on testing the knowledge and lower rungs of the Miller's Pyramid. Subsequent to the development of the Learning Management Systems (LMS) such as Moodle and Blackboard allowed medical educators to design, administer, and evaluate assessments seamlessly and in a better manner. The early 2000s saw a proliferation of Massive Open Online Courses (MOOCs), further popularizing online assessments as a scalable solution for a global audience. The advent of Zoom,

Google forms, and LMS gave a big boost to the online teaching learning and assessment in the medical education.

Currently, different types of the assessment tools exist which can independently test individual domains including that of clinical reasoning, skill testing, as well as soft skill assessment.[3] Some of the online assessment tools are listed in **Table 1**. The brief detail of the common ones is being described below.

TABLE 1: Common online assessment tools used in medical education.

Name of the tool	*Description*
Hotspot questions	• Interactive quiz questions • Stem is given and student is asked to label the area on the provided image • For example, mark the tricuspid area on image
Computer-assisted e-assessments	• Most commonly used tool • MCQ, matching, True/False type questions • Can assess from rote recall to higher level of cognitive domain
Confidence-based marking	• More used in basic sciences • The students mark their answers digitally • In addition, they also indicate level of their confidence
Open labyrinth	• Web application-based platform • Clinical virtual patients and virtual scenarios are present • Interactive content is provided • Scenario-based questions are present • Based upon the previous answer, the platform provides next question • Multiple options could be the best answer • Tests higher level of knowledge domain
Moodle	• Open-source LMS • Medical educators design personalized courses • Activities like quizzes, simulations, and peer assessments • Self-paced learning • Provides instant feedback on clinical skills assessments
Clickers	• Best used for group quizzes or group discussions • Audience response systems • Immediate feedback can be judged • Immediate self-assessment is possible.
Calibrated peer review	• Web-based writing development program • Students upload their notes or scripts • Others can comment and give feedback.
Digital "open book" examination	• Students are allowed to use any resource material • They can then submit their responses • Critical thinking scenarios can be given to the students
Context-rich short answer questions assessment system	• Essay-based answers can be checked based upon the content • Words and images are prefilled in the software • Presence or absence of those gives grading of the student

Contd...

Contd...

Name of the tool	*Description*
Remote assessment via video evaluation (RAVVE)	• Communication skills and clinical performance can be virtually evaluated • Recorded or direct videos are evaluated • Feedback is then provided based upon the performance • Affective domain and psychomotor domains are assessed
Video-based communication assessment	• Video-based vignettes are given by the software • The communication in response to the vignettes is recorded by the subject responses are then evaluated and feedback is given • Affective domain is being assessed
Objective structured video examination (OSVE)	• Stations similar to OSCE are placed in video format • Standardized patient findings and communication skills can be assessed
Online progress testing	• Formative assessment • Assessment over a period of time can be tracked. • Good tool for self-evaluation
Clinical image and video assessment	• Assessment of clinical competencies can be done • Useful for classroom assessment • Clinical vignettes, images, or small videos are given
Virtual patient simulation	• Online simulation is provided using software and artificial intelligence • High-end mannequins can be used to assess complex clinical and surgical scenarios in the students • Mannequins communicate and provide information based upon the demand of the students • The clinical responses and thinking are evaluated while comparing with the standard answers • Virtual clinical rounds are also available
HireVue, Spark Hire, Paradlx, Woo, Ideal, Willo	• AI tools for assessment of soft skills • Analyze the speech and semantic analysis • Facial coding, tone, and expression can be analyzed

ADVANTAGES AND CHALLENGES OF ONLINE ASSESSMENT

The advantages of the online assessment methods include enhanced learning opportunity by the students, administrative ease, scope of continuous improvement, more accessibility and flexibility, and improved assessment quality when the tool is well designed. The challenges include difficulty in integration in the traditional assessment methods, lack of subjective holistic grading, unintended bias in assessment, and the deviation from achieving the intended outcomes.[4] The advantages and the challenges are listed in **Table 2**.

INTEGRATION OF THE ONLINE ASSESSMENT IN THE EXISTING CURRICULUM

Integrating online assessments in medical education requires a holistic approach to meet the academic, technical, and ethical standards of evaluating. The stakeholders should be mentally prepared to accept it as a

TABLE 2: Advantages and challenges of online assessment.

Advantage	*Challenges*
Enhanced learning opportunities: • Provides personalized learning pathways • Immediate feedback is permissible as results are instantaneous • Usage of multimedia engages the students more effectively • Use of simulated virtual clinical cases bridges the gap between theoretical knowledge and practical applications	*Difficulty in integration in existing system:* • Gaps in acquiring digital skills in students and faculty • Inequity/disparities in access of technology • Computers, stable internet speed • Financial obligations on institute • Complexity of technical systems • Training to navigate digital platforms • Privacy and security risks • Communication barriers
More accessible and flexible: • No geographical barriers • Can be used across time zones • Specially-abled friendly • Student friendly • Continued assessment even when traditional methods get disrupted	*Biases in digital assessments:* • Less-than-ideal testing space • Auditory and visual distractions • Unclear communication • Cheating • Lack of holistic assessment due to non-human assessing tools
Improved assessment quality in well-designed tool: • Rules out subjectively • Reliable • Valid • Variety can be added • Collaboration between multiple assessors easier	*Efficacy gap:* • Suboptimal assessment of the complex competencies • Less than thorough knowledge of the digital platforms leads to subaligned goal achievement • Higher-order thinking analysis difficult
Administrative efficiency: • Time-saving • Scalable • Cost-effective • Streamlined procedure, less goof ups • Quicker to mark and declare result • Environment friendly	*Need for infrastructure:* • More need of computers • More need of laboratory tests • Continuous training • Understanding of technology • Stable internet connection
Continuous improvement: • Score metrics can be analyzed to decide learning goals • Actionable insights possible to deduce	*Psychological impact:* • Examination anxiety • Failure of disruption of internet • Nonhuman environment • Emotional distress due to privacy issues

tool for assessment. The first and the foremost step to incorporate this is by providing the resources both for the learners and the educators for designing as well as utilizing the digital assessment tools effectively. Faculty must receive comprehensive training to use analytics tools for tracking student progress, identifying knowledge gaps, and tailoring feedback. They should be able to understand the nuances of this method, understand the technical nitty-gritty, should have an easy access to the training. Their proficiency should be supplemented by performing mock run of the assessment tool.

Having adequate technical infrastructure is critical for the online assessment and includes reliable servers with high uptime, secure data encryption, integration with tools like plagiarism checkers and proctoring software. The website should be user-friendly, with intuitive navigation, clear instructions, and a design that minimizes cognitive load. Additionally, ensuring equitable access is vital; the platform must be compatible with various devices and offer offline options for students with limited internet connectivity.

Once the faculty and the students are ready for the online assessment and the infrastructure is there, due credit should be given to select the appropriate digital tool to run the show. The foundation lies in selecting a reliable LMS capable of supporting diverse assessment formats, including theoretical questions, clinical case analyses, virtual simulations, and OSCE-style evaluations. Content upload capabilities should accommodate multimedia resources such as clinical images, videos, and interactive modules essential for medical training. The platform should incorporate advanced assessment features such as adaptive testing, which adjusts question difficulty based on student performance, and tools to measure higher-order thinking, like critical reasoning and diagnostic skills. It should also be equipped with robust security measures to safeguard the integrity of the exam and the privacy of the students. A dedicated support team should be available for troubleshooting technical issues during assessments.

The actual carrying out of assessment needs a well-drafted assessment which is efficient and is aligned to the objectives of the curriculum. More than one type of assessment tools should be used to increase the integrity, validity, and reliability of the assessment method.

Finally, ongoing monitoring of the data analytics should give an insight about the student's performance in different domains. The assessments should be customized based upon the strengths and weakness of the students. Feedback from all stakeholders including the students, assessors and external evaluators and continuous refinement of the process should be taken up frequently. Regular audits should be performed and feedback shared among various stakeholders.

TECHNOLOGICAL ADVANCEMENTS IN ONLINE ASSESSMENT

Artificial Intelligence and Machine Learning

Artificial intelligence (AI) and machine learning have revolutionized online assessments. Automated essay grading systems, for example, analyze linguistic patterns and coherence to assign scores. Similarly, AI-driven plagiarism detection tools ensure the originality of submitted work.

Adaptive Testing

Adaptive testing tailors the difficulty level of questions based on the test-taker's responses. This personalized approach not only provides a more accurate measure of abilities but also enhances the test-taking experience by reducing frustration or boredom.

Proctoring Solutions

Advanced proctoring solutions have addressed many of the security concerns associated with online assessments. AI-driven tools monitor test-takers through facial recognition, eye-tracking, and behavior analysis, flagging any suspicious activities in real time.

Integration with Gamification

Gamification elements, such as leaderboards, badges, and interactive quizzes, make online assessments more engaging. Platforms like Kahoot and Quizizz have successfully incorporated these elements, turning assessments into enjoyable learning experiences.

Blockchain for Credential Verification

Blockchain technology is being used to securely store and verify assessment credentials. This ensures that certificates and transcripts are tamper-proof and can be easily authenticated by employers or educational institutions.

FUTURE OF ONLINE ASSESSMENT

The future of online assessment is poised for significant advancements, driven by emerging technologies and an increasing focus on inclusivity. Virtual reality (VR) and augmented reality are expected to redefine assessments, enabling immersive simulations that assess practical skills in real-world scenarios. For instance, medical students could perform virtual surgeries or invasive procedures using high end simulation equipment.

Big data analytics will play a crucial role in predictive analysis, helping educators identify at-risk low performers and will provide timely interventions. In coming times, efforts to bridge the digital divide and enhance accessibility features will ensure that online assessments are equitable for all participants. Global standardization of assessments will also become a reality, enabling seamless cross-border recognition of qualifications. This will be particularly beneficial in a world where remote work and global mobility are becoming the norm.

CONCLUSION

Online assessments have revolutionized the way medical knowledge and skills are evaluated. By offering flexibility, efficiency, and scalability, they address many of the limitations of traditional assessment methods. However, challenges such as technical reliability, security concerns, and accessibility barriers must be addressed to realize their full potential. As technology continues to evolve, online assessments are likely to become even more sophisticated, incorporating elements of AI, VR, and blockchain. The focus must remain on balancing innovation with ethical considerations and inclusivity, ensuring that online assessments serve as a tool for empowerment and growth in an increasingly digital world.

Therefore, online assessments are not merely a trend but a transformative force that is reshaping medical education and professional development. With continuous advancements and a commitment to equity, they hold the promise of a future where evaluation is not only efficient but also enriching and inclusive. The teachers and the students need to be trained to make the best use of this tool.

REFERENCES

1. Ang CS, Ito S, Cleland J. Navigating digital assessments in medical education: Findings from a scoping review. Med Teach. 2024;1-16.
2. Walsh K. Oxford Textbook of Medical Education. Oxford: Oxford University Press; 2013.
3. Singh T, Anshu. Principles of Assessment in Medical Education, 2nd edition. New Delhi: Jaypee Brothers Medical Publishers; 2022.
4. Fatima SS, Idrees R, Jabeen K, Sabzwari S, Khan S. Online assessment in undergraduate medical education: Challenges and solutions from a LMIC university. Pak J Med Sci. 2021;37(4):945-51.

CHAPTER 28

Student-Doctor Program

Priyanka Gupta

INTRODUCTION

A key innovation in the updated competency-based curriculum for Indian Medical Graduates (IMG) training, implemented from 2019, is the introduction of the "Learner-Doctor or Student-Doctor Program."[1] This "longitudinal immersive learning during clinical rotations" provides students with the experience of being part of longitudinal patient care in both inpatient and outpatient settings. This initiative is designed to offer medical students sustained, and hands-on experience in patient care within a supervised clinical environment. This forward-thinking experiential learning approach integrates hands-on practice, personalized guidance, and skills enhancement to nurture confident and competent doctors.

CLINICAL TEACHING VERSUS TEACHING IN CLINICS

Clinical teaching is the cornerstone of the MBBS curriculum, encompassing all three domains of learning—cognitive, psychomotor, and affective. However, there is a subtle yet significant distinction between "clinical teaching" and "teaching in clinics."[2]

"Clinical teaching" refers to a broad spectrum of educational strategies that may occur in various settings, such as clinics, skill laboratories, or demonstration rooms. It does not necessarily require the presence of a patient. For instance, it might involve simulations, case-based discussions, or practice on models, allowing students to acquire skills in a controlled environment.

In contrast, *"teaching in clinics"* is specifically tied to real-life clinical settings, directly involving patient's interactions. This method is focused on learning through observation, examination, and management of actual patients, enabling students to develop hands-on skills and patient-centered approaches.

While clinical teaching provides foundational knowledge and simulated practice opportunities, teaching in clinics offers experiential learning crucial for understanding patient's care in real-world scenarios. Both approaches are essential and complementary in medical education.

OBJECTIVES OF THE STUDENT-DOCTOR PROGRAM

The student-doctor program aims to:

- Integrate students into healthcare teams as supervised members.
- Expose medical students to longitudinal patient care.
- Provide practical, hands-on patient's care experience in both outpatient departments (OPDs) and inpatient settings.
- Foster the development of critical thinking, empathy, and communication skills.
- Prepare students for professional roles by emphasizing accountability and lifelong learning.

ADVANTAGES OF THE LEARNER-DOCTOR METHOD

The learner-doctor method offers numerous benefits:

- *Application of theoretical knowledge:* It allows students to apply classroom knowledge in real-world patient's care settings, fostering a deeper understanding of medical concepts.
- *Skill development:* Enhances critical skills, such as history-taking, physical examination, clinical reasoning, and decision-making.
- *Patient-centered care:* Encourages students to prioritize patients' emotions, preferences, and overall well-being, promoting holistic care.
- *Effective communication:* Helps students to master communication skills essential for accurate diagnoses, fostering patient's trust, and ensuring adherence to treatment plans.
- *Teamwork and collaboration:* Introduces students to the dynamics of working in multidisciplinary healthcare teams, highlighting the importance of collaboration with other professionals.
- *Professional growth:* Enables gradual development of professional attributes such as empathy, accountability, and ethical practice.
- *Residency readiness:* Prepares students for the challenges of residency by familiarizing them with clinical workflows and responsibilities, easing the transition to postgraduate training.
- *Self-directed learning and reflection:* Encourages habits of continuous improvement through feedback, self-assessment, and reflection.
- *Lifelong learning:* Promotes curiosity and adaptability, critical for staying updated in medical science.

STRUCTURE AND IMPLEMENTATION

The learner-doctor program is systematically integrated into the MBBS curriculum to ensure progressive skill development:

- *Early integration:* This becomes an integral component of clinical rotations in the MBBS curriculum from the very beginning second phase of MBBS onwards. Students are assigned to departmental units and begin functioning as supervised members of the healthcare team until 6 pm except during the designated class hours.
- *Patient's interaction:* Students are assigned patients in the OPD or the wards, tasked with the history taking, examining, and working up patients under supervision.
- *Rounds and feedback:* Students present cases during rounds on designated days and receive feedback from faculty and residents to enhance their learning.
- *Documentation:* All tasks and learning experiences are documented in a logbook or portfolio, assessed formatively by supervising faculty for its completeness and the quality of the report.
- *Assessment:* Logbooks and supporting case records for the respective subject are reviewed periodically and submitted as part of the examination requirements to ensure sincerity and proper learning.

LEVELS OF LEARNING DURING THE STUDENT-DOCTOR PROGRAM

During the first phase of MBBS, students are introduced to the hospital environment through early clinical exposure. This helps them to understand the patient's perspective on illness and familiarizes them with clinical settings. Afterward, the clinical training in the MBBS curriculum should be structured to match the student's stage of learning, progressively building knowledge and skills appropriate for their level. This stepwise progression ensures that students acquire the necessary skills and confidence to provide comprehensive and patient-centered care as they advance through their medical training.

The learner-doctor program should ensure a stepwise progression. This progression ensures that students acquire the necessary skills and confidence to provide comprehensive and patient-centered care as they advance in their training.

- *Second phase:* Students learn foundational clinical skills, including patient history taking, physical examination skills, assessing and evaluation of changes in a patient's clinical status during daily rounds, and communicating effectively with patients.
- *Third Phase Part 1:* Building on earlier skills, students are introduced to choosing appropriate investigations based on clinical scenarios, performing procedures, and further understanding the importance of continuity of care.
- *Third Phase Part 2:* In the final phase, students focus on advanced clinical competencies, including decision-making in patient's care, developing and implementing management plans, and understanding and evaluating patient's outcomes.

CHALLENGES IN THE IMPLEMENTING THE STUDENT-DOCTOR PROGRAM AND SOLUTIONS TO OVERCOME THEM

Implementing the Student-Doctor Program, which aims to provide medical students with hands-on clinical experience under the guidance of physicians, can face several challenges. By addressing these challenges with clear strategies and continuous evaluation, the student-Doctor Program can be successfully integrated into medical education, enhancing both student's learning and patient's care.

Below are some common challenges and their potential solutions:

Limited Clinical Exposure

Challenge: Inadequate clinical settings or a shortage of patients for students to observe and interact with can limit their learning opportunities.

Solution: Collaborate with multiple healthcare facilities to expand the range of clinical experiences. Utilize simulation-based training, role-playing, and virtual patient platforms to provide additional learning opportunities.

Inadequate Faculty Support

Challenge: There may not be enough trained faculty members to mentor students effectively, especially in high-demand specialties.

Solution: Provide faculty development programs to train more faculty members in mentorship and teaching clinical skills. Encourage interdisciplinary collaboration, allowing faculty from different specialties to share the mentorship burden.

Lack of Structured Curriculum

Challenge: The absence of a clear and structured curriculum may result in inconsistencies in what students are taught or miss out on essential skills.

Solution: Develop a standardized curriculum for the program that outlines key learning objectives, clinical skills, and competencies.

Regularly assess and update the curriculum to ensure it aligns with current medical practices.

Time Constraints

Challenge: Balancing the Student-Doctor Program with academic responsibilities, clinical duties, and personal commitments can overwhelm students and faculty.

Solution: Introduce a flexible schedule for clinical placements, allowing students to manage their time effectively.

Variation in Student Engagement

Challenge: Students may show varying levels of interest, initiative, or readiness to engage in the program, impacting the overall success of the learning experience. Students may lack engagement due to unclear expectations or a lack of interest.

Solution: Implement strategies to foster intrinsic motivation, such as personalized learning goals and a supportive and nonjudgmental environment. Include reflective practices where students self-assess their involvement and progress. Clearly define responsibilities, encourage curiosity, and create a structured learning environment that rewards active participation.

Institutional Barriers

Challenge: Institutional resistance to change or new teaching methods may limit the implementation of the program.

Solution: Engage key stakeholders (administrators, faculty, and students) early in the planning process to ensure buy-in and support. Demonstrate the benefits of the program through pilot studies or success stories from other institutions.

Attendance in Scheduled Classes

Challenge: Students may misuse clinical postings to skip scheduled classes.

Solution: Monitor attendance and enforce accountability to ensure balanced participation in both academic and clinical responsibilities.

Evaluation and Feedback Challenges

Challenge: Inadequate or inconsistent evaluation methods may hinder the identification of areas where students need improvement.

Solution: Implement a robust feedback mechanism, including formative assessments, peer reviews, and faculty evaluations. Conduct regular one-on-one feedback sessions between students and faculty to provide actionable insights.

Patient's Cooperation and Consent

Challenge: Patients may be reluctant to involve students in their care.

Solution: Emphasize the importance of obtaining informed consent and respecting patient's autonomy to maintain trust and ethical standards.

Access to Patient Records

Challenge: Institutional policies might limit students' access to records.

Solution: Develop clear policies and supervision mechanisms to balance patient's privacy with educational needs.

Overstepping Boundaries

Challenge: Students may attempt tasks beyond their training in their eagerness to learn.

Solution: Implement strict supervision and establish clear guidelines to ensure safe practices.

Patient's Behavior

Challenge: Patients misbehaving with students can undermine their confidence.

Solution: Establish support systems to address such incidents promptly and provide emotional support to students.

Professional Identity of Students

Challenge: Patients may undervalue the role of students, perceiving them as less significant due to their "medical student" label.

Solution: Introduce a professional designation like "student-doctor" to enhance their perceived role and foster a more respectful environment.

CONCLUSION

- The learner-doctor program represents a paradigm shift in medical education, prioritizing experiential and longitudinal learning.
- By addressing implementation challenges and leveraging its inherent advantages, this approach has the potential to transform medical graduates into competent, compassionate, and confident professionals.
- Its emphasis on continuity, teamwork, and active patient's engagement aligns seamlessly with the goals of modern medical education—to produce doctors who are not only skilled but also empathetic and ethically grounded.
- This program not only prepares students for the demands of residency but also instills in a culture of lifelong learning essential for success in the ever-evolving field of medicine.

REFERENCES

1. Shrivastava SR, Shrivastava PS, Pise R, et al. Practice makes perfect: The learner-doctor blueprint for proficient physicians. J Family Med Prim Care. 2024;13:1156-9.
2. Burgess A, van Diggele C, Roberts C, et al. Key tips for teaching in the clinical setting. BMC Med Educ. 2020;20(2):463.

CHAPTER 29

Mentor–Mentee Programs

Girish Chandra Baniya

INTRODUCTION

Mentorship, a bedrock of medical education, has always been the conduit between academic knowledge and practical application. It is the catalyst for individual and professional growth, ethical decision-making, and clinical competence.[1] The evolution of mentorship from traditional apprenticeship systems to structured programs has responded to the increasing complexities of the medical field. This evolution has transformed mentorship into a collaborative process that nurtures leadership, emotional intelligence, and resilience, making all involved feel engaged and part of a team.[2]

Mentorship originated in the 18th and 19th centuries as apprenticeship models in which prospective physicians trained through observation and hands-on experience.[3] While these interactions were helpful for skill acquisition, they could have promoted overall intellectual and emotional development. The renaissance and enlightenment brought formal education, which combined mentorship and structured learning to foster critical thinking and intellectual curiosity.[4,5]

During the 19th century, mentorship was formalized alongside the establishment of medical schools and residency programs. The Flexner Report of 1910 highlighted the need for scientific rigor and ethical standards, positioning mentorship as an essential component of professional education.[6] By the mid-20th century, technological breakthroughs and specialization broadened mentorship to encompass leadership development, research guidance, and cross-cultural collaboration.[7]

In the late 20th century, Competency-based Medical Education (CBME) strongly emphasized mentorship, particularly in developing abilities, such as communication and professionalism.[8] With the advent of digital resources, such as e-mentorship platforms, the contemporary form of mentorship has transcended geographical boundaries, making it accessible worldwide. This global accessibility not only promotes inclusivity but also equips mentees for interprofessional collaboration among medical, nursing, and pharmacy fields, fostering a sense of unity in the medical community.[9,10]

In the future, artificial intelligence (AI) and virtual reality will transform mentorship. Virtual reality offers immersive training for intricate procedures, while AI systems customize education based on data. The significance of mentorship is acknowledged, included in curricula, and maintained through resource distribution and international cooperation.[11]

Mentorship in medical education transcends mere skill transfer; it is a transformative process that equips healthcare workers to adeptly manage the complexity of an interconnected and continuously expanding environment.[12] Through the promotion of diversity, the utilization of technology, and the mitigation of structural hurdles, mentorship will persist in influencing the future of medical education.[13]

MODELS OF MENTORSHIP

Mentorship in medical education is not a universal method. Various approaches have been developed to address the distinct requirements of mentees, mentors, and institutions. Each model has different benefits and tackles certain obstacles, rendering mentorship a versatile and responsive instrument for promoting growth and development.[14]

Formal Mentorship

Formal mentorship is defined by organized, institutional interactions with specific objectives, timetables, and assessment methods. These programs are executed by academic institutions, residency programs, or professional organizations to guarantee that mentees have focused mentorship following institutional goals.[15]

- *Key features:*
  - *Structured goals:* Both mentors and mentees collaborate to establish clear, measurable objectives, such as improving clinical skills, publishing research, or preparing for licensing examinations.
  - *Scheduled meetings:* Regularly planned interactions ensure continuity and progress.
  - *Evaluation mechanisms:* Periodic assessments help gauge the relationship's effectiveness and identify areas for improvement.
- *Examples in practice:*
  - Formal mentoring aids trainees in navigating tough clinical training in residency programs. For example, a surgical resident could collaborate with a senior surgeon to improve technical abilities and patient management.
  - Medical students are supervised by improving their academic performance, career options, and research.
- *Advantages*
  - Formal mentoring provides clear accountability for both mentors and mentees.
  - It aligns mentorship with institutional goals, resulting in an organized learning environment.
  - It facilitates measurable outcomes, enabling institutions to evaluate program success.

Informal Mentorship

Informal mentorship emerges naturally through shared interests, reciprocal respect, or interpersonal relationships. In contrast to formal programs, informal mentorship is characterized by the absence of inflexible structures and predetermined goals, facilitating enhanced flexibility and adaptability.[8]

- *Key features:*
  - *Spontaneous formation:* These relationships often develop naturally, such as between a medical student and a faculty member during clinical rotations.
  - *Personalized guidance:* Informal mentors offer tailored advice based on their experiences and the mentee's needs.
  - *Broad scope:* Discussions may go beyond academic or professional difficulties to address work-life balance, emotional resilience, and negotiating workplace dynamics.
- *Examples in practice:*
  - A senior faculty member mentors a junior colleague informally, guiding

how to balance teaching and research tasks.
- A resident forms a mentorship relationship with a consultant throughout rounds, seeking advice on complicated cases and career planning.

- *Advantages:*
  - Informal mentorship encourages open, relaxed dialogue, fostering more profound connections.
  - It allows mentees to seek advice on diverse topics without institutional constraints.
  - Adapts to the evolving needs of the mentee, providing holistic support.

One-on-One Mentorship

One-on-one mentorship is the most classic and well-known model. This strategy involves a mentor focusing solely on the needs and goals of a particular mentee and providing personalized guidance and help.[16]

- *Key features:*
  - *Individualized attention:* Mentors dedicate their time and experience to helping mentees achieve their goals and overcome problems.
  - *Tailored plans:* Learning paths are tailored to the mentee's career goals, whether pursuing a subspecialty, succeeding in research, or developing leadership abilities.
- *Examples in practice:*
  - A medical student interested in oncology may be matched with an oncologist to get insights into the discipline, investigate research opportunities, and develop clinical proficiency.
  - A postgraduate student engaged in thesis work benefits from individualized mentorship with an experienced researcher, getting help in study design, data analysis, and manuscript preparation.
- *Advantages:*
  - Establish a robust, trust-based relationship between mentor and mentee
  - Facilitates a concentrated and comprehensive review of the mentee's objectives
  - Delivers customized feedback and constructive critique

Group Mentorship

In group mentoring, a single mentor guides multiple mentees simultaneously. This collaborative paradigm promotes peer learning by encouraging mentees to share their experiences, viewpoints, and resources.[17]

- *Key features:*
  - *Collaborative learning:* Mentees learn from each other and the mentor, enriching the overall experience.
  - *Diverse perspectives:* Group discussions expose mentees to various perspectives and problem-solving methods.
  - *Efficient use of resources:* One mentor can impact several mentees, making this model ideal for institutions with limited faculty availability.
- *Examples in practice:*
  - A faculty member helps a group of medical students prepare for competitive exams by discussing study strategies and dealing with everyday issues.
  - A senior doctor conducts a session for residents on patient communication skills, which includes group discussions and role-playing scenarios.
- *Advantages:*
  - Promotes teamwork and networking among mentees

- Encourages collaborative problem-solving and peer-driven support
- Provides mentees with multiple avenues for guidance and learning

Peer Mentorship

Peer mentorship includes senior students, junior faculty, or residents guiding less experienced persons. Everyday experiences, relatability, and a nurturing environment frequently define such partnerships.[18]

- *Key features:*
  - *Relatable experiences:* Peer mentors use their recent experiences to provide practical guidance and empathy.
  - *Accessibility:* Peer mentors are often more approachable than senior teachers, particularly when discussing casual or sensitive topics.
  - *Supportive environment:* Peer mentorship develops a sense of community and inclusivity.
- *Examples in practice:*
  - Senior medical students mentor first-year students, advising on academic responsibilities, clinical rotations, and stress management.
  - Residents mentor interns in managing the challenges of their first year.
- *Advantages:*
  - Minimizes hierarchical pressure, facilitating transparent communication
  - Supports mentees in confronting urgent difficulties through pertinent guidance
  - It fosters a mentorship circle, as mentees frequently evolve into future mentors.

E-Mentorship

E-mentorship uses digital tools to connect mentors and mentees worldwide. This paradigm has acquired popularity with technological developments, particularly in neglected or remote areas.[19]

- *Key features:*
  - *Technology-driven:* Virtual encounters can be facilitated through Zoom, Skype, and mentorship applications.
  - *Global reach:* Mentors and mentees can communicate regardless of location, providing access to various perspectives and knowledge.
  - *Flexibility:* Asynchronous communication allows individuals to interact at their own pace.
- *Examples in practice:*
  - An Indian medical student receives mentorship from a global epidemiology expert via an online platform.
  - An international mentorship program that allows residents from other countries to exchange ideas and learn about each other's healthcare systems.
- *Advantages:*
  - Overcomes geographical and logistical hurdles
  - Encourages intercultural learning and worldwide collaboration
  - Mentorship is more adaptable and scalable using this technique.

KEY COMPONENTS OF EFFECTIVE MENTORSHIP

Effective mentorship is based on several essential components promoting meaningful and fruitful interaction between mentors and mentees. These aspects are the foundation for a mentorship program, fostering trust, collaboration, and mutual progress.

Selection and Matching

Mentorship success begins with matching mentors and mentees who are compatible. A mismatch in goals, personalities, or communication styles might jeopardize a relationship, whereas a well-matched couple can thrive and reach key milestones.[20]

- *Criteria for selection:*
    - *Mentors* must show proficiency in their area, exceptional interpersonal abilities, and a sincere dedication to mentoring others.
    - *Mentees* must exhibit receptiveness to input, clarity in objectives, and a proactive attitude.
- *Matching strategies:*
    - *Shared interests:* Matching mentors and mentees according to similar academic or professional interests ensures consistency in the aim.
    - *Compatibility assessments*: Tools, such as personality inventories or goal-alignment questionnaires help identify potential matches.
    - *Dynamic matching:* Institutions may facilitate regular evaluations of mentor–mentee to accommodate changing requirements.

Example: A mentee wishing to specialize in pediatric cardiology may be paired with an experienced mentor to guide the mentee's objectives.

Communication

Clear and effective communication is the backbone of any mentorship relationship. It fosters understanding, builds trust, and ensures that both parties meet their expectations and objectives.[21]

Key elements:

- *Active listening:* Mentors should attentively listen to mentees' concerns, aspirations, and challenges, creating a supportive environment.
- *Feedback delivery:* Constructive, actionable feedback is essential for mentees to understand their strengths and areas for improvement.
- *Open dialogue:* Encouraging open and honest conversations helps address misunderstandings and ensures the relationship remains productive.

Strategies for effective communication are:

- Regular check-ins to discuss progress, challenges, and plans.
- Use technology for flexible communication, such as video calls or messaging platforms.
- Setting clear expectations for communication frequency and preferred modes.

Example: A mentor might provide weekly feedback on a mentee's clinical performance, highlighting areas of excellence while offering specific advice for improvement.

Goal Setting

Defining clear and achievable goals at the outset of the mentorship relationship ensures that mentors and mentees have a roadmap for collaboration. Goals provide focus, motivate action, and enable measurable progress.[22]

Types of Goals

Types of goals are as follows:

- *Short-term:* Objectives achievable within weeks or months, such as mastering a specific clinical procedure
- *Long-term:* Broader aspirations, such as completing a research project or preparing for board exams

SMART Goals Framework

The SMART goals framework is composed of the following:

- *Specific:* Clearly define the goal (e.g., "Publish a case study on rare pediatric conditions").
- *Measurable:* Include metrics to track progress (e.g., "Submit the manuscript within 6 months").

- *Achievable:* Ensure the goal is realistic, given the mentee's current skills and resources.
- *Relevant:* Align the goal with the mentee's academic or career aspirations.
- *Time-bound:* Establish deadlines to maintain momentum.

Example: A mentee aiming to improve public speaking skills might set a goal to present at 3 departmental meetings within the next 6 months.

Trust and Mutual Respect

Effective mentorship requires trust to allow mentees to disclose their vulnerabilities, struggles, and goals. Mutual respect ensures mentors and mentees value each other's time, knowledge, and opinions.[18]

Building Trust

Building trust involves the following:

- Maintaining confidentiality and honoring commitments.
- Being empathetic and nonjudgmental in interactions.
- Demonstrating reliability through consistent support.

Fostering Mutual Respect

Fostering mutual respect includes:

- Mentors should acknowledge the mentee's unique strengths and potential.
- Mentees should show appreciation for the mentor's guidance and effort.

Example: A mentor consistently provides timely feedback and supports a mentee's career decisions, fostering a relationship of trust and respect.

Feedback and Reflection

Feedback is a cornerstone of mentorship, enabling continuous improvement and self-awareness. Effective feedback is constructive, actionable, and delivered in a supportive manner.[23]

Effective feedback practices are:

- Focus on specific behaviors or outcomes rather than personal attributes.
- Balance positive reinforcement with areas for improvement.
- Encourage mentees to reflect on feedback and identify their solutions.

Reflection: Mentorship is a two-way process; mentors and mentees benefit from regular reflection. Mentees should evaluate their progress, while mentors can assess their approach to ensure alignment with the mentee's needs.

Example: A mentor might praise a mentee's clear presentation during rounds while suggesting ways to enhance patient interaction skills.

Commitment and Accountability

Mentorship requires dedication from both parties to ensure that goals are achieved and the relationship remains effective.[24]

Mentor responsibilities:

- Dedicate sufficient time and resources to support the mentee.
- Provide timely feedback and follow through on commitments.

Mentee responsibilities:

- Actively participate in meetings and discussions.
- Take ownership of their learning and progress.

Example: A mentee preparing for residency interviews consistently attends mock sessions arranged by their mentor and applies the feedback received.

Adaptability

Every mentorship relationship is unique and requires flexibility to address evolving goals, challenges, and dynamics.

Effective mentors adapt their approach to suit the mentee's learning style, pace, and changing circumstances.[25]

Adaptation strategies:

- Adjusting goals as the mentee progresses
- Exploring alternative methods to address challenges (e.g., incorporating e-mentorship tools during busy periods)
- Being open to feedback from the mentee to refine the mentoring approach

Example: When a mentee expresses difficulty balancing research with clinical responsibilities, the mentor helps them prioritize tasks and adjusts meeting schedules.

CHALLENGES IN MENTORSHIP

While mentorship is an invaluable tool in medical education, it is not without challenges. Both mentors and mentees face barriers that can hinder the effectiveness of the relationship, and addressing these challenges requires thoughtful strategies and institutional support **(Table 1)**.[26]

IMPLEMENTATION STRATEGIES

Effective implementation of mentorship programs in medical education requires a well-thought-out approach, combining strategic planning, resource allocation, and ongoing evaluation. Institutions must create frameworks that cater to the diverse needs of mentees and mentors while ensuring sustainability and alignment with educational goals.

Establishing Program Goals

The foundation of a successful mentorship program lies in defining its objectives. Clear goals help align the efforts of all stakeholders and provide a roadmap for implementation.[27]

Key objectives:

- Foster the personal and professional growth of mentees.
- Enhance academic performance, clinical skills, and research capabilities.
- Promote inclusivity and diversity within medical education.
- Cultivate leadership and teaching skills among mentors.

Example: A residency mentorship program might improve surgical residents' competency in advanced laparoscopic techniques while supporting their career development.

Selection and Matching of Participants

The process of selecting and pairing mentors with mentees is critical to the success of a mentorship program. Effective matching ensures compatibility, enhances communication and fosters meaningful relationships.[28]

- *Mentor selection criteria:*
    - Expertise in the relevant field or specialty
    - Strong interpersonal and communication skills
    - Commitment to mentorship and a willingness to dedicate time and resources.
- *Mentee selection criteria:*
    - Clarity in goals and expectations
    - Openness to feedback and a proactive attitude toward learning
    - Compatibility with the mentorship program's objectives
- *Matching techniques:*
    - *Interest alignment:* Pair mentors and mentees with shared academic or professional interests.
    - *Personality assessments:* Tools, such as Myers–Briggs Type Indicator (MBTI) or DiSC assessments can help identify compatible personalities.
    - *Dynamic matching:* Allow for reassessment and rematching as goals or circumstances evolve.

TABLE 1: Challenges in mentorship.

Challenge	*Impact*	*Solutions*	*Example*
Time constraints	• Limited time for interactions • Delayed feedback, mentees feel neglected	• Allocate dedicated time for mentorship • Efficient scheduling • Leverage technology for virtual interactions	The residency program designates weekly slots for mentor–mentee meetings
Mismatched expectations	• Misaligned goals cause dissatisfaction • Mentors may perceive disengagement	• Set clear expectations at the start • Use written agreements • Conduct periodic check-ins to realign goals	A mentor–mentee pair focuses on career planning initially, transitioning to research guidance
Power dynamics	• Stifled communication and lack of trust. • Over-imposition of mentor's perspectives	• Create a safe space for dialogue • Offer training on power dynamics • Enable anonymous feedback mechanisms	A mentor ensures mentees can share feedback without fear of repercussions
Cultural and gender barriers	• Exclusion of underrepresented groups • Miscommunication because of cultural differences	• Recruit mentors from diverse backgrounds • Conduct cultural sensitivity training • Implement peer mentorship for relatability	A mentorship program includes faculty from diverse professional and cultural backgrounds
Lack of institutional support	• Mentors feel overburdened • Programs become unsustainable	• Allocate protected time for mentorship activities • Provide administrative and academic recognition • Integrate mentorship into faculty performance appraisal	A university includes mentorship in faculty performance evaluations
Emotional burnout	• Reduced quality of interactions • Disengagement or strained relationships	• Organize support networks • Encourage mindfulness practices • Balance workloads to allow meaningful engagement	Hospitals offer monthly wellness workshops to reduce burnout among mentors
Virtual mentorship challenges	• Impersonal interactions and scheduling conflicts • Technical difficulties	• Use hybrid mentorship models • Train participants in digital tools • Set clear communication agendas and follow-ups	An e-mentorship program includes annual in-person workshops to enhance relationships

Example: An academic institution might pair a medical student interested in cardiology with a faculty member specializing in interventional cardiology, ensuring alignment of goals and expertise.

Mentor and Mentee Training

Training is essential to prepare mentors and mentees for their roles and responsibilities within the program. Practical training equips participants with the skills and knowledge needed to navigate challenges and maximize the benefits of the relationship.[29]

- *Training for mentors:*
    - Communication and active listening techniques
    - Strategies for providing constructive feedback
    - Cultural competency and inclusivity training to address diversity in mentees
- *Training for mentees:*
    - Setting realistic expectations and goals
    - Strategies for effective communication and active participation
    - Understanding the importance of accountability and feedback

Example: A university might conduct workshops for mentors on fostering inclusivity, ensuring that underrepresented medical groups feel supported and empowered.

Creating Structured Frameworks

Structured frameworks provide clarity and consistency, ensuring that mentorship relationships remain focused and productive.[24]

Key elements of a structured framework:

- *SMART goals:* Mentorship objectives should be specific, measurable, achievable, relevant, and time-bound.
- *Regular meetings:* Scheduled interactions (e.g., biweekly or monthly) to maintain continuity and momentum.
- *Defined roles:* Clearly outline mentors' and mentees' roles and responsibilities.
- *Documentation:* Use mentorship logs to track progress, challenges, and milestones.

Example: A mentorship program for medical students might include monthly goal-setting sessions, followed by progress evaluations at the end of each semester.

Providing Institutional Support

Institutional backing is essential for the success and sustainability of mentorship programs. Mentors may feel overburdened without adequate support, and mentees may struggle to access resources.[30]

Types of institutional support:

- *Time allocation:* Provide protected time for mentors and mentees to engage in mentorship activities.
- *Funding:* Allocate resources for workshops, technology, and program administration.
- *Recognition:* Acknowledge and reward mentors for their contributions through awards, promotions, or academic credits.

Example: A hospital might include mentorship activities as a key performance indicator in faculty evaluations, recognizing the time and effort invested by mentors.

Leveraging Technology

Technology can enhance mentorship programs by facilitating communication, tracking progress, and expanding access to mentors.[31]

Technological tools:

- *Video conferencing platforms:* Tools like Zoom and Microsoft Teams enable virtual mentorship, overcoming geographical barriers.
- *Mentorship applications:* Platforms, such as Chronus or Mentorloop help manage

mentorship relationships, track goals, and provide feedback.

- *Learning management systems (LMS):* Integrate mentorship with coursework and training modules for a seamless learning experience.

Example: An e-mentorship program might use an application to connect mentors and mentees globally, allowing them to set goals, share resources, and monitor progress digitally.

Feedback and Evaluation Mechanisms

Regular feedback and program evaluations ensure continuous improvement and alignment with goals. Both mentors and mentees should provide input on their experiences to identify areas for enhancement.[32]

Feedback mechanisms:

- *Self-assessments:* Encourage mentors and mentees to reflect on their progress and challenges.
- *Surveys:* Use anonymous surveys to gather candid feedback on the program's structure and effectiveness.
- *Periodic reviews:* Conduct formal evaluations at defined intervals to assess outcomes and adjust strategies.

Evaluation metrics:

- Academic achievements (e.g., grades and research outputs)
- Career milestones (e.g., residency matches and job placements)
- Personal growth indicators (e.g., confidence, resilience, and communication skills)

Example: A residency mentorship program might evaluate success by tracking mentees' board exam pass rates and feedback on their preparedness for independent practice.

Promoting Inclusivity and Diversity

Inclusivity is a cornerstone of effective mentorship. Programs must ensure fair access to opportunities for all participants, regardless of gender, ethnicity, socioeconomic background, or other factors.[33]

Strategies for promoting inclusivity:

- Recruit mentors from diverse backgrounds to reflect the mentee population.
- Address implicit biases through training programs.
- Create peer mentorship opportunities for underrepresented groups.

Example: A medical school might establish a mentorship program specifically for women in surgery, providing tailored support and addressing unique challenges.

FUTURE DIRECTIONS IN MENTORSHIP

The future of mentorship in medical education lies in embracing innovation, inclusivity, and global collaboration. Emerging trends and technologies are poised to transform how mentorship is delivered, expanding its reach and impact.

Technology-Driven Mentorship

Advancements in technology have already revolutionized mentorship by enabling virtual and asynchronous interactions. Future developments will further enhance the mentorship experience.[34]

Artificial Intelligence

Artificial intelligence-powered platforms can personalize mentorship by analyzing mentees' strengths, weaknesses, and goals. Predictive analytics may suggest tailored learning paths and resources, ensuring mentees receive highly individualized guidance.

Example: An AI-based mentorship application might recommend specific training modules or research opportunities based on a mentee's career interests and skill gaps.

Virtual and Augmented Reality

Virtual reality (VR) and augmented reality (AR) technologies can create immersive learning environments, allowing mentees to practice clinical procedures or simulate patient interactions under the guidance of a mentor.

Example: A surgical mentor could use AR tools to provide real-time feedback during a virtual simulation of a complex operation.

E-mentorship platforms: Dedicated platforms, such as Mentorloop or Chronus streamline mentorship by facilitating goal-setting, tracking progress, and maintaining communication. These tools make mentorship accessible to individuals in remote or underserved areas.

Interprofessional Mentorship

As healthcare becomes increasingly collaborative, interprofessional mentorship is gaining prominence. This approach involves mentors guiding teams of learners from different disciplines, such as medicine, nursing, and pharmacy.[35]

Key features:

- Encourages teamwork and interdisciplinary communication
- Prepares mentees for collaborative healthcare settings
- Expands mentees' understanding of diverse roles in patient care

Example: An interprofessional mentorship program might pair medical students with nursing and pharmacy students to work on case studies, fostering mutual respect and collaboration.

Emphasis on Diversity and Inclusion

The mentorship landscape is becoming more inclusive, reflecting the growing recognition of diversity as a strength in medical education. Programs are designed increasingly to address the unique challenges faced by underrepresented groups, such as women, minorities, and individuals from low-income backgrounds.[36]

Strategies for inclusivity:

- Recruiting mentors from diverse backgrounds to reflect mentee demographics
- Creating mentorship programs tailored to specific groups, such as women in surgery or LGBTQ+ medical students
- Offering scholarships or stipends to remove financial barriers to participation

Example: A mentorship initiative for women in orthopedic surgery might focus on addressing gender biases, supporting career progression, and fostering a sense of community.

Global Collaborations

The future of mentorship lies in fostering global networks that connect mentors and mentees across borders. These collaborations provide access to diverse perspectives, innovative practices, and unique learning opportunities.[37]

Key features:

- Cross-cultural exchanges that enrich learning experiences
- Opportunities for mentees to engage in international research or clinical rotations
- Shared best practices among mentors from different healthcare systems

Example: A global mentorship program might pair a medical student in Africa with a mentor in Europe, exposing the mentee to advanced diagnostic tools while providing the mentor insights into resource-limited settings.

Sustainability and Scalability

For mentorship programs to remain effective long-term, they must be sustainable and scalable. Institutions must invest in mentorship infrastructure, including training, funding, and administrative support.[18]

Strategies for sustainability:

- Establishing mentorship as a core institutional value
- Providing ongoing training and support for mentors
- Leveraging technology to reduce costs and expand access

Example: A university might develop a mentorship application to connect its alumni network with current students, ensuring a steady pool of mentors while scaling the program's reach.

ETHICAL CONSIDERATIONS IN MENTORSHIP

Ethics form the backbone of effective mentorship in medical education. The mentor–mentee relationship is built on trust, respect, and a shared commitment to professional and personal growth. However, the inherent power dynamics and varying expectations can lead to ethical challenges, making it essential to establish clear guidelines and foster a culture of integrity.

Power Dynamics in Mentorship

The hierarchical nature of medical education can create power imbalances, potentially leading to exploitation, favoritism, or conflicts of interest. Mentors hold significant authority, often influencing mentees' academic performance, career prospects, and overall confidence.[38]

- *Challenges:*
    - *Intimidation:* Mentees may hesitate to voice concerns or provide feedback because of fear of retaliation.
    - *Favoritism:* Mentors may unconsciously prioritize specific mentees, leading to feelings of exclusion among others.
    - *Dependency:* Over-reliance on a mentor can hinder a mentee's ability to make independent decisions.
- *Strategies:*
    - *Transparency:* Clearly defining the scope and boundaries of the mentor–mentee relationship minimizes misunderstandings.
    - *Empowering mentees:* Encouraging mentees to express their opinions and concerns promotes open dialogue.
    - *Mentor training:* Providing mentors with training on power dynamics and implicit biases ensures a fairer approach.

Example: A mentor explicitly communicates that mentees are encouraged to share honest feedback about their interactions, ensuring a safe and respectful environment.

Confidentiality and Privacy

Confidentiality is a cornerstone of ethical mentorship. Mentees often share sensitive information, such as personal challenges, career insecurities, or academic struggles, trusting that it will remain private.[39]

- *Challenges:*
    - Breaches of confidentiality can damage trust and harm the mentee's reputation or relationships.
    - Mismanagement of sensitive information may lead to unintended consequences.

- *Strategies:*
  - *Explicit agreements:* Mentors and mentees should establish confidentiality agreements at the beginning of the relationship.
  - *Data protection:* For digital platform programs, ensuring secure storage and communication of sensitive data is crucial.
  - *Ethical disclosure:* If disclosure of information is necessary (e.g., in cases of harm or misconduct), mentors should discuss it with the mentee beforehand.

Example: A mentor assures a mentee that their discussions about challenges in balancing residency and family life will remain private unless the mentee consents to share them.

Boundary Management

Blurring the boundaries between personal and professional aspects of the mentor–mentee relationship can lead to ethical dilemmas. While mentorship often involves holistic guidance, it is crucial to maintain professionalism.[40]

- *Challenges:*
  - Overstepping boundaries may cause inappropriate or overly personal interactions.
  - Unclear boundaries can confuse mentees about the relationship.
- *Strategies:*
  - *Setting expectations:* Clearly define the limits of the relationship at the outset.
  - *Professional conduct:* Mentors should model professional behavior and avoid engaging in activities that could compromise the relationship.
  - *Third-party mediation:* In cases of boundary violations, institutions should provide mechanisms for resolution.

Example: A mentor refrains from involving a mentee in personal disputes or decision-making, focusing solely on their academic and professional growth.

Ethical Decision-Making in Mentorship

Mentorship often involves navigating complex ethical scenarios, such as conflicts of interest, mentee underperformance, or cultural misunderstandings.[41]

- *Challenges:*
  - Mentors may face dilemmas when balancing their professional goals with their commitment to the mentee.
  - Mentees may struggle with ethical issues, such as reporting errors or handling conflicts with peers.
- *Strategies:*
  - *Ethical frameworks:* Use established ethical frameworks, such as the "Four Principles" of biomedical ethics (autonomy, beneficence, nonmaleficence, and justice), to guide decision-making.
  - *Scenario-based training:* Role-playing exercises can help mentors and mentees develop ethical problem-solving skills.
  - *Mentorship committees:* Institutions can establish committees to guide on complex ethical issues.

Example: A mentor advises a mentee on addressing a clinical error by emphasizing transparency, accountability, and patient safety.

Addressing Favoritism and Bias

Favoritism and unconscious biases can undermine the fairness and inclusivity of mentorship programs. These issues often stem from cultural, gender, or professional stereotypes.[38,42]

- *Challenges:*
    - Favoritism may alienate other mentees and reduce the program's effectiveness.
    - Biases can limit opportunities for underrepresented groups.
- *Strategies:*
    - *Bias awareness training:* Educate mentors on recognizing and mitigating implicit biases.
    - *Structured evaluations:* Use objective criteria to evaluate mentee progress and achievements.
    - *Promoting diversity:* Recruit mentors and mentees from diverse backgrounds to ensure inclusivity.

Example: A mentorship program ensures that mentees from underrepresented minorities are paired with mentors who understand and address their unique challenges.

Grievance Redressal Mechanisms

Establishing systems to address grievances is essential for maintaining trust and accountability in mentorship programs.[43]

- *Challenges:*
    - Mentees may hesitate to report issues because of fear of repercussions.
    - Lack of clear policies can exacerbate conflicts or misunderstandings.
- *Strategies:*
    - *Anonymous reporting:* Allow mentees to raise concerns anonymously without fear of retaliation.
    - *Conflict resolution training:* Equip mentors with the skills to address disputes constructively.
    - *Institutional policies:* Clearly outline procedures for handling grievances, ensuring fairness and transparency.

Example: An academic institution establishes a mentorship advisory board to mediate conflicts and provide guidance on ethical concerns.

Fostering a Culture of Integrity

Ethical mentorship thrives on a culture of integrity, respect, and professionalism. Institutions play a key role in cultivating this environment.[41]

Strategies:

- *Leadership commitment:* Institutional leaders should model ethical behavior and prioritize mentorship as a core value.
- *Recognition and rewards:* Celebrate mentors who show exemplary ethical conduct.
- *Ethics education:* Integrate ethical principles into mentorship training and curricula.

Example: A medical school includes a session on ethical mentorship in its faculty development program, highlighting case studies and best practices.

CONCLUSION

Mentorship bridges theoretical knowledge and practical application, fostering growth for mentees, fulfillment of mentors, and systemic improvement for institutions. It enhances competencies, leadership, and collaboration while addressing challenges, such as time constraints and cultural barriers through institutional support and innovative tools, such as AI and virtual platforms. Diverse mentorship models cater to varied needs, emphasizing communication, trust, and inclusivity. Ethical considerations ensure integrity in mentor–mentee relationships. By investing in mentorship, medical education institutions and professionals create a legacy of excellence and innovation, preparing healthcare providers to meet the complexities of an evolving global landscape.

REFERENCES

1. Toklu HZ, Fuller JC. Mentor-mentee relationship: A win-win contract in graduate medical education. Cureus. 2017;9(12):e1908.
2. Commons DS. Who needs mentoring in case management? Prof Case Manag. 2010;15(1):49.
3. Osborn TM, Waeckerle JF, Perina D, et al. Mentorship: Through the looking glass into our future. Ann Emerg Med. 1999;34(2):285-9.
4. Peng P, Kievit RA. The development of academic achievement and cognitive abilities: A bidirectional perspective. Child Dev Perspect. 2020;14(1):15-20.
5. Johnson S. The neuroscience of the mentor-learner relationship. NDACE. 2006;2006(110):63-9.
6. Beck AH. The Flexner report and the standardization of American medical education. JAMA. 2004;291(17):2139-40.
7. National Academies of Sciences, Engineering, and Medicine; Policy and Global Affairs; Board on Higher Education and Workforce; Committee on Effective Mentoring in STEMM; Dahlberg ML, Byars-Winston A (Eds). Introduction: Why Does Mentoring Matter? In: The Science of Effective Mentorship in STEMM. Washington (DC): National Academies Press (US); 2019.
8. Rose GL, Rukstalis MR, Schuckit MA. Informal mentoring between faculty and medical students. Acad Med. 2005;80(4):344-8.
9. Hill SEM, Ward WL, Seay A, et al. The nature and evolution of the mentoring relationship in academic health centers. J Clin Psychol Med Settings. 2022;29(3):557-69.
10. Newsome AS, Ku PM, Murray B, et al. Kindling the fire: The power of mentorship. J Health Syst Pharm. 2021;78(24):2271-6.
11. Pottle J. Virtual reality and the transformation of medical education. Future Healthc J. 2019;6(3):181-5.
12. Goosby EP, von Zinkernagel D. The medical and nursing education partnership initiatives. Acad Med. 2014;89(8):S5-7.
13. Otaki F, Naidoo N, Heialy SA, et al. Shaping the future-ready doctor: A first-aid kit to address a gap in medical education. Int J Med Educ. 2020;11:248-9.
14. Galbraith MW, Cohen NH. Issues and challenges confronting mentoring. NDACE. 1996;66:89-93.
15. Nemani V, Park CN, Nawabi DH. What makes a "great resident": The resident perspective. Curr Rev Musculoskelet Med. 2014;7(2).
16. Ward EC, Hargrave C, Brown E, et al. Achieving success in clinically based research: the importance of mentoring. J Med Radiat Sci. 2017;64(4):315-20.
17. Tom W, Albarran D, Salman N, et al. Ensuring mentorship of new physicians in their first year: Constructs for new mentoring processes. Perm J. 2019;23(2).
18. Hart EW. In focus—mentoring—nurturing relationships provide many benefits. In: Leadershit in Action. 2009. [online] Available from https://onlinelibrary.wiley.com/doi/10.1002/lia.1279 [Last accessed January, 2026].
19. Keynejad RC. Global health partnership for student peer-to-peer psychiatry e-learning: Lessons learned. Global Health. 2016;12(1):82.
20. Leier CV, Auseon AJ, Binkley PF. Selecting a mentor: A guide for residents, fellows, and young physicians. Am J Med. 2011;124(10):893-5.
21. Patel K, Gupta Y, Patel A. Key communication skills for mentors. JACR. 2022;19(7):903-4.
22. Sensmeier J. Developing guidelines for mentorship. CIN.. 2014;32(8):359.
23. Sundgren PC. Mentoring radiology residents in clinical and translational research. Acad Radiol. 2012;19(9):1110-3.
24. Rabatin JS, Lipkin M, Rubin AS, et al. A year of mentoring in academic medicine: Case report and qualitative analysis of fifteen hours of meetings between a junior and senior faculty member. J Gen Intern Med. 2004;19(5):569-73.
25. Gillespie SM, Thornburg LL, Caprio TV, et al. Love letters: An anthology of constructive relationship advice shared between junior mentees and their mentors. J Grad Med Educ. 2012;4(3):287-9.

26. Fallatah HI, Farsi J, Tekian A, et al. Mentoring clinical-year medical students: Factors contributing to effective mentoring. 2018.
27. Dougherty PJ. Surgical mentoring: Building tomorrow's leaders. JAMA. 2011;305(4):410-1.
28. Eltorai AE, Daniels A. National medical school matching program: Optimizing outcomes. Adv Med Educ Pract. 2016;7:371-3.
29. Osman NY, Gottlieb B. Mentoring Across Differences. MedEdPORTAL. 2018;14:10743.
30. Nick JM, Delahoyde TM, Prato DD, et al. Best practices in academic mentoring: A model for excellence. Nurs Res Pract. 2012;2012:937906.
31. Tinoco-Giraldo H, Torrecilla Sánchez EM, García-Peñalvo FJ. E-Mentoring in Higher Education: A Structured Literature Review and Implications for Future Research. Sustain. 2020;12(11):4344.
32. Torbeck L, Canal DF, Choi J. Is our residency program successful? Structuring an outcomes assessment system as a component of program evaluation. J Surg Educ. 2014;71(1):73-8.
33. Mark S, Link H, Morahan PS, et al. Innovative mentoring programs to promote gender equity in academic medicine. Acad Med. 2001;76(1):39.
34. McReynolds MR, Termini CM, Hinton AO, et al. The art of virtual mentoring in the twenty-first century for STEM majors and beyond. Nat Biotechnol. 2020;38(12):1477-82.
35. Marshall M, Gordon F. Exploring the role of the interprofessional mentor. J Interprof Care. 2010;24(4):362-74.
36. Bettis J, Thrush CR, Slotcavage RL, et al. What makes them different? An exploration of mentoring for female faculty, residents, and medical students pursuing a career in surgery. Am J Surg. 2019;218(4):767-71.
37. Manzi A, Hirschhorn LR, Sherr K, et al. Mentorship and coaching to support strengthening healthcare systems: Lessons learned across the five Population Health Implementation and Training partnership projects in sub-Saharan Africa. BMC Health Services Research. 2017;17(3):831.
38. Olson DA, Jackson D. Expanding leadership diversity through formal mentoring programs. J Leadersh Stud. 2009;3(1):47-60.
39. Steinberg A. Disclosure of information and informed consent: Ethical and practical considerations. J Child Neurol. 2009;24(12).
40. Barnett JE. Mentoring, boundaries, and multiple relationships: Opportunities and challenges. Mentor Tutoring Partnersh Learn. 2008;16:3-16.
41. Rose GL, Rukstalis MR. Imparting medical ethics: The role of mentorship in clinical training. Mentor Tutoring Partnersh Learn. [Internet]. 2008:16(1):77-89.
42. 2030STEM Collaboration; Adams JD, Asai D, Cohen R, et al. (2023). Accelerating and scaling mentoring strategies to build infrastructure that supports underrepresented groups in STEM. [online] Available from https://arxiv.org/pdf/2302.13691 [Last accessed January, 2026].
43. Crotts JC. The college gets its act together: Cutting the costs of disputes in organizations. JCEL. 2021;25(1).

CHAPTER 30

Faculty Development Programs

Satvik Bansal

Learning Objectives

After reading this chapter, learners will be able to:

- Define faculty development and explain its importance in enhancing educator competencies and institutional quality in medical education.
- Describe the core components of faculty development programs including teaching skills, research, leadership, ethics, curriculum planning, digital tools, and assessment literacy.
- Trace the historical evolution of faculty development in India from NTTC establishment (1975) to current NMC-mandated programs.
- Apply evaluation frameworks (Kirkpatrick's, ARCS, CIPP models) to assess faculty development program effectiveness.
- Recommend strategies to strengthen faculty development at policy, programmatic, and institutional levels in India.

INTRODUCTION

Faculty development refers to a structured set of initiatives aimed at enhancing the competencies, effectiveness, and professional growth of academic staff in their diverse roles as educators, researchers, and institutional leaders. It serves as a foundational support system, enabling faculty to adapt to the evolving demands of modern education system.

Faculty development encompasses both *personal* and *professional* growth. *Personal development* includes nurturing ethical values, cultivating a positive attitude toward research, and promoting global engagement. *Professional development*, on the other hand, involves deepening one's understanding of educational philosophies, pedagogical principles, subject expertise, teaching methodologies, communication, assessment practices, feedback, and reflective teaching.

In India, medical education is undergoing significant transformation. These include a shift from the traditional teacher-centric approach to a more facilitative role, adoption of diverse learning styles, innovative curriculum structures, and a reevaluation of assessment strategies and tools. It becomes necessary, therefore, for the present-day medical teachers to familiarize themselves and become part of these far-reaching updates.

HISTORY OF FACULTY DEVELOPMENT PROGRAMS

The foundation for international faculty development in medical education was laid in 1969 with the establishment of two international regional teacher training centers (IRTTCs)—one at the Centre for Medical Educational Development, University of Illinois College of Medicine, Chicago, and the other at the Department of Medical Education, University of Southern California, Los Angeles. These initiatives were the result of 1968 World Health Organization (WHO) resolution, which acknowledged the urgent need for in-service training of medical school faculty to enhance the quality of medical education.[1]

The IRTTCs played a pivotal role in preparing educational leaders and specialists who subsequently supported the formation of regional teacher training centers (RTTCs) in the six WHO regions. The RTTCs, in collaboration with IRTTCs, worked toward building national capacity by training academic leaders to establish national teacher training centers (NTTCs). The NTTCs, in turn, were tasked with developing medical education units (MEUs) at individual medical colleges, aimed at training faculty in pedagogy and curriculum delivery.

A major global milestone followed in 1988 with the Edinburgh Declaration, adopted during the World Conference on Medical Education organized by the World Federation for Medical Education (WFME). The declaration laid out 12 core principles for reforming medical education, advocating for curriculum relevance, lifelong learning, social accountability, ethical training, and the need for ongoing evaluation and adaptation of educational programs.

In the new millennium, the scope of faculty development programs (FDPs) has now become significantly broadened.[2] Experts have begun to emphasize the importance of including areas such as educational research, academic leadership, and structured career development in FDPs.[3] This shift probably reflects a growing recognition that the developmental needs of medical faculty evolve over different stages of their careers. Consequently, contemporary

TABLE 1: Faculty development needs across stages.

Career stage	*FDP focus areas*
Early career	Teaching basics, time management, and mentorship
Mid career	Research skills, leadership, and academic writing
Senior faculty	Policy development, strategic planning, and mentoring

FDPs are designed to be diverse, multilevel, and modular, accommodating the varied professional roles and growth trajectories of medical educators **(Table 1)**.[4]

CORE COMPONENTS OF FACULTY DEVELOPMENT PROGRAMS

Faculty development programs should be designed to be comprehensive and adaptable, addressing the unique needs of both individual faculty members and their institutions. The core objective of these programs is to improve the overall standard of education by equipping educators with the necessary skills to teach effectively, assess learners appropriately, provide mentorship, and contribute to educational innovation.[2] At the same time, faculty development initiatives should also support personal growth and facilitate career progression, ensuring well-rounded professional advancement.

Enhancement of Teaching and Learning Skills

Promoting adult learning principles, active student engagement, experiential learning, reflective practices, and effective communication is essential in modern medical education. This need becomes even more critical with the growing integration of digital tools and simulation technologies, which call for more innovative and flexible teaching approaches. Faculty should also be supported in developing skills for managing classrooms effectively, fostering respectful and inclusive learning environments, responding to diverse student needs, and utilizing feedback mechanisms such as student evaluations and reflective teaching journals to continuously enhance their teaching capabilities. Innovative teaching strategies such as problem-based learning (PBL), case-based learning (CBL), simulation-based education, blended learning, small group facilitation, and flipped classrooms are widely recognized for promoting critical thinking and the application of knowledge in real-life contexts.[5]

Promoting Research Aptitude

Developing research competence is an essential aspect of a medical educator's professional growth, and FDPs play a key role in building these capabilities. Faculty are introduced to the fundamentals of research methodology, including qualitative, quantitative, and mixed-methods approaches. They receive guidance on formulating research questions, designing study protocols, seeking ethical clearance, and performing data analysis using statistical tools such as SPSS. Training also covers academic writing skills, such as drafting research papers, conducting literature reviews, and preparing grant proposals. In addition, FDPs emphasize the importance of academic integrity by addressing issues related to plagiarism, ethical conduct in research, the peer review process, and responsible publication practices.

Fostering Leadership, Mentorship, and Academic Management

An important focus of FDPs is to prepare faculty members for leadership roles within academic departments, regulatory bodies, and institutional administration. Educators are encouraged to actively participate in departmental decision-making, curriculum development, and governance processes. FDPs also provide training in various mentorship models, including peer, group, and individual mentoring, emphasizing the importance of trust, career support, and professional development of mentees. In addition, topics such as time management, stress reduction, and overall faculty well-being are incorporated into the training. These leadership and personal development skills are essential for cultivating a supportive academic culture, enhancing faculty satisfaction and retention, and developing the next generation of leaders in medical education.

Facilitating Professionalism and Ethics

The introduction of the Attitude Ethics and Communication (AETCOM) module by the Medical Council of India in 2018 marked a significant shift in the landscape of medical education in India.[6] By formally incorporating the teaching of ethics, professionalism, and communication into the undergraduate curriculum, it addressed a long-standing gap in value-based education. Implemented from the 2019 MBBS batch as part of the competency-based medical education (CBME) framework, the module underscored the importance of preparing faculty to serve as role models—demonstrating integrity, empathy, ethical decision-making, and respect for patient rights. Faculty development workshops have been designed to build capacity in facilitating small group discussions and promoting ethical reasoning. Educators are also made aware of the hidden curriculum and its subtle influence on student attitudes and behaviors.

In addition, FDPs emphasize communication skills, particularly in areas such as delivering constructive feedback and handling emotionally sensitive situations, often using role-plays and reflective exercises.

Curriculum Planning and Implementation

Effective curriculum planning and implementation are crucial for ensuring that teaching and assessment are aligned with clearly defined learning outcomes. FDPs play a vital role in preparing educators to understand and apply national educational frameworks such as CBME and the National Education Policy (NEP) 2020. The shift from a traditional, time-based curriculum to a competency-based model demands specific skills and a clear understanding of outcome-driven education—skills that require dedicated training and cannot be assumed. FDPs aim to build faculty competence in areas such as curriculum design, blueprinting, integration of disciplines, competency mapping, and the development and evaluation of innovative assessment strategies. Additionally, these programs emphasize the importance of incorporating feedback systems, ongoing quality enhancement processes, and regular curriculum reviews to maintain relevance and effectiveness.

Effective Navigation of Digital Tools

Faculty development programs play a critical role in equipping educators to effectively adapt to the ongoing digital transformation in medical education. These programs enable faculty to incorporate emerging technologies such as artificial intelligence, data analytics, and e-learning platforms into their teaching methodologies. In doing so, FDPs serve as a vital link that promotes equitable access to professional development across institutions with varying levels of resources. Educators are introduced to learning management systems (LMS) such as Moodle, Canvas, and Google Classroom, which support both blended and fully online modes of instruction. Training includes the creation of diverse digital learning materials—such as e-modules, podcasts, screencasts, and interactive videos—to accommodate different learner preferences. Increasing emphasis is also placed on simulation-based education using low- and high-fidelity manikins, along with immersive technologies such as virtual reality (VR) and augmented reality (AR). Faculty are encouraged to explore AI-driven tools that enhance adaptive learning, enable real-time analytics, and facilitate personalized feedback. These innovations contribute not only to improved student engagement and learning outcomes but also to greater teaching efficiency and flexibility for faculty members.

Familiarization with New Assessment Methods and Tools

Assessment literacy forms a fundamental aspect of faculty development, aimed at equipping educators with the skills required to design, implement, and evaluate meaningful assessment strategies. Faculty are introduced to core assessment principles such as reliability, validity, feasibility, and educational impact, which underpin sound evaluation practices. Training includes the use of a range of competency-based assessment tools, including objective structured clinical and practical examinations (OSCEs/OSPEs), the objective structured long examination record (OSLER), mini-clinical evaluation exercises (Mini-CEX), direct observation of procedural skills (DOPS), multisource feedback, and learner portfolios. These tools are designed to assess both cognitive and clinical competencies in diverse learning environments. In addition, faculty are trained in psychometric concepts such as blueprinting, item analysis, and the development of assessment rubrics, all of which contribute to the creation of robust and valid assessment systems. The overarching aim is to ensure that assessments are not merely evaluative but also serve as tools to enhance learning through constructive feedback and informed educational decisions.

GUIDING FRAMEWORKS

The design and evaluation of FDPs are supported by several well-established theoretical frameworks that help align training with educator competencies and institutional goals.

- *National Medical Commission (NMC) Framework (India):* This model underpins structured basic and advanced courses in medical education technology, which are mandatory for faculty career progression. It emphasizes standardizing core teaching competencies across medical colleges in India.
- *Miller's Pyramid of Clinical Competence:* Commonly adapted for teaching skills, this model provides a stepwise structure—ranging from knowing (knowledge) to showing how and ultimately doing (performance)—which helps assess and guide faculty development from theory to practice.
- *Dreyfus Model of Skill Acquisition:* This framework categorizes learners into five stages—novice, advanced beginner, competent, proficient, and expert—allowing FDPs to be customized based on individual faculty members' stages of professional development.

TYPES OF FACULTY DEVELOPMENT PROGRAMS

Faculty development programs can be classified based on their scope, format, and intended objectives:[7]

- *Induction and orientation programs:* Typically short-term in nature, these programs are designed for newly appointed faculty. They aim to introduce participants to the institutional structure, educational philosophy, academic responsibilities, and expectations related to teaching and student engagement.
- *In-service or continuing FDPs:* These are periodic, skill-based programs intended for practicing faculty. They help educators stay updated with evolving pedagogical techniques, technological tools, curriculum reforms, and research methodologies.
- *Workshops and seminars:* Focused and time-bound, these sessions address specific areas such as assessment design, OSCE planning, reflective teaching, or digital content creation. They are often conducted in collaboration with MEUs or regulatory bodies.
- *Certificate, diploma, or postgraduate programs:* These long-duration courses, including fellowships and postgraduate diplomas, are offered by recognized institutions or professional bodies. They provide in-depth training in medical education, educational leadership, or research.
- *Mentorship programs:* Structured mentoring initiatives aim to enhance faculty performance, professional growth, and retention. These programs may include peer observation, feedback, coteaching, and career guidance.
- *Online FDPs:* Delivered via digital platforms, these flexible, self-paced programs offer accessibility and

TABLE 2: Faculty development programs in the Indian context.

FDP type	*Example*	*Duration*	*Target group*	*Focus area*
Short-term	Revised Basic Course Workshop (rBCW)	3 days	All faculty	Teaching-learning methods, assessment, and adult learning
Short-term	Curriculum Implementation Support Program (CISP)	2–3 days	All faculty	CBME, AETCOM, and curriculum planning
Short-term	AETCOM Orientation Workshop	1–2 days	All faculty	Ethics, communication, and professionalism
Short-term	Simulation Training Workshops	2–5 days	Clinical educators	Clinical skills and simulation-based learning
Longitudinal	Advanced Course in Medical Education (ACME)	6 months	Senior faculty	Curriculum design, assessment, and educational research
Longitudinal	FAIMER Fellowship (PSG/GSMC)	2 years	Medical educators	Leadership, innovation, and scholarship
Longitudinal	NTTC Course at JIPMER	Several weeks	New faculty	Teaching skills, curriculum, and assessment
Online/hybrid	NMC Online FDPs (2020–21)	Varies	All faculty	Online teaching and digital assessment
Online/hybrid	Swayam/Nptel FDPs	4–8 weeks	All faculty	Educational technology and instructional design
Online/hybrid	IGNOU Certificate in Medical Education	Flexible	Health science educators	Foundations of teaching and learning
Specialized	Leadership for Academicians Programme (LEAP)	Several weeks	Senior administrators	Leadership and academic governance
Specialized	Medical Education Research Workshops (ICMR)	3–5 days	Interested faculty	Research methods in medical education

TABLE 3: Comparison between short-term and long-term FDP.

	Short-term	*Long-term*
Duration	1–5 days	Weeks-years
Focus	Skill based and orientation	Reflective practice and research
Impact	Immediate and procedural	Sustained and conceptual
Evaluation	Feedback and MCQs	Portfolios and scholarly output
Example	BCME course	ACME course, FAIMER

microcredentialing through certificates or digital badges. Platforms such as SWAYAM, NPTEL, and university-based MOOCs are common facilitators.

A summary of commonly implemented FDPs in India is provided in **Table 2**, while **Table 3** presents a comparison between short-term and long-term faculty development initiatives.

EVALUATION OF FACULTY DEVELOPMENT PROGRAMS

Several theoretical models are commonly employed to guide the evaluation and design of faculty development programs:

- *ARCS model:* Developed by John Keller, this model emphasizes enhancing learner motivation through four key components—attention, relevance, confidence, and satisfaction. It is particularly useful in designing engaging and learner-centered educational experiences.
- *Kirkpatrick's four-level model:* Widely used for evaluating training effectiveness, this model assesses outcomes across four levels: Reaction (participant satisfaction), learning (knowledge or skills gained), behavior (changes in teaching practices), and results (impact on learners or institutional outcomes).[9]
- *CIPP model:* This comprehensive evaluation framework includes context, input, process, and product. It supports decision-making at various stages of program planning, implementation, and impact assessment.
- *Logic model:* A planning and evaluation tool that connects inputs, activities, outputs, and intended outcomes or impacts. It provides a structured approach for visualizing how program resources and activities lead to short- and long-term goals.

FUTURE OF FDPs

Highlighting successful examples of faculty development—particularly those that resulted in improved student engagement, curriculum innovation, and assessment practices—can provide valuable insights for future planning. Looking ahead, several trends are expected to shape the future of FDPs:

- *Personalized and flexible learning:*[10] Faculty development is likely to adopt a modular approach, offering customizable learning paths based on individual needs and interests. Online and hybrid models will enhance accessibility and accommodate diverse schedules.
- *Global collaboration:* Increasing international partnerships will offer faculty exposure to varied educational practices and research methodologies, fostering cross-cultural learning and collaboration.
- *Focus on emerging trends:* FDPs will incorporate training in cutting-edge areas such as artificial intelligence, data literacy, and digital pedagogy, preparing educators for the evolving demands of medical education.
- *Integration of technology:* The use of virtual reality (VR), augmented reality (AR), and artificial intelligence (AI) will enhance interactivity and engagement in faculty training, creating more immersive learning environments.
- *Lifelong learning:* Faculty development will progressively support lifelong learning, encouraging continuous skill enhancement and adaptability throughout an educator's career.

THE INDIAN SCENARIO

The Evolution of Faculty Development in India

Establishment of NTTC and the Beginnings of Faculty Development in India

Formal faculty development in India began with the establishment of the first National Teacher Training Centre (NTTC) at the Jawaharlal Institute of Postgraduate Medical Education and Research (JIPMER), Puducherry, in 1975. Inspired by its early success, the Ministry of Health and Family Welfare set up three additional NTTCs at the Postgraduate Institute of Medical Education and Research (PGIMER), Chandigarh; the Institute of Medical Sciences, Banaras Hindu University (BHU), Varanasi; and Maulana Azad Medical College, New Delhi. These centers were instrumental in developing the initial cadre of educational leaders and trained faculty members during the 1980s and 1990s. Their contributions laid the foundation for the structured growth of faculty development across the country. However, in 2002 when government funding was withdrawn, it led to the discontinuation of national training programs at these centers due to financial constraints. A timeline of faculty development in India is provided in **Figure 1**.

Establishment of KL Wig Center for Medical Education and Technology

Another significant milestone in the early advancement of faculty development in India was the establishment of the KL Wig Centre for Medical Education and Technology at the All India Institute of Medical Sciences (AIIMS), New Delhi, during 1989–1990. The center emerged as a major proponent of educational reform and innovation in medical teaching. Beyond its contributions to faculty training, it played a leading role in shaping national policy by actively participating in the revision of MBBS regulations undertaken by the Medical Council of India in 1997. Its efforts helped lay the foundation for more structured and forward-looking medical education practices in the country.[11]

Role of consortium of Medical Education

The Consortium of Medical Institutions for Reform of Medical Education significantly contributed to the evolution of faculty development programs in India between 1989 and 1995. Initially comprising four key institutions—All India Institute of Medical Sciences (AIIMS), New Delhi; Christian Medical College (CMC), Vellore; Jawaharlal Institute of Postgraduate Medical Education and Research (JIPMER), Puducherry; and the Institute of Medical Sciences, Banaras Hindu University (IMS-BHU), Varanasi—along with the Department of Medical Education at the College of Medicine, University of Illinois, Chicago, the consortium later expanded to include 16 medical colleges. This collaborative effort was instrumental in promoting curriculum reform and introducing structured classification of competencies. One of its notable contributions was the categorization of essential skills into "must know" and "good

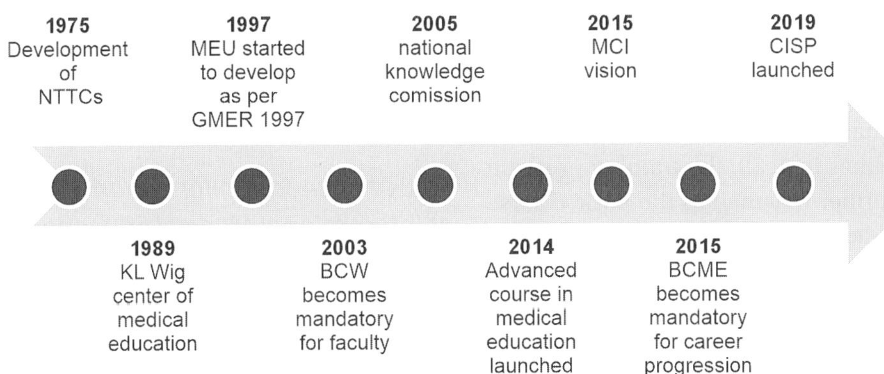

Fig. 1: Timeline of faculty development in India.

to know," helping institutions prioritize and streamline medical training content.

Various Medical Council of India Initiatives

- A major step toward structured faculty development in India began with the Graduate Medical Education Regulations of 1997, issued by the Medical Council of India (MCI), which mandated the establishment of MEUs in all medical colleges. To implement this directive, MCI developed a multitiered framework by setting up regional and nodal centers across the country. These centers were responsible for training faculty members from MEUs, who would, in turn, facilitate faculty development activities within their own institutions.
- At the foundational level, MCI introduced the Basic Medical Education Technology Workshop (BCW), a three-day intensive program aimed at building core competencies in teaching and learning. In 2003, the MCI Board of Governors accepted the Academic Council's recommendation that faculty should undergo this training either before joining, upon selection, or during the probation period. However, at that time, it was advisory in nature and not strictly enforced. This workshop was revised and renamed as Revised Basic Medical Education Technology Workshop (rBCW), aligning its content with the upcoming reforms. With the rollout of the National Medical Commission (NMC) guidelines in 2019, the training program was further renamed as the Basic Course in Medical Education (BCME), reflecting its alignment with CBME.
- The MCI Vision 2015 document served as a major driver of faculty development in India. It institutionalized a nationwide system for continuous training of medical educators by mandating the creation of MEUs, standardizing faculty development practices, and linking participation in these programs to eligibility for academic promotion. While faculty development was encouraged as early as 2009, it was only in 2015 that completion of the basic medical education course became a mandatory requirement for promotion to the rank of associate professor and beyond and was implemented consistently across all institutions.[12]
- In 2014, MCI further advanced faculty training by introducing the Advanced Course in Medical Education Technology (ACME) across 10 designated nodal centers. The course spanned 1 year and included two contact sessions—1 of 3 days and another of 2 days—held in September and March. During the intersession period, participants engaged in online discussions and were required to complete a project to demonstrate application of the learned principles. Recently, the duration of ACME has been revised to 6 months.
- Finally, just before the official launch of CBME in 2019, the curriculum implementation support program (CISP) workshops were introduced. These were developed to equip faculty with the skills needed for effective CBME implementation, focusing on curriculum delivery, integration, assessment design, and feedback strategies.

Role of Foundation for Advancement of International Medical Education and Research

The Foundation for Advancement of International Medical Education and Research (FAIMER), a nonprofit organization established by the Educational Commission for Foreign Medical Graduates (ECFMG), USA, plays a significant role in promoting faculty development globally. One of its key initiatives is a 2-year, part-time fellowship program that focuses on building leadership and managerial competencies among medical educators. The program also fosters innovation in medical education through collaborative learning and international networking. As part of its global outreach, FAIMER established a network of regional institutes, including three in India—located at Seth GS Medical College, Mumbai; Christian Medical College, Ludhiana; and PSG Institute of Medical Sciences, Coimbatore. These centers have contributed to strengthening educational leadership and promoting academic excellence within the Indian medical education system.

SITUATION ANALYSIS AND SHORTCOMINGS OF FDPs IN INDIA

- *Faculty shortage:* A significant concern in medical education is the shortage of qualified faculty, currently estimated at around 30% across medical colleges in India. This gap presents a major challenge in scaling up faculty development efforts within a limited timeframe to ensure quality education.
- *Lack of a formal policy framework:* Although the basic course in medical education became mandatory for academic promotion starting in 2015, there is still no national policy mandating formal faculty development training at the time of appointment. The absence of such a requirement affects the consistency and preparedness of newly recruited educators.
- *Short-term and cross-sectional programs:* Most faculty development initiatives, such as the basic course in medical education and the curriculum implementation support program (CISP), are brief and one-time interventions. These workshops often lack structured follow-up, limiting opportunities for sustained behavior change, practice, reflection, and reinforcement of skills.
- *Inadequate program evaluation:* Robust evaluation mechanisms are lacking at the institutional level. In the absence of ongoing assessment and feedback, the skills and knowledge gained through FDPs may diminish over time. Additionally, peer and student feedback on faculty teaching performance is not systematically implemented, as it is resource intensive and not mandated by regulatory authorities.
- *Limited skill depth in current FDP structure:* Existing programs primarily address the lower tiers of Miller's pyramid—namely the "knows," "knows how," and occasionally "shows how" levels. However, they fall short of preparing faculty to reach the "does" level, which involves consistent application and integration of competencies in real-world teaching contexts.
- *Faculty resistance and cultural barriers:* Resistance to change, traditional mindsets, skepticism toward new teaching approaches, and low motivation—particularly among senior faculty—pose significant barriers to the successful implementation and acceptance of faculty development initiatives.
- *Resource and time limitations:* Faculty members are often burdened with clinical, academic, and administrative responsibilities, leaving limited time for professional development. Additionally, a lack of trained facilitators, inadequate infrastructure, limited access to technology, and insufficient institutional funding further constrain the effective implementation of FDPs.

RECOMMENDATIONS FOR INDIA

The following recommendations for strengthening faculty development in India can be broadly categorized into three areas: *Policy-level changes, programmatic improvements in FDPs,* and *institutional-level strategies.* A visual summary of these recommendations is presented in **Figure 2.**

Policy-level Recommendations

Formulation of a National Health Professions Education Policy

In alignment with the revised National Education Policy of 2020, there is an urgent need to draft a comprehensive policy focused specifically on health professions education. This should be undertaken collaboratively by regulatory councils such as the National Medical Commission (NMC), Dental Council, Nursing Council, and other relevant bodies, along with academic experts and health education stakeholders. The policy should provide strategic direction for faculty development, curriculum innovation, and quality assurance in medical and allied health education.

Shift Toward Accreditation-focused Quality Assurance

The current system of recognizing medical colleges primarily emphasizes quantitative metrics such as faculty numbers, infrastructure, and facilities. There is a need to move beyond this checklist approach and adopt a robust accreditation model that prioritizes educational quality. Quality assurance should incorporate indicators such as curriculum effectiveness, faculty competency, student outcomes, and institutional learning culture.

Integration of Medical Education Training in Postgraduate Curriculum

Since postgraduate trainees are potential future educators, it is important to introduce structured training modules on teaching methodologies, assessment practices, e-learning, medical ethics, and scholarly writing. This approach will ensure that future

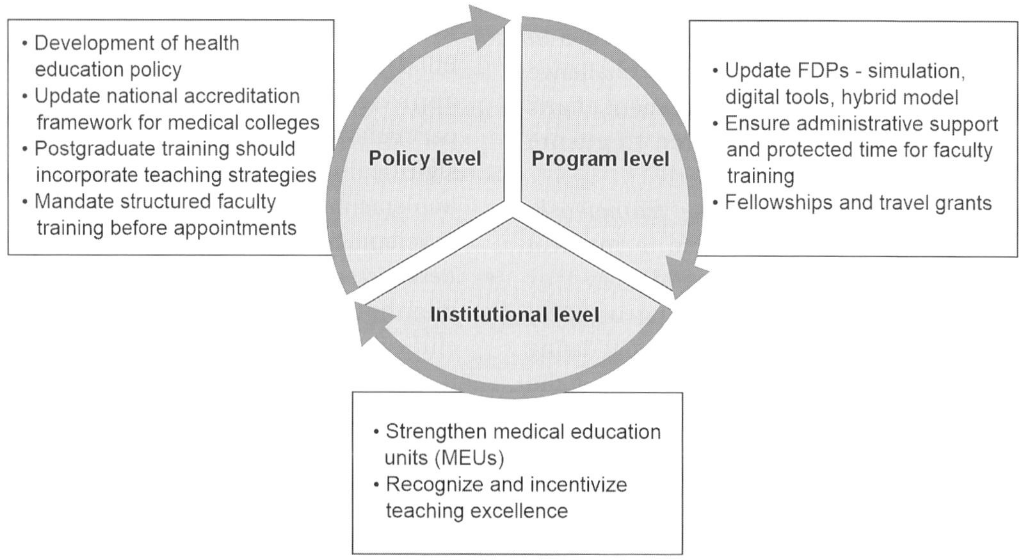

Fig. 2: Summary of recommendations for India.

faculty are adequately prepared for academic roles, especially in contexts where prior training in education is not a prerequisite for faculty appointments.

Expansion of Medical Education Units into Interprofessional Centers

Given the shared challenges and limited resources across health professions, it is advisable to broaden the scope of existing MEUs into Centers for Health Professions Education. These centers could serve as common platforms for training faculty from medicine, nursing, dentistry, physiotherapy, and allied health fields, promoting an interprofessional and integrated approach to faculty development.

Recommendations for FDPs

- *Reforms in FDP workshop structure:*
    - **Integrated workshop delivery:** The Basic Course in Medical Education (BCME) and the Curriculum Implementation Support Program (CISP) workshops can be combined into a single, integrated module. As these programs often cover overlapping content, merging them would streamline administrative efforts, reduce redundancy, and support more cohesive learning. Integrated objectives would also enhance conceptual understanding and prevent cognitive overload or disengagement among participants.
    - **Adoption of a hybrid model:** FDPs should evolve to a blended learning format. Didactic presentations and foundational content can be delivered through online platforms, with supplementary reading materials made available beforehand. In-person sessions can then focus on group activities, discussions, and application-based learning, offering a more engaging and flexible experience for faculty.
    - **Development of online refresher modules:** To support continuous learning, refresher courses should be developed and hosted online. These can be offered through nodal centers in collaboration with platforms such as NPTEL or other national educational portals. This would allow faculty to update their knowledge at their own pace.
    - **Longitudinal faculty development approaches:** Rather than one-time workshops, FDPs should adopt a longitudinal format using tools such as objective structured teaching encounters (OSTEs). Establishing microteaching laboratories in medical colleges—managed by the Medical Education Unit and Curriculum Committee—can provide faculty with regular opportunities for feedback, reflection, and improvement.
- *Revival of fellowships and travel support:* National and international organizations, including the World Health Organization and Indian health education bodies, should reinstate fellowship programs that allow educators to train at renowned medical education centers within India and abroad. Travel grants should also be made available to promote wider participation and exposure.
- *Institutional support for faculty development:* Faculty development should be recognized as an essential component of academic progression. Regular participation in FDPs should be linked to promotions, empanelment as examiners,

and eligibility for academic leadership roles. Institutions should actively support faculty by offering leave of absence, funding for travel and registration, and administrative facilitation for participation in training events.

- *Ongoing quality enhancement:* To ensure relevance and effectiveness, regular evaluation of FDPs should be conducted using established models such as Kirkpatrick's framework. This will enable evidence-based course revisions and the identification of areas requiring improvement, thus maintaining the educational quality and alignment with current needs.

At the Institutional Level

- *Establishment and strengthening of functional MEUs:* Medical colleges—both private and government—should ensure that their medical education units are not only established but actively engaged in core academic functions. These units should be involved in organizing faculty development programs, driving curricular reforms, supporting assessment innovations, and promoting educational research. To sustain such efforts, it is recommended that institutions allocate a minimum of 1% of their annual budget specifically for MEU activities. Additionally, flexible staffing policies should be implemented to ensure that MEUs are adequately staffed and supported, especially in newly established colleges.
- *Recognition and support for teaching excellence:* Institutions should implement systems for the regular evaluation of faculty performance, emphasizing accountability and academic contribution. Faculty engagement in teaching should be recognized as a scholarly pursuit, characterized by continuous reflection, active participation, collaboration, and evidence-based practice. Encouraging a culture of teaching excellence through awards, public recognition, and opportunities for academic leadership can serve as strong motivators for faculty involvement in educational innovation.
- *Assessment of faculty readiness and motivation:* It is essential to evaluate faculty preparedness for implementing new curricular approaches such as CBME.[13] Tools such as the Measuring Organizational Readiness for Change (MORC) questionnaire can be employed to assess both motivation and perceived institutional support. This can help identify specific barriers and guide targeted interventions to enhance the success of educational reforms.

CONCLUSION

Faculty development programs play a vital role in ensuring the quality and relevance of medical technology education. As educational paradigms shift and newer pedagogical approaches emerge, it becomes essential for faculty to receive continuous support, training, and professional development. Well-designed FDPs not only enhance the skills and effectiveness of individual educators but also contribute significantly to institutional growth and improved student learning outcomes.

Looking ahead, FDPs must evolve to become more inclusive, interdisciplinary, technology-integrated, and results focused. There is a growing need to transition from traditional, passive training models to reflective and transformative faculty development approaches that align closely with institutional priorities and global educational standards. To realize this vision, strong policy frameworks, sustained institutional support, and proactive academic leadership are crucial. With these enablers in place, FDPs in India are well equipped to meet the evolving demands of health professions education in the 21st century.

Summary Points

- Faculty development programs enhance teaching, assessment, leadership, and research skills in medical educators.
- India's journey in FDPs evolved from NTTC and CMET to structured programs under MCI Vision 2015 and NMC.
- Core domains include pedagogy, assessment, curriculum planning, technology use, professionalism, and mentorship.
- FDPs can be short term, longitudinal, online, or specialized, tailored to different faculty needs.
- Evaluation models such as Kirkpatrick's and CIPP help assess impact on teaching behavior and learner outcomes.
- MCI Vision 2015 made FDPs mandatory for career progression, leading to widespread adoption across institutions.
- Innovations such as digital FDPs, simulation training, and interprofessional education are gaining ground.
- Strengthening MEUs, institutional support, and national policy alignment is key to sustaining impact.

REFERENCES

1. WHO. Transforming and scaling up health professionals' education and training. 2013. Available from: https://apps.who.int/iris/handle/10665/93635
2. Steinert Y, Mann K, Centeno A, Dolmans D, Spencer J, Gelula M, et al. A systematic review of faculty development initiatives designed to improve teaching effectiveness in medical education. Med Teach. 2006;28(6):497-526. doi:10.1080/01421590600902976
3. O'Sullivan PS, Irby DM, Levine RE. Faculty development: from program effectiveness to impact. Acad Med. 2022;97(9):1280-85. doi:10.1097/ACM.0000000000004756
4. Leslie K, Baker L, Egan-Lee E, Esdaile M, Kaczorowski J, Kilminster S, et al. Advancing faculty development in medical education: a systematic review. Med Educ. 2021;55(3):239-52. doi:10.1111/medu.14307
5. Harden RM, Crosby JR. AMEE Guide No. 20: The good teacher is more than a lecturer—the twelve roles of the teacher. Med Teach. 2000;22(4):334-47. doi:10.1080/014215900409429
6. National Medical Commission (NMC), India. Competency-Based Undergraduate Curriculum for the Indian Medical Graduate. 2019. Available from: https://www.nmc.org.in
7. Srinivasan M, Li ST, Meyers FJ, Pratt DD, Collins JB, Braddock C, et al. "Teaching as a competency": competencies for medical educators. Acad Med. 2011;86(10):1211-20. doi:10.1097/ACM.0b013e31822c5b9a
8. Maiti M, Priyaadharshini M, S H. Design and evaluation of a revised ARCS motivational model for online classes in higher education. Heliyon. 2023 Dec 1;9(12):e22729. doi:10.1016/j.heliyon.2023.e22729
9. Kirkpatrick DL, Kirkpatrick JD. Evaluating Training Programs: The Four Levels. San Francisco: Berrett-Koehler Publishers; 2006.
10. Shin H, Kim MJ. Faculty development: the need to ensure educational excellence and health care quality. Kosin Med J. 2023;38(1):4-11.
11. Zodpey S, Sharma A, Zahiruddin QS, Gaidhane A, Shrikhande S. Faculty development programs for medical teachers in India. J Adv Med Educ Prof. 2016;4(2):97-101. PMID:27104205; PMCID:PMC4827763
12. Dash D, Mohanty A, Pattnaik SK. Impact of faculty development programs on teaching competency: an Indian perspective. J Educ Eval Health Prof. 2023;20:3. doi:10.3352/jeehp.2023.20.3
13. Garg R, Singh S, Bansal P. Faculty development in India: past, present, and future. Indian J Community Med. 2020;45(1):10-14. doi:10.4103/ijcm.IJCM_45_19

CHAPTER 31

Feedback in Medical Education

Sanghamitra Ray

INTRODUCTION

The literary meaning of feedback is useful information or criticism that is given to someone to explain what can be done to improve a performance. As medical education is expanding its horizon in order to gain deeper knowledge regarding effective learning, educational feedback has gained renewed attention of medical academicians and effective feedback has been a core component of learning even in medical education.[1]

Feedback is very critical to medical education in promoting deep learning and ensuring the quality care.[2] It can be further classified as positive feedback and negative feedback. Ideally, the feedback should also be given to the facilitator of the learning—the teacher, so that teaching method is further improvized and improved as per the need of the students. Numerous studies emphasize its role in bridging the gap between actual and desired performance, fostering self-regulation, and enhancing the clinical skills.

CHARACTERISTICS OF EFFECTIVE FEEDBACK

For feedback to be effective in medical education, certain characteristics are essential:

- *Promotes reflective practice:* Effective feedback encourages learners to reflect on their clinical performance, leading to better self-awareness and professional growth.[3]
- *Enhances competency development:* Feedback allows learners to align their clinical skills with established competencies, providing targeted guidance on areas of improvement.[4]
- *Timeliness:* Feedback provided soon after an event allows learners to relate the comments to their specific actions, making the feedback more relevant.[5]
- *Specificity:* Specific and concrete suggestions enable learners to focus on distinct areas for improvement. Vague feedback is often unhelpful.[6]
- *Actionability:* Learners benefit most from feedback that includes an actionable recommendation, which they can implement in subsequent clinical practice.[7]
- *Balanced:* Feedback should include both strengths and areas for improvement, avoiding an overly negative or positive bias.
- *Learner engagement:* Effective feedback engages the learner in a dialogue, encouraging questions and clarifying uncertainties.

CLOSED AND OPEN SYSTEM OF TEACHING-LEARNING METHOD

Teaching-learning system without feedback is incomplete in true sense and is called open system, while the system with effective

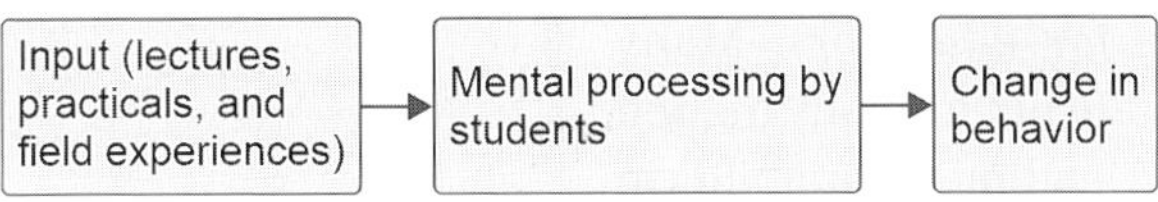

Fig. 1: Open system of teaching-learning method.

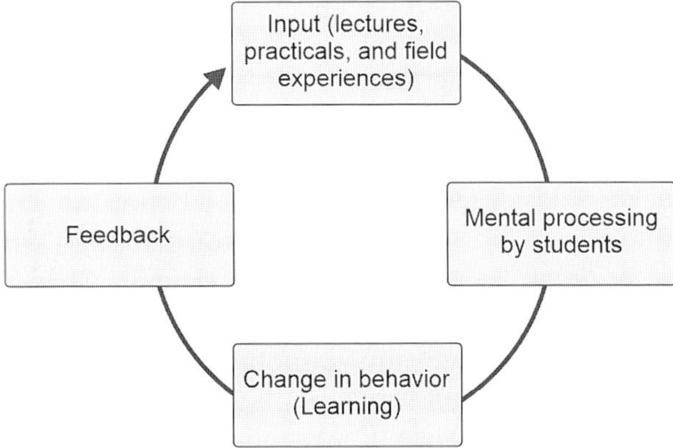

Fig. 2: Closed system of teaching-learning method.

feedback process is known as closed system **(Figs. 1 and 2)**.

Importance of feedback: It has been seen that closed system of learning is better than open system without feedback. Feedback delivered in a nonjudgmental and systematic way in a positive environment makes learning effective and also creates a motivational bond between teachers and students. It emphasizes positive or negative reinforcement to behavior, diagnosing gaps between demonstrated and expected standards, finds ways to fill the gaps, and addressing ways to support development and attainment of competencies according to the phase of learning. Feedback allows learners to align their clinical skills with established competencies, providing targeted guidance on areas of improvement.[3]

The required qualities of teachers for providing effective feedback are:

- To have sound knowledge of the subject.
- To observe the student meticulously for providing useful feedbacks.
- He/she should be familiar with different scientific methods of feedback in medical education.
- Should be able to apply the best method of feedback depending on the situation and type of learners.
- The teacher should be trained in effective communication skills, and should be able to establish rapport with the students/trainees.
- Should be able to handle ambiguity and difficult situations.

COMMON PROBLEMS FACED IN GIVING FEEDBACK

- Students are often not ready to accept negative comments.
- Often feedback is given in a demeaning way or with humiliation.
- Negative feedback often dominates over positive feedback in most of the case.
- Despite the well-established benefits of feedback, its implementation in medical education faces several challenges. Common barriers include: *Time constraints:* Clinical educators often cite time limitations as a barrier to providing detailed feedback.[8]

- *Lack of training for educators:* Many clinical educators are not formally trained in giving feedback, leading to variability in feedback quality and effectiveness.[1,9]
- *Learner resistance:* Some learners may be defensive or resistant to feedback, especially if it is perceived as overly critical or if it challenges their self-assessment.[9,10]
- *Faulty timing of feedback:* Delay in giving feedback often makes it less useful and less accurate too.
- *Generalization of feedback:* In most of the cases feedback is not individualized and common feedback is given to the entire batch of students. This is not very effective and loses the very purpose of improvement of performance and it is not well received by the group.

MODELS OF FEEDBACK

Feedback of Sandwich Model

Feedback begins and ends with appreciative and positive feedback (about what the student has done well); the crucial feedback component (constructive criticism for the area of improvement) is "sandwiched" between the positive aspects. This approach is useful for learners with low esteem; however, if used frequently, its effectiveness can be lost, as the students start ignoring the crucial middle component of feedback **(Fig. 3)**.[11]

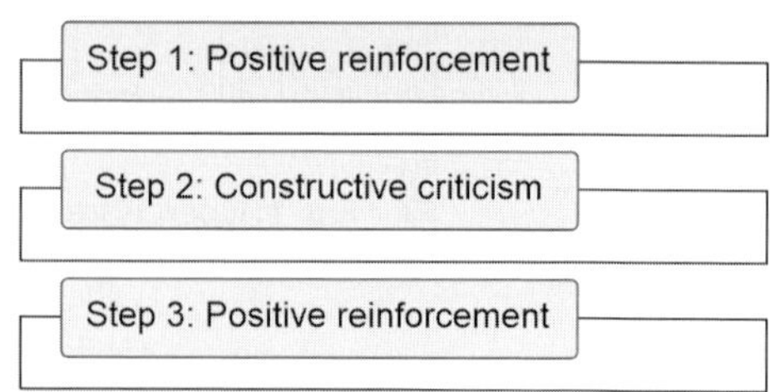

Fig. 3: Sandwich model of feedback.

Pendleton's Model

Pendleton rules are so designed that the learner's strengths are discussed first, avoiding discussing weaknesses right at the beginning. The learner is encouraged to reflect on the positive areas (What was done well?) followed by discussion on positive aspects. The facilitator reinforces those positive areas. Further, the person is asked regarding what should have been done in a better way and then the learning facilitator discusses what should be done for betterment. This method focuses on positive aspects and so it is more acceptable among learners **(Fig. 4)**. One interesting point of this method is that the learner is encouraged to reflect on own strengths and weaknesses.[12]

TYPES OF FEEDBACK

There are several methods for providing feedback, each suited to different learning environments and objectives. Feedback can be broadly categorized as formative or summative. Formative feedback is ongoing and developmental, intended to guide learners toward improvement. Summative feedback, on the other hand, is evaluative and is often used at the end of a learning cycle or assessment.

Formative Feedback

The literature stresses the importance of frequent and constructive formative feedback, which fosters a culture of continuous learning. Van de Ridder et al.[13] highlighted that formative feedback should be timely, specific, and actionable to be the most effective.

Purpose: To help learners improve during the learning process.

Example: Frequent feedback during clinical rotations or simulation sessions, highlighting strengths and areas for improvement in real time.

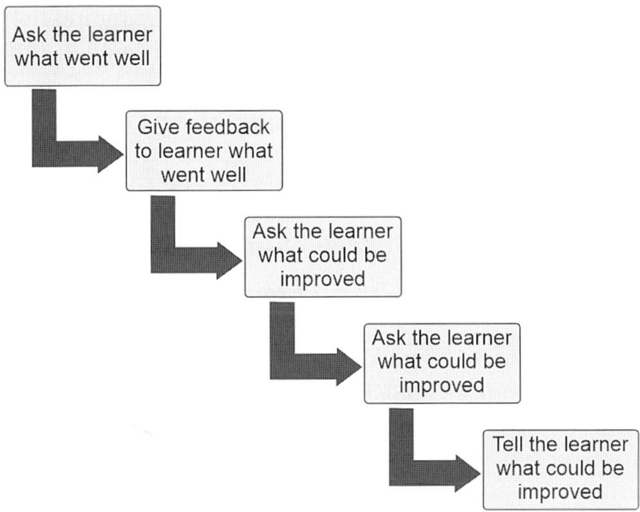

Fig. 4: Pendleton's model of feedback.

Summative Feedback

Although summative feedback is important in assessing learner's performance, it is often less useful for fostering growth, as it may lack the specific guidance needed to enhance future performance.[14]

Purpose: To evaluate performance at the end of a learning period, often linked to grading or certification.

Example: Feedback provided after a final clinical examination or end-of-rotation evaluation.

Direct Observation Feedback

Purpose: Immediate feedback based on direct observation of a learner's performance.

Example: A teacher observes a student performing a patient's counseling and provides feedback immediately after the interaction.

360° Feedback

Purpose: Feedback from multiple sources (peers, patients, nurses, and supervisors) to provide a well-rounded assessment of the learner's performance.

Example: A resident receives feedback from colleagues, teachers, and patients on communication skills, teamwork, and professionalism.

Peer Feedback

Purpose: Feedback provided by peers, which encourages collaborative learning and reflection.

Example: Medical students or residents provide constructive feedback to one another after working together in a clinical team.

Self-assessment and Feedback

Purpose: Learners assess their own performance and compare it to feedback from others, promoting self-reflection and autonomy.

Example: A resident reviews their performance on a procedure and compares their self-assessment with feedback from their attending.

Verbal Feedback

Purpose: Quick, informal feedback that is often provided in real-time during patient care or skills training.

Example: An instructor gives brief pointers or praise while observing a student performing a clinical skill.

Written Feedback

Purpose: Detailed and structured feedback often provided in evaluations or after assessments, allowing for reflection and review.

Example: Written comments on an "Objective Structured Clinical Examination (OSCE)" evaluation form.

Feed-forward

Purpose: Instead of only commenting on past performance, this method focuses on providing guidance for future learning and improvement.

Example: A feedback session after a clinical case that includes suggestions for improvement in the next case or rotation.

1-Minute Preceptor Model

Purpose: A structured and quick method to provide targeted feedback in clinical settings.

Example: During clinical rounds, the teacher identifies what the learner did right, explains the clinical reasoning behind it, and points out what they could do differently next time.

Debriefing Feedback (in Simulation)

Purpose: A postsimulation feedback method where learners reflect on their performance, often guided by an instructor.

Example: After a simulated clinical scenario, the instructor leads a debrief, highlighting the learners' decisions, teamwork, and areas for future focus.

Each method has its strengths and can be applied based on the learning context, the needs of the learner, and the goals of the educational program.

FEEDBACK FOR TEACHERS/ LEARNING FACILITATORS

One of the tested methods of feedback for teachers is microteaching. This method focuses on improving a small part of teaching at a time **(Fig. 5)**.

THE METHOD OF MICROTEACHING

The teacher prepares a small presentation and presents in front of a small group of

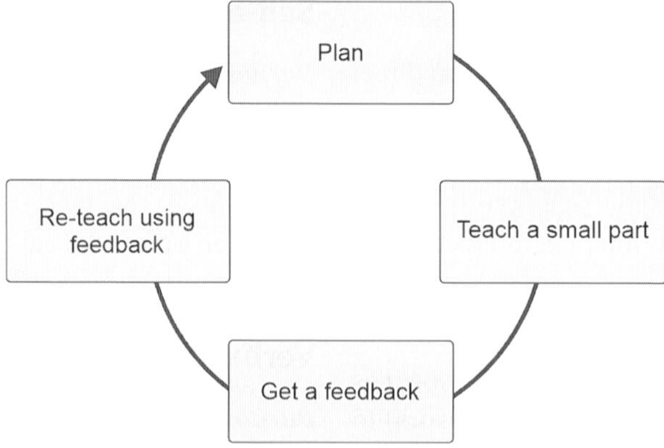

Fig. 5: Cycle of microteaching.

colleagues or students. After teaching, the group gives feedback regarding the overall teaching process. The teacher takes all feedbacks and incorporates them in the same teaching topic. He or she again presents the same topic in front of the same group for documentation of the improvement. Thus, change of behavior of teacher is based on feedback from the learner.

Other methods of feedback for teachers are:

- *Electronic feedback:* Recording the teaching process and reflecting on it afterward for improvement in teaching methodology and for better facilitation of learning.
- *Self-evaluation:* A teacher can self-evaluate oneself by retrospection of the teaching session. This can be collaborated with the electronic feedback when recorded teaching session is critically assessed by the teacher himself or herself.
- *Peer feedback:* This is also a method used for giving feedback to teachers where colleagues/fellow teachers give feedback.

STRATEGIES FOR IMPROVING FEEDBACK

To address these barriers and optimize feedback in medical education, several strategies have been proposed:

1. *Educator training:* Providing feedback training for clinical educators can improve the quality of feedback delivery. Studies suggest that structured feedback models, such as Pendleton's Rules and the "Situation-Behavior-Impact (SBI)" model, can help educators to give more effective feedback.[15]
2. *Feedback culture:* Establishing a culture of feedback within medical education, where feedback is expected and valued, encourages both learners and educators to engage more openly in the feedback process.[16]
3. *Use of technology:* The integration of digital platforms can facilitate feedback by offering asynchronous feedback options and real-time tracking of learner progress.

CONCLUSION

- Feedback is an integral part of effective teaching.
- Individualized feedback is better than generalized feedback.
- Feedback is essential for both learners and teachers for improvement in quality of teaching-learning exercise.
- Role of feedback needs to be re-emphasized in medical education.

REFERENCES

1. Hewson MG, Little ML. Giving feedback in medical education: verification of recommended techniques. J Gen Intern Med. 1998;13(2):111-6.
2. El Boghdady M, Alijani A. Feedback in surgical education. Surgeon. 2017;15(2):98-103.
3. Cantillon P, Sargeant J. Giving feedback in clinical settings. BMJ. 2008;337:a1961.
4. Archer JC. State of the science in health professional education: effective feedback. Med Educ. 2010;44(1):101-8.
5. Shute VJ. Focus on Formative Feedback. Rev Edu Res. 2008;78(1):153-89.
6. Hattie J, Timperley H. The Power of Feedback. Rev Edu Res. 2007;77(1):81-112.
7. Bing-You RG, Paterson J, Levine MA. Feedback falling on deaf ears: Residents' receptivity to feedback tempered by sender credibility. Medical Teacher. 1997;19(1):40-4.
8. Chun M. Taking teaching to (performance) task: Linking pedagogical and assessment practices. Change: The Magazine of Higher Learning. J Innovat Teach Learn. 2010;42(2):22-9.
9. Molloy E, Boud D. Feedback models for learning, teaching and performance. In: Spector JM, Merrill D, Elen J, Bishop MJ (Eds). Handbook of Research on Educational Communications and Technology, 4th

Edition. New York: Springer; 2013. pp. 413-24.
10. Eva KW, Armson H, Holmboe E, et al. Factors influencing responsiveness to feedback: On the interplay between fear, confidence, and reasoning processes. Advan Health Sci Edu. 2012;17(1):15-26.
11. Dohrenwend A. Serving up the feedback sandwich. Fam Pract Manag. 2002;9(10):43-6.
12. Hardavella G, Aamli-Gaagnat A, Saad N, et al. How to give and receive feedback effectively. Breathe (Sheff). 2017;13(4):327-33.
13. Van de Ridder JM, Stokking KM, McGaghie WC, et al. What is feedback in clinical education? Med Educ. 2008;42(2):189-97.
14. Schuwirth LW, van der Vleuten CP. Programmatic assessment and Kane's validity perspective. Med Educ. 2012;46(1): 38-48.
15. Veloski J, Boex JR, Grasberger MJ, et al. Systematic review of the literature on assessment, feedback and physicians' clinical performance: BEME Guide No. 7. Med Teach. 2006;28(2):117-28.
16. Watling C, Driessen E, van der Vleuten CP, et al. Learning culture and feedback: an international study of medical athletes and musicians. Med Educ. 2014;48(7):713-23.

CHAPTER 32

Reflection Writing

Vikra Bhaskar

INTRODUCTION

The emphasis on the use of reflection in both undergraduate and postgraduate teaching has increased in past few decades. Reflective writing in the field of medicine allows physicians to take a step back, review their performance, and recognize how their thoughts, feelings, and emotions affect their decision-making, clinical reasoning, and professionalism. Medical students are often asked to write reflection paper as part of their clinical posting to increase empathic interaction with their patients.

The term "reflection" is widely used in different contexts, from physics to medical education. This Latin word literally means "to bend" or "to turn back". Reflection in the education can be seen as a process in which thoughts or feelings are "turned back" so that they can be interpreted or analyzed.[1]

Reflection writing is the most common form of reflective practice in medical education. It is one of the distinct approaches to achieve integrated learning. Reflective writing plays a crucial role in medical education, bridging theoretical, and practical knowledge. As the field of medicine continues to evolve, medical teachers and healthcare professionals recognize the importance of reflection in fostering critical thinking, enhancing clinical skills, and promoting lifelong learning.

IMPORTANCE OF REFLECTIVE WRITING

The main aim of reflective writing is to assist students to internalize their learning in both cognitive and affective domains. It is particularly important for medical students as it not only integrates theoretical learning and clinical practice, but it also prepares students for dealing with messy, ill-defined, and unexpected issues. It is a part of student-centered learning, action research, and experiential learning. Some of the important features of reflective writing are discussed here.

Enhanced Learning

Reflective writing serves as a tool for students to engage with their experiences actively. It encourages them to analyze their thought processes, emotions, and actions during clinical encounters. By reflecting on events, students gain deeper insights into their learning, which can enhance their understanding of medical concepts and patient care.

Development of Critical Thinking Skills

In medical education, critical thinking is paramount. A person who is not sufficiently critical, might arrive at hasty conclusions, without analyzing all the possibilities.

Reflective writing helps students to not only articulate their clinical experiences but also to question their assumptions and evaluate their clinical decisions. This process fosters higher-order thinking skills, enabling students to make informed decisions in complex clinical situations.

Provide Different Perspective

Medical practitioners require a high level of emotional intelligence and empathy. Reflective writing allows students to contemplate their interactions with patients, recognize their feelings, and articulate the impact of those interactions on their personal and professional growth. This introspection promotes empathy, which is essential for patient-centered care. Also, the students learn to understand that problems can be viewed in many different ways depending on the perspective of the person/patient involved.

Continued Learning

The practice of reflection cultivates a habit of continuous learning. As students become accustomed to evaluating their experiences, they develop skills that encourage ongoing self-assessment throughout their careers. This mindset is critical in a fast-evolving field like medicine, where lifelong education is necessary to stay updated with new developments and practices.

THE PROCESS OF REFLECTIVE WRITING

Step 1: Experience

The first step in reflective writing is the experience itself. This can include patient interactions, clinical rotations, lectures, or simulations. Students are encouraged to actively participate and fully engage in their experiences to lay the foundation for meaningful reflection.[2]

Step 2: Reflection

After the experience, students should take time to reflect. This involves considering what happened, the actions taken, and the emotions felt during the experience.[3] Reflection can be guided by specific questions, such as:

- What was the situation?
- What was my role?
- How did I feel during this experience?
- What did I learn?

Step 3: Analysis

Analysis involves delving deeper into the reflection. Students should consider the significance of their experiences in the context of their training and future practice. This means linking theory to practice, discussing what went well, what challenges were faced, and how these experiences shape their understanding of medical practice.

Step 4: Learning and Action Plan

The final step of the reflective writing process is to formulate a learning and action plan based on the insights gained from the reflection and analysis. This includes identifying areas for improvement, setting goals for future practice, and considering how to apply the lessons learned in upcoming clinical encounters.

IMPLEMENTATION OF REFLECTIVE WRITING IN MEDICAL EDUCATION

Curriculum Integration

Incorporating reflective writing into the medical school curriculum requires intentional design. Faculty can integrate reflective writing assignments into various courses, such as clinical skills, ethics, and patient care. These assignments can take the form of journals, essays, or structured reflections following clinical experiences.

Structured Reflection Frameworks

Providing students with structured reflection frameworks can enhance the effectiveness of the reflective writing process. Frameworks, such as Gibbs' Reflective Cycle or Schön's Reflection-in-Action can guide students through the stages of reflection and analysis, making the process more systematic and meaningful.[4]

Peer and Faculty Feedback

Encouraging peer reviews and faculty feedback can enrich the reflective writing experience. Sharing reflections in small groups fosters a supportive environment where students can learn from each other's experiences. Faculty feedback can provide guidance and encouragement, helping students to articulate their thoughts more clearly and effectively.

E-Portfolios

The use of e-portfolios in medical education offers a platform for students to document their reflective writing alongside their academic and clinical achievements. E-portfolios can serve as a comprehensive record of their learning journey, allowing them to track their progress and reflect on their growth over time.

BENEFITS OF REFLECTIVE WRITING IN MEDICAL EDUCATION

Improved Clinical Competence

Research shows that reflective writing correlates with improved clinical competence. As students engage in reflective practice, they become more adept at problem-solving, decision-making, and applying theoretical knowledge to real-world contexts.[5]

Enhanced Communication Skills

Writing reflections fosters better communication skills. Medical professionals must convey complex information clearly and empathetically to patients and colleagues. Reflective writing helps students practice articulating their thoughts, ultimately enhancing their ability to communicate effectively in the clinical setting.

Increased Self-Awareness

Reflective writing encourages self-awareness by prompting students to explore their values, motivations, and biases. This self-awareness is critical in fostering an understanding of how personal experiences and beliefs influence clinical practice, thereby promoting more mindful and considerate patient care.

Psychological Well-Being

The act of reflecting can serve as a stress-relief mechanism. Medical education is often associated with high levels of stress and emotional turmoil. Reflective writing provides an outlet for students to process their feelings, helping them to manage stress and prevent burnout.

CHALLENGES OF REFLECTIVE WRITING

Time Constraints

One of the significant challenges in implementing reflective writing in medical education is the time required for students to engage meaningfully in the process. The demanding nature of medical studies often leaves little room for self-reflection, making it difficult for students to prioritize reflective writing among their many responsibilities.

Variability in Reflection Quality

The quality of reflective writing can vary significantly among students. Some may struggle to articulate their thoughts, while others may provide superficial reflections. Educators play a crucial role in guiding students to develop their reflective writing skills and encouraging deep and meaningful engagement with the process.

Resistance to Reflective Practices

Some medical students may resist reflective writing, viewing it as an additional burden rather than a valuable learning tool. Overcoming this skepticism involves highlighting the benefits and providing clear guidance on how to approach reflective writing effectively.

THE ROLE OF EDUCATORS IN REFLECTIVE WRITING

Facilitating Reflection

Educators must take an active role in facilitating reflective writing by creating a safe and supportive environment that encourages open dialogue about experiences. This can involve providing prompts, guiding questions, and examples of effective reflective writing.

Offering Support and Guidance

Providing support and guidance is essential for helping students navigate the reflective writing process. This can include workshops on reflective writing techniques, feedback on written reflections, and individual meetings to discuss students' thoughts and insights.

Modeling Reflective Practice

Educators themselves must model reflective practice. By sharing their own reflections on teaching and clinical experiences, faculty can demonstrate the value of reflection and inspire students to engage in their reflective writing.

CONCLUSION

Reflective writing is an invaluable component of medical education, promoting critical thinking, empathy, and lifelong learning among future healthcare professionals. By intentionally integrating reflective writing into the curriculum, providing structured frameworks for reflection, and offering support for students, educators can cultivate a culture of reflection that enhances both personal and professional growth.

As the medical landscape continues to change, the ability to reflect on experiences will remain a vital skill for healthcare providers. By committing to reflective practices, medical students can become more competent, compassionate, and self-aware practitioners, ultimately improving patient care and contributing positively to the healthcare system. The journey of medical education is not solely about acquiring knowledge; it is also about developing the reflective capacity to apply that knowledge effectively in the service of others.

Summary points

- Reflection writing is the most common form of reflective practice in medical education. It is one of the distinct approaches to achieve integrated learning.
- It is a part of student-centered learning, action research, and experiential learning.
- Incorporating reflective writing into the medical school curriculum requires intentional design.
- Research shows that reflective writing correlates with improved clinical competence.
- By committing to reflective practices, medical students can become more competent, compassionate, and self-aware practitioners.

REFERENCES

1. Wear D, Zarconi J, Garden R, et al. Reflection in/and writing: pedagogy and practice in medical education. Acad Med. 2012;87(5):603-9.
2. Shapiro J, Kasman D, Shafer A. Words and wards: a model of reflective writing and its uses in medical education. J Med Humanit. 2006;27(4):231-44.
3. Lim JY, Ong SY, Ng CY, et al. A systematic scoping review of reflective writing in medical education. BMC Med Educ. 2023;23(1):12.
4. Song P, Stewart R. Reflective writing in medical education. Med Teach. 2012;34(11):955-6.
5. Wald HS, Reis SP. Beyond the margins: reflective writing and development of reflective capacity in medical education. J Gen Intern Med. 2010;25:746-9.

CHAPTER 33

Educational Network and Growth

Chandra Mohan Kumar, Richie Dalai

INTRODUCTION

Recent advancements in technology have influenced teaching and learning methods. This has led to an amalgamation of older techniques of dissemination of knowledge with the newer techniques that make use of social media for educational purposes. Social networking refers to content creation and dissemination by the users to a group of people using applications which are internet based.[1] It consists of people with shared interests. Using this social networking with the aim of providing education is called "Educational Networking". This leads to mutual benefit for all those who are involved, the teachers as well as the students. Networking in medical education is, however, not just limited to usage of social media alone. It can refer to any platform where there occurs interconnection between students, teachers, and others, either directly or indirectly, with the common goal of dissemination of knowledge. Moreover, such platforms allow medical educators to also take help from experts in their respective fields for professional growth and development.

COMMON PLATFORMS FOR NETWORKING AND GROWTH IN MEDICAL EDUCATION

Blogs

These refer to "web logs" which are either written by a single author or a group of authors regarding a particular field. These may contain embedded videos, links, literature review, images, and interactive polls or puzzles. They are stored chronologically, with the latest information appearing on the top. They allow interaction between the authors and the readers who can post comments. One of the modern world examples is the British Medical Journal blogs (https://blogs.bmj.com/). These blogs provide an insight into the minds of the readers of the journal articles and their point of view. These posts help the dissemination of current materials and hot topics. However, there can be a few limitations of blogs, these being propagation of information that may be biased, presence of materials that have not been updated for a long time, and accuracy of the information provided.[2]

Wikis

These refer to websites which allow the content to be altered by anyone. They can help in dissemination of knowledge but are prone to inaccuracies due to lack of peer review. One of the examples for medical educational purposes, includes flu-wiki (https://www.fluwikie.com/) that provided myriad subtopics related to symptoms, vaccination, and treatment of various forms of influenza.[2]

Podcasts/YouTube

These platforms help in dissemination of multimedia content created to cater to a specific audience. One of the modern world examples is the YouTube channel "Preterm Baby Package" which has over 216 videos on various aspects of care of a preterm neonate, including topics on essential and sick newborn care (https://www.youtube.com/@pretermbabypackage6710). Various experts in the field of neonatology teach different topics in a pointwise manner and as short videos which are easy to recall. The main advantage is that the learners can access these videos at their own convenience and run them at their own pace of understanding by pausing wherever necessary. However, there is limited scope for interaction between the learners and the teachers.[2]

Social Bookmarking

These platforms like Mendeley (https://www.mendeley.com/?interaction_required=true) are meant for researchers and teachers to upload, share, and store data in the form of research papers, blog articles, news articles, etc., and disseminate the same in their community.[2]

Social Media

These refer to web-based platforms which allow interaction between like-minded people and to share content in a brief manner. Examples include "Twitter" and "Facebook" which are similar but yet different from each other. Twitter allows microblogging up to 140 characters, and the followers (people who follow a person) can see the contents. The account holder has no control over who can follow them. Facebook on the other hand has specific people called "friends" who can access the content posted by a specific person, based on the level of visibility of the post.[3] Both platforms have played a great role in recent times for dissemination of current research topics, multimedia, educational links, etc. The main advantage is that the learners can freely interact with the content creators or teachers for quick clarification of their questions. Major registries and journals also have now developed their Facebook and Twitter accounts. One such example is the International Standard Randomized Control Trial Number (ISRCTN) registry's account on twitter which posts small microblogs on recent trial protocols which are registered in the registry (https://x.com/ISRCTN). The ISRCTN is an international registry for randomized trials which is recognized by the World Health Organization (WHO) and the International Committee of Medical Journal Editors (ICMJE) (https://www.isrctn.com/). Its Twitter handle helps clinicians to remain updated with the ongoing trials in their respective fields.

Another platform called "Sermo" is a social media platform which is basically designed for doctors. Its usage is however limited to physicians in the United States of America.[2] LinkedIn is another such platform which is open for usage but is mainly used for business interactions rather than for dissemination of knowledge. "Curofy", "Docplexus", and "DailyRounds" are other such platforms developed for doctors for discussing critical cases.

Mobile Applications

Communities, such as "WhatsApp Groups" and "Telegram Groups" have paved the way forward to fast and easy interaction between various stakeholders of medical education and help in easy sharing of teaching materials. These methods allow interactions and debates between various experts of a field. The major problem is limited interaction due to the small physical size of a mobile screen.

However, importing these applications to computers is now possible for better interaction.

E-Learning

In the post-COVID era, many online courses and modules have come into picture which have revolutionized remote learning. One of these courses is ONTOP-IN (Online Neonatal Training Orientation Program-In India) which is meant for dissemination of evidence-based practices among pediatricians and nursing officers for continuing medical education in neonatology.

Some online software also allow live interaction between teachers and students. One of the examples is "CANVAS" which combines the features of live online teaching sessions with recorded lectures, and other multimedia content on specific learning topics (https://www.instructure.com/en-au/canvas). It also allows comments from the students and teachers. It allows integration of other software like "iThenticate", "Zoom", and various resource links into itself for better accessibility by the participants on a single learning platform.

Also, there is a lot of scope of taking online assessments or e-assessments. These are computer-aided tests which may be in the form of multiple choice questions, virtual OSCE stations, behavior/attitude based assessments, etc. The advantages of such a form of assessment include less need for physical travel, the participants can also appear for these assessments from the ease of their homes. They can allow instant marking and feedback. However, the disadvantages include a risk of technical failure and inadequate invigilation.[4]

Other resources include e-libraries, like HOLLIS which is the e-library of Harvard Medical School, that has access to multiple databases and online educational materials at a common platform. However, it is open only for students who are enrolled in any courses in the Harvard Medical School (https://library.harvard.edu/).

Virtual Simulations

Computer-based simulations of patients and scenarios are increasingly being used to improve the problem-solving abilities and practical skills of medical students who act on various roles and make virtual decisions.[4] These platforms are also being employed to allow the medical students to perform various procedures, such as central like insertion and intubation virtually and act as adjuncts to the classical method of bedside teaching for procedures. A few examples of such virtual reality simulations among many include "MediSimVR", "MEDVR", "GAPER", etc. The advantages include learning through virtual scenarios without any actual real-life threat to the patients. The main disadvantage is that this field is still in its infancy. Many models, especially for smaller infants and neonates for various procedures, are yet not available.

Research Collaboration Networks

These include a consortium of medical educational institutions with the main aim of facilitation of multisite research. Important examples of such networks include the following:

- *Center for the Advancement of Healthcare Education and delivery (C-AHEAD)*: It consists of three medical schools, which mainly focuses on family medicine.
- *Continuity Research Network (CORNET)*: Sponsored by the Academic Pediatric Association, with focus on pediatrics resident education.

- *Longitudinal Educational Assessment Research Network (APPD LEARN)*: Sponsored by the Association of Pediatric Program Directors, with focus on pediatric education in the United States.[5]

Another such network is the ResearchGate Network which allows scientists and researchers of various fields to post their articles (journal articles, book chapters, and conference presentation) to a common platform and allows interaction to a certain extent in the form of options for sending messages or full-text requests to the concerned authors (https://www.researchgate.net/). It has a specific feature of creating a "Research Spotlight", which allows the users to prominently exhibit their articles to their followers, which earns these articles more readership and citations.

POTENTIAL PITFALLS

The different forms of platforms for dissemination of medical education through web have their own pitfalls, which have been described under individual headings discussed earlier. Apart from these there remains the problem of accessibility to these platforms which still remains a major problem for various medical educators and students, due to differences in age, race, ethnicity, social class, gender, and specifically in the low resource settings in low-middle income countries.[6] Additionally, cost may act as an impediment in accessing educational networks that are not free. Hence, to allow equality in dissemination of knowledge, it is important that educators of the current era understand these difficulties and promote usage of their educational networks by the students in the low economic or remotest areas through free or subsidized educational resource materials and provide scholarships to the meritorious students from poverty-stricken backgrounds. One such example is FAIMER (Foundation for Advancement of International Medical Education and Research), which allows participants to have a part-time fellowship in medical education methods and leadership. It has a 3-week residential session in the United States followed by a 11-month distance learning program. The participants can also apply for scholarships.[7]

Another issue that plagues usage of these platforms is the "conflict of interest" and the same should be disclosed, if any. Ethical concerns including informed patients' consents should also be obtained if their medical information is being shared for educational purposes.

CONCLUSION

The various networking platforms in the modern day have upscaled learning and dissemination of knowledge in medical education. This has not only lead to improvement in the knowledge of the students but also in that of the medical educators. Though accessibility still remains a major concern, availability of scholarships can bridge the gap in developing countries and allow a more large-scale audience of medical professionals.

Statements

- *Ethics statement*: This article does not involve any human participants. It does not require any ethics approval.

- *Conflict of interest*: None declared.
- *Funding*: None declared.

REFERENCES

1. Latif M, Hussain I, Saeed R, et al. Use of Smart Phones and Social Media in Medical Education: Trends, Advantages, Challenges and Barriers. Acta Inform Med. 2019;27(2):133.

2. Sparks MA, O'Seaghdha CM, Sethi SK, et al. Embracing the Internet as a Means of Enhancing Medical Education in Nephrology. Am J Kidney Dis. 2011;58(4):512-8.
3. Mishra S. Looking for Medical Advice in Everyday Digital Spaces: A Qualitative Study of Indians Connecting with Physicians on Facebook. Vikalpa. 2021;46(2):86-98.
4. Ellaway R, Masters K. AMEE Guide 32: e-Learning in medical education Part 1: Learning, teaching and assessment. Med Teach. 2008;30(5):455-73.
5. Schwartz A, Young R, Hicks PJ, et al. Medical education practice-based research networks: Facilitating collaborative research. Med Teach. 2016;38(1):64-74.
6. Salib S, Hudson FP. Networking in Academic Medicine: Keeping an Eye on Equity. J Grad Med Educ. 2023;15(3):306-8.
7. Burdick W, Morahan P, Norcini J. Capacity Building in Medical Education and Health Outcomes in Developing Countries: The Missing Link. Educ Health. 2007;20(3):65.

CHAPTER

34 Scholarship and Publications

Akash Bang, Anant Khot

INTRODUCTION

Academic advancement is an ongoing, cyclical process that encompasses gaining subject expertise, engaging in continuous and critical self-evaluation of one's professional practices, and actively contributing to the health professions education (HPE) community. Scholarship in HPE refers to a rigorous and reflective process of inquiry aimed at improving the teaching, learning, and assessment in HPE.[1] Traditionally, skills needed for scholarship in medical education are not a part of medical training.[2] Hence, this chapter aims to discuss scholarship in itself, and publications as the outcome of scholarship.

WHAT IS SCHOLARSHIP?

To be considered as a scholarly activity, it must satisfy five criteria, called the **five Ps**:

1. *Product* of high quality
2. Whose *Process* is explained
3. *Peer*-reviewed
4. Placed under the *Public* domain
5. Which serves as a *Platform* for further work.

In the past, research was the sole criterion that met all the necessary standards and was deemed the pinnacle of scholarly achievement.[3] Boyer challenged this notion, questioning why research alone was considered scholarship and no other equally important activities like teaching or clinical work. He subsequently proposed four distinct categories of scholarship.

1. *Scholarship of discovery*: In medical education, the scholarship of discovery is an invigorating endeavor that employs scientific methodology to reveal new insights. This approach is characterized by its hypothesis-driven nature and deductive reasoning. Findings from such research are typically disseminated through peer-reviewed publications, academic presentations, and research grants.
2. *Scholarship of teaching and learning (SoTL)*: The methodical examination of education and knowledge acquisition employs established scholarly criteria to explore how instruction (including beliefs, actions, mindsets, and principles) can enhance learning outcomes and foster a deeper comprehension of the learning process. This approach yields outcomes that are openly disseminated for evaluation and application by relevant professional communities.[4]
3. *Scholarship of application*: The application scholarship involves activities that bridge the gap between theoretical knowledge and practical implementation, or employ expertise to tackle real-world issues. This form of scholarship can be demonstrated through various means, such as giving public talks, providing

academic advice, managing a simulation center, or directing a clinical internship or graduate-level residency program.

4. *Scholarship of integration*: The scholarship of integration encompasses innovative syntheses, evaluations, or examinations that establish "links between disciplines" or apply fresh perspectives to existing research. This scholarship form aims to interpret, examine, and consolidate original research outcomes or creative endeavors. Examples of integrative scholarship include review articles, reports on clinical cases, and chapters or entire books.

   Combining the writings of noted scholars like Shulman L, Barker DWM, Willox AC, and Dale provides a more expansive discussion, including a fifth component —the Scholarships of Engagement and Learning, to the above list of four categories pf scholarships.

5. *Engagement (public scholarship)*: Public scholarship refers to academic endeavors that generate novel insights through scholarly reflection on community engagement. This approach combines research, teaching, and service, challenging the notion that valuable knowledge only flows from universities to the broader community. Instead, it acknowledges that practical application in real-world settings and creates new understanding, enhancing the educational and investigative missions of academic institutions. The goal of public scholarship extends beyond publishing in specialized academic journals or accumulating citations in faculty works, aiming for a more widespread impact.

These categories of scholarships can be remembered with the acronym "DETAIL" which stands for Discovery, Engagement, Teaching, Application, Integration and Learning.

PRODUCTS OF SCHOLARSHIP

The products of scholarship in HPE range widely. While a peer-reviewed research article is widely recognized as the primary scholarly output, HPE offers various other avenues for significant academic contributions. These include authoring book chapters, full-length books, monographs, or edited volumes. Additionally, scholars can produce essays, opinion pieces, editorials, book reviews, and letters. In the educational realm, case reports, conference summaries, teaching materials, descriptions of instructional methods, and curriculum outlines are valuable. Furthermore, alternative publication formats such as videos, simulators, and online tutorials also serve as important scholarly works in HPE. All scholarships should be guided and judged by following Glassick's six core principles of excellence for scholarship.[5,6]

Glassick's Criteria for Scholarship

1. *Clear goals*:
   a. Has the study's primary purpose been clearly defined by the investigator?
   b. Are the researcher's objectives both feasible and realistic?
   c. Does the study tackle important questions within the researcher's area of expertise?
2. *Adequate preparation, to include understanding of prior scholarship*:
   a. Is the researcher demonstrating a grasp of current academic literature in their field?
   b. Has the researcher acquired the appropriate expertise for their study?
   c. Is the researcher able to gather the essential resources to advance their project?

3. *Approaches aligned with the objectives and building upon previous research*:
   a. Are the researcher's methodologies aligned with their objectives?
   b. Is the researcher implementing the chosen methods effectively?
   c. Does the researcher adapt their procedures when faced with changing circumstances?
4. *Results that are meaningful and honest*:
   a. Has the researcher accomplished their intended objectives?
   b. Does the researcher's contribution significantly advance the field of study?
   c. Does the researcher's work create new avenues for future investigation?
5. *Dissemination of results with clear, organized presentation*:
   a. Is the academic's writing style and organizational approach appropriate for presenting their research?
   b. Has the researcher chosen suitable platforms to communicate their findings to the intended audience?
   c. Does the scholar convey their message clearly and with academic integrity?
6. *Reflective critique in the context of prior scholarship and study limitations*:
   a. Can the investigator objectively evaluate their own study?
   b. Does the researcher consider a wide enough spectrum of data in their examination?
   c. Does the researcher use assessment to improve the standard of their subsequent work?

According to Glassick's scholarship criteria, it is essential to examine existing research and select methods that align with your project's objectives in relation to previous work. This necessitates planning for scholarly activities before implementing new curricula, evaluation tools, faculty training sessions, or initiatives to promote well-being.

THINK PROSPECTIVELY, NOT RETROSPECTIVELY

Attempting to retroactively apply assessments or outcomes to an already completed educational activity or survey can result in significant shortcomings.[7] The issues that may arise in such situations include:

- Lack of power analysis
- Selection of outcome measures based on convenience rather than appropriateness for the intervention
- Improper classification of open-ended responses as qualitative research without following rigorous methodologies
- Insufficient testing of self-developed surveys
- Failure to analyze individuals who did not respond or participate

Micro-scholarship: It is characterized as the method of revealing the tiniest accessible and evaluable steps that chronicle an academic journey, which can subsequently be compiled and exhibited as a product of scholarly work. This concept functions as both a result and a procedure, involving the repetitive and gradual creation of various micro-assets that can be united and regarded as conventional "scholarship".[8]

CONDUCTING SCHOLARLY RESEARCH

Academic research follows a cyclical and repetitive pattern rather than a linear progression. This ongoing process involves continuous review, evaluation, and examination, often requiring multiple iterations. While this approach can be time-consuming and demanding, scholars can gain in-depth knowledge of their field and

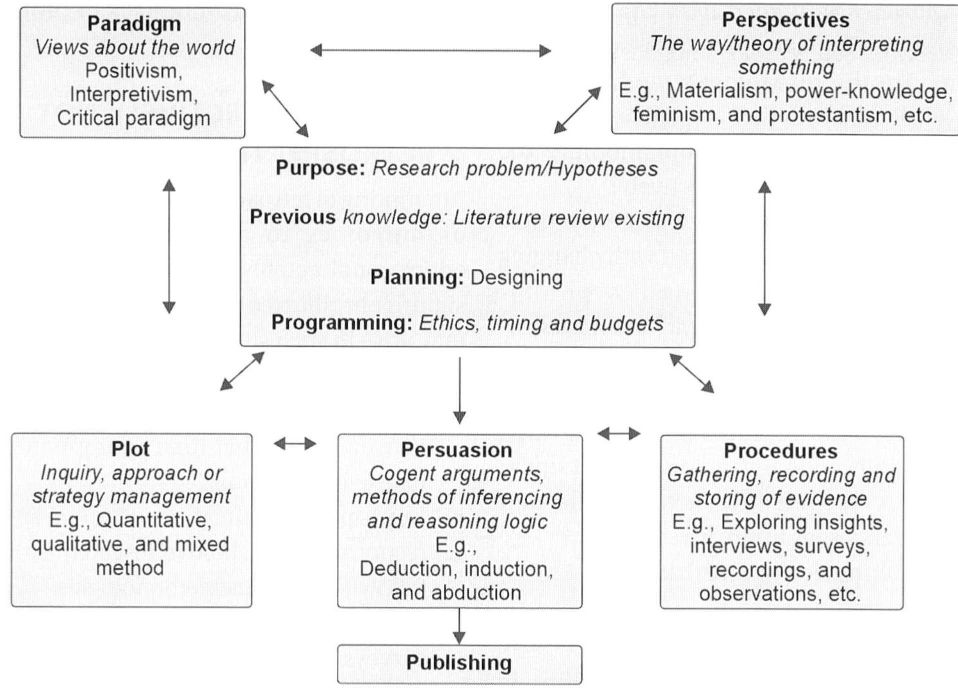

Fig. 1: The 10 elements of the research process (10Ps)

Source: Reproduced with permission from the author; Saliya CA. Doing Social Research and Publishing Results: A Guide to Non-Native English Speakers. Singapore: Springer Nature Singapore; 2022.

produce publishable works such as articles, commentaries, or case studies. The rigorous nature of this method is crucial for generating high-quality academic output. The circular nature of research necessitates constant refinement and reassessment, contributing to the development of expertise and the creation of scholarly contributions that meet publication standards.[14] The ten elements in the research process are summarized in **Figure 1**.

Medical Education Research (MER) can address five types of research questions:[2]

1. *Descriptive*: Descriptive research aims to document and characterize phenomena as they exist without manipulation. It answers the "what" questions and provides a foundation for further research. Descriptive studies often use surveys, observational methods, or secondary data analysis to generate baseline data; e.g., how do medical students view the incorporation of artificial intelligence (AI) into their educational program?
2. *Explanatory*: Explanatory research aims to uncover the causal relationships and underlying mechanisms of observed phenomena. It explores the "why" and "how" behind the processes and outcomes in education. These studies frequently utilize experimental designs, such as randomized controlled trials and longitudinal studies; e.g., how does mentorship impact the career choices of postgraduate medical trainees?
3. *Exploratory*: Exploratory research is used to investigate new or poorly understood areas, often generating hypotheses for

future studies. It seeks to understand potential connections and the uncharted regions of medical education. Exploratory research frequently employs qualitative approaches, including one-on-one interviews, group discussions, and analysis of recurring themes; e.g., what are the challenges faculty face in adopting competency-based medical education (CBME) frameworks?

4. *Predictive*: It focuses on forecasting outcomes based on existing data or variables. It often answers "what will happen if" scenarios and involves statistical modeling or machine learning approaches. Predictive studies often utilize regression analysis, predictive modeling, or AI-based tools; e.g., can academic performance in the first year predict success in clinical rotations?
5. *Evaluative*: It examines the effectiveness or impact of educational programs, interventions, or policies. It addresses questions such as "Does it work?" or "How effective is it?"; e.g., does introducing a flipped classroom model improve examination scores among medical students? This type of research typically uses mixed methods, incorporating both qualitative and quantitative approaches to assess outcomes.[10]

All scholarly work must be publicly disseminated to make it accessible to the broader academic community and beyond. Effective dissemination strategies include:

- Publishing in peer-reviewed journals
- Presenting at conferences
- Writing books and book chapters
- *Engaging in public outreach*: Sharing research findings with the general public through popular media outlets, promoting public understanding of scientific research and its societal impact
- *Using social media and online platforms*: Leveraging online tools to reach a wider audience and engage in dialogue with peers, disseminating research findings in accessible and engaging formats; the chosen dissemination strategy should align with the research topic, the target audience, and the intended impact of the work.

The types of articles commonly published in biomedical journals are depicted in **Figure 2**.

According to the AMEE (Association of Medical Education in Europe) guidelines, publishing scholarly work in HPE requires specific knowledge, skills, and actions.

- *What is important and reportable*: When determining whether a manuscript should progress in the editorial process, editors often employ the "Who cares?" criterion. This assessment evaluates whether the paper offers a meaningful contribution to the field or merely reiterates existing information.
- *Planning and preparation*: A meticulously designed and implemented research study typically results in a high-quality manuscript. Aspiring authors should investigate whether their intended research or review article type has established reporting guidelines to follow; e.g., Strengthening the Reporting of Observational Studies in Epidemiology (STROBE) Statement for observational studies and PRISMA (Preferred Reporting Items for Systematic Reviews and Meta-Analyses) statement for reporting systematic reviews.
- *Discipline of writing*: Academic writing requires a set of skill sets, and they will aim for clarity and simplicity. Academic writing is often done in three stages:
  1. Framing the structure of a report or manuscript: Most published articles

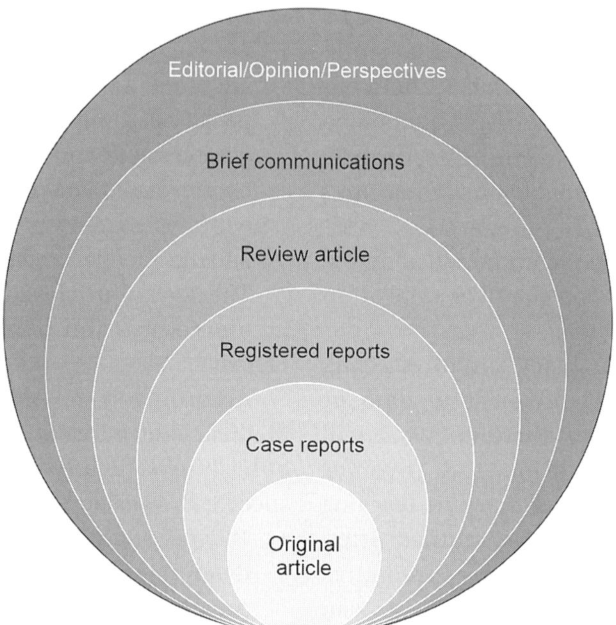

Fig. 2: Types of articles published in the scientific journals.

follow the Introduction, Materials and Methods, Results and Discussion (IMRaD) structure as suggested by Sir Austin Bradford Hill, and journal length limits.

2. Formulate the arguments by writing the "big picture" about the topic of a manuscript.
3. Edit and improve an early draft.

- *Manuscript quality*: The composition of a high-quality manuscript is not a fortuitous occurrence. It is the result of diligent effort, structured writing practices, and peer review. Authors should meticulously attend to manuscript details before submission for publication consideration. Furthermore, authors are advised to peruse and adhere to the recommendations for the Conduct, Reporting, Editing and Publication of Scholarly Work in Medical Journals (ICMJE Recommendations).
- *Manuscript submission and sequelae*: Once a manuscript is finished, the next step involves choosing a suitable journal and submitting the work. The dissemination of academic knowledge depends on publishing articles in scholarly journals, which is also essential for researchers' professional growth. Thus, when deciding on a publication venue, researchers must carefully consider various aspects, such as the journal's focus, availability of open-access options, and impact indicators. In December 2016, the International Committee of Medical Journal Editors (ICMJE) issued updated guidelines for authors: "An increasing number of organizations are marketing themselves as 'medical journals' without functioning as such *predatory journals*."[11] These pseudo-journals accept and publish nearly all submissions and impose article processing (or publication) fees, often

notifying authors about these charges after accepting a paper. They frequently claim to conduct peer review but fail to do so and may intentionally use names resembling those of established journals. The ICMJE advised authors: "When submitting manuscripts, researchers have an obligation to assess the credibility, background, methods, and standing of the journals they choose. It is incumbent upon writers to scrutinize these aspects of potential publication venues before sending their work." It is also best to avoid unsolicited mails with inadequate information regarding the journal or its publishing policies. Seeking advice from experienced colleagues/mentors or the institute's academic wing may be useful in this regard. Various resources which can help an author in identifying predatory journals have been listed below along with weblink for few of them.

- Beall's list: https://beallslist.net/
- Cabell's Scholarly Analytics platform: https://cabells.com/
- Checklists: https://thinkchecksubmit.org/
- https://www.wame.org/identifying-predatory-or-pseudo-journals
- https://ugccare.unipune.ac.in/Apps1/Home/Index

The publishing process of a submitted manuscript varies from publisher to publisher. Most of the journals are using Journal Manuscript Management Systems for submission and peer review of the articles. After choosing the journal, do the formatting of the manuscript according to the journal style requirement. It may be helpful to have a similarity test before submitting a manuscript to a journal. Prepare the covering letter and submit the version of the manuscript agreed by all the authors.

- *Manuscript review*: Once a manuscript is submitted to a journal by its corresponding author, it will be sent for peer-reviewing if the editor decides it is worth reviewing. If the editor identifies the underlying problem, the manuscript will be rejected. This is called desk review and desk rejection. If the editor finds that the basic criteria of a manuscript have been met and it does not have major deficiencies, he decides to select peer-reviewers. Peer reviewers often consist of one member of the journal's editorial board or recently published scholars. Single-blind review is sometimes used if the author is more powerful than the reviewer. Other forms of peer review include double-blind review and open review. Peer reviewers read the manuscript and critically review its novelty, contribution, clarity, relevance, originality, scholarly findings, validity of the methodology, interesting analysis, and strong arguments. Reviewers recommend whether the publication of the manuscript should be accepted or rejected.
- *Writing in English*: "How to write an English medical manuscript that will be published and have an impact" by Tompson A[12] has the following suggestions for writing the articles:
    - Convey one concept per sentence.
    - Group related ideas into paragraphs to improve readability.
    - Eliminate unnecessary words and phrases.
    - Choose the most succinct and clear expressions.
    - Write assertively, preferring active voice.
    - Avoid ambiguity.
    - Maintain consistent grammar throughout.

- Use verb tenses uniformly.
- Refrain from redundant repetition of facts and data in your manuscript.
- Opt for concise yet precise language.
- Craft your abstract after analyzing and interpreting your results.
- Devote special attention to your title, as it is the most crucial word arrangement in your entire paper.

An essential but overlooked aspect of the scholarly publication is publication ethics. Ethics of scientific publications is a system of norms of professional behavior in the relations between authors, reviewers, editors, publishers, and readers in creating, distributing, and using scientific publications.[13] Key ethical considerations in scholarly publication include:

- Plagiarism
- Data fabrication and falsification
- Authorship issues or disputes
- Conflict of interest
- Redundant and duplicate publication
- Publication in predatory journals

Ethical standards for research conduct and publication are now established through guidelines that aim to foster and uphold integrity in research practices and scholarly output.[8] Some organizations give recommendations and develop guidelines to assist authors, editors, and reviewers. The organizations involved with publication ethics are ICMJE, the World Association of Medical Editors (WAME) and the Committee on Publication Ethics (COPE). In India, the Indian Council of Medical Research (ICMR) policy on research integrity and publication ethics is in place to ensure the highest professional and ethical standards for biomedical and health research at all stages right from its inception, conduct, review, reporting and publication.

Measuring scholarly impact: Metrics used to assess scholarly impact include:

- *Citations*: The number of times a publication is cited by other researchers, indicating its influence and relevance within the field.
- *Altmetrics*: Alternative metrics that capture the broader impact of research, such as social media mentions, news coverage, and policy documents.
- *Fuzzy metrics*: Noncitation-based bibliometrics
- *Research grants and funding*: The level of funding secured for research projects, demonstrating the value and importance of the work[12]
- *Awards and recognition*: Receiving awards or recognition from professional organizations or institutions, indicating the quality and impact of research contributions
- *Public engagement and outreach*: The extent to which research findings are disseminated to the public and their impact on policy decisions or public discourse.[14]

Common Barriers to Scholarship and Publication

- Lack of clarity in the research question
- Inadequate methodology to assess the study question
- Losing momentum
- Lack of follow through
- Lack of expertise and formal training in research methodology
- Lack of financial support

Methods to Overcome those Barriers in Scholarship and Publication

- Identifying collaborators, either within your institution or outside the institution. Also, consider learners as potential collaborators.

- *Identify a team of mentors*: Effective mentorship results in faculty who are more scholarly, promoted more quickly, and more likely to stay at their academic institution.
- *Develop your expertise*: Expand your knowledge and scholarly activity by attending workshops on scholarship-related topics, faculty development, education fellowships, and online courses.
- *Secure funding through funding agencies*: Funding sources for medical education scholarships include:[15]
  - International organizations:
    - Association of American Medical Colleges (AAMC)—Group on Educational Affairs (GEA) and Regional GEAs
    - National Board of Medical Examiners (NBME) Stemmler Grant
    - Patient-Centered Outcomes Research Institute (PCORI)
    - American Educational Research Association (AERA)
  - Foundations:
    - Josiah Macy Jr. Foundation
    - Arthur P. Gold Foundation
    - Alfred P. Sloan Foundation
    - W.K. Kellogg Foundation
    - Robert Wood Johnson (RWJ) Foundation
    - Spencer Foundation
- Providing training on case report writing earlier in the medical school curriculum could foster greater interest among medical students in writing case reports during their clinical clerkships.
- *Get involved in national organizations*: Professional organizations allow you to present your work, network, learn what others are doing, and reenergize and motivate you to achieve in your areas of interest.

CONCLUSION

- Scholarship in HPE is a reflective and systematic process to enhance teaching, learning, and assessment.
- It encompasses rigorous inquiry and dissemination of results while adhering to criteria such as quality, peer review, public accessibility, and fostering further exploration.
- HPE scholarship produces diverse outputs, from peer-reviewed research articles to innovative educational tools and reviews.
- Practical scholarship is guided by Glassick's six principles, emphasising clarity of goals, rigorous methodology, and meaningful dissemination.
- Publication success hinges on disciplined planning, adherence to structured formats like IMRaD, and ethical conduct, including avoidance of predatory journals. Peer review serves as a critical quality filter.
- Dissemination strategies span journals, conferences, and public outreach, focusing on maximising societal and academic impact.
- Scholarly metrics such as citations, altmetrics, and grants measure impact, while barriers like methodological gaps and lack of mentorship can hinder progress.
- Overcoming these requires collaboration, mentorship, skill-building workshops, and institutional support.
- High ethical standards ensure the credibility of scholarship in advancing medical education.

REFERENCES

1. Mcgaghie WC. Scholarship, publication, and career advancement in health professions

education: AMEE Guide No. 43. Med Teach. 2009;31(7):574-90.
2. Adkoli BV. Educational Research and Scholarship in India: The Way Forward. Indian Pediatr. 2023;60(7):577-80.
3. Cleland JA, Jamieson S, Kusurkar RA, et al. Redefining scholarship for health professions education: AMEE Guide No. 142. Med. Teach. 2021;43(7):824-38.
4. Cameron MW, Crowther LN, Huang GC. Faculty Development and Infrastructure to Support Educational Scholarship: A Scoping Review on Author Development. Acad Med. 2023;98(1):112-22.
5. Bockrath R, Osman C, Trainor J, Wang HC, Phatak UP, Richards DG, et al. Education Scholarship Assessment Reconsidered: Expansion of Glassick's Criteria to Incorporate Health Equity. Academic Medicine. 2024 May 1;99(5):487–92.
6. Crites GE, Gaines JK, Cottrell S, Kalishman S, Gusic M, Mavis B, et al. Medical education scholarship: An introductory guide: AMEE Guide No. 89. Med. Teach. 2014;36(8):657–74.
7. Sullivan GM. A Toolkit for Medical Education Scholarship. J. Grad. Med. Educ. 2018 Feb;10(1):1–5.
8. Goh PS, Roberts-Lieb S, Sandars J. Micro-Scholarship: An innovative approach for the first steps for Scholarship in Health Professions Education. Med. Teach. 2023;45(3):307–12.
9. Saliya CA. The 10 Elements of Academic Research (10Ps). In: Saliya CA, editor. Doing Social Research and Publishing Results: A Guide to Non-native English Speakers [Internet]. Singapore: Springer Nature Singapore; 2022. p. 45–52. Available from: https://doi.org/10.1007/978-981-19-3780-4_5.
10. Ringsted C, Hodges B, Scherpbier A. "The research compass": An introduction to research in medical education: AMEE Guide No. 56. Med. Teach. 2011 Sep;33(9):695–709.
11. Singhal S, Kalra BS. Publication ethics: Role and responsibility of authors. Indian J Gastroenterol. 2021 Feb;40(1):65-71
12. Tompson A. How to write an English medical manuscript that will be published and have impact. Surg Today. 2006;36(5):407-9. doi: 10.1007/s00595-005-3170-9. PMID: 16633745.
13. Yadav SK. Publication ethics. In: Yadav SK editor. Research and Publication Ethics. New Delhi: Springer with Ane Books Pvt. Ltd; 2023.p.109-209.
14. Gruppen LD, Durning SJ. Needles and haystacks: finding funding for medical education research. Acad Med 2016;91:480–4.
15. Ross PT. Pursuing Scholarship: Educating Faculty and Students on How to Publish Their Academic Work. In: Markovac J, Kleinman M, Englesbe M, editors. Medical and Scientific Publishing [Internet]. Academic Press; 2018. p. 69–77. Available from: https://www.sciencedirect.com/science/article/pii/B9780128099698000085.

CHAPTER 35

Introduction to Artificial Intelligence

Kush D Jhunjhunwala, Aarushee Jhunjhunwala

INTRODUCTION

We all know that our medical education is a lifelong learning process, stretching from undergraduate to postgraduate, specialty training, superspecialty training, and beyond. Therefore, it is essential to acknowledge the immense role of artificial intelligence (AI) in medical education in this era of rapidly advancing technology.

Artificial intelligence is emerging as a powerful force in shaping the future of healthcare. With rapid technological advancements and the evolution of AI, it is becoming increasingly easier to detect diseases and develop more effective, advanced treatments. As healthcare methods continue to evolve, and the need to enhance medical education grows, there is an increasing demand to integrate newer technologies and innovative approaches to better prepare future healthcare professionals.

The field of AI and research is widely considered to have begun in the fifth decade by immense contribution of Dr Alan Turing and Dr John McCarthy. At that time, there were various names for the field of "thinking machines," including cybernetics and automata theory.

This concept and the ideas behind it inspired scientists to begin discussing the possibility of building an electronic artificial brain. The artificial brain was supposed to work like both software and hardware with cognitive abilities similar to those of the animal or human brain. Thus, "Artificial Intelligence" is a broad term that refers to technology that helps robots and computers to mimic human intellect. It is based on the belief that the functioning of humanly thoughts can be mechanized. It is a technology that primarily employs computer systems to imitate human thought processes.

The prominence of the field ebbed and flowed over the ensuing years, but by the late 1990s and early 2000s, AI had returned to the forefront by focusing on finding-specific solutions to specific problems rather than pursuing the original goal of creating versatile, fully intelligent machines. Today, faster computers and access to large amounts of data have enabled advances in machine learning and data-driven deep learning methods.

The rise of AI in last couple of years, carried by the ideas of development and transformation in architecture, leads to the rapid scaling and public release of large language models (LLMs) like ChatGPT and Chatbots. These models exhibit human-like traits of knowledge, attention, and creativity and have been integrated into various sectors, fueling exponential investment in AI. However, concerns about the potential risks and ethical implications of advanced AI have also emerged, which has sparked discussions about the future of AI and its effects on society.

As medical field cannot remain aloof in this ever-changing fast-pace world of technology, AI technology is rapidly evolving and reshaping the magnificent field of medicine, particularly through developments accelerated by COVID-19 pandemic, wherein telemedicine, online teaching, and online sharing of knowledge became a new normal.

The integration of AI in medicine and research offers significant potential, not just for enhancing educational approaches, but also for elevating patient care and quality of life. AI not only helps in diagnosis and treatment but also enhances the learning power of undergraduate students by providing personalized study materials, virtual simulations, through interactive 3D models, instant feedback, and more effective ways to understand complex concepts.

The application of AI includes chatbots, intelligent tutoring systems (ITSs), virtual reality system (VRS), enhanced engagement, medical distance learning and management, telemedicine, recording teaching videos in medical colleges, gamification, virtual patients, and simulation-based teaching and adaptive learning systems. Now, the medical students have all the information related to their education on their palms in the form of AI-driven smartphones and I-Pads.

Nowadays, programs like 3D organon provide highly detailed 3D model of the human body. All the emergency procedures routinely taught in emergency rooms can be virtually simulated, allowing medical students to gain hands-on experience in techniques, such as cardiopulmonary resuscitation and emergency medical care. AI has also transformed the field of radiology through applications like echopixel, which generate virtual 3D images, enabling X-rays and CT/MRI scans to be viewed at the click of a button. Even AIIMS, Delhi has developed AI software named MadhuNetrAI, wherein very early diagnosis of diabetic retinopathy with high accuracy can be done even before the development of signs and symptoms of the disease. Not a single branch of medical field has remained untouched by revolutionary world of AI technology.

Surgical robots are another fine example of supra-human precision using AI-driven technology, which has changed the world of surgical world in all super specialties. Now is the right time to incorporate this technology in our medical curriculum both in postgraduate and superspecialty courses. Advantages of incorporating AI in medical education are much more then quick evaluation of students, active learning strategies, learning at own leisure pace through distant learning, learning to handle emergencies effectively through simulation, horning skills multiple times on mannequins, and so on.

According to the National Medical Council (NMC), it is mandatory for all the medical colleges to have a Simulation Virtual Lab (SVL), where the students are trained on high-fidelity mannequins using AI-based algorithms and simulation technology. They can fine tune their skills on high-end mannequins multiple times.

Artificial intelligence has also helped in preparing multiple questions and answers bank where thousands of MCQ according to their difficulty levels as level 1, level 2, and level 3 are parked, so the educators can set question papers in click of button and at the same time assess them using optical mark recognition, thus evaluating large number of answer sheets in very short time. Over the past decade, AI has addressed several challenges in education, including language processing, planning, and cognitive modeling.

Traditional methods of assessment and evaluation can be time-consuming, involving manual grading and extensive feedback, which may hinder timely learning and make it difficult to cater to individual student needs. In contrast, AI streamlines these tasks by automating assessments, providing instant feedback, and efficiently tracking student progress, thereby enhancing learning outcomes. AI can also help in performing summative and formative assessment of the students in very effective way as per the curriculum of NMC-guided comprehensive-based medical education system. Rather than relying solely on traditional fact-based learning and clinical internships, academic institutions must also prioritize innovation and research. Skills like data literacy, statistical reasoning, and human empathy are becoming just as essential as clinical knowledge.

Artificial intelligence has significantly enhanced research in medical colleges by streamlining data collection, analysis, clinical trials, and the writing of theses and publications. As a result, traditional teaching methods, such as didactic lectures are being replaced by more interactive and learner-centered approaches. This shift has facilitated the comprehensive implementation of Competency-Based Medical Education (CBME) in medical colleges across the country.

Gaining adequate knowledge and skills regarding AI applications in medicine is crucial for both medical students as well as for medical teachers who may even have to use applications that did not exist during their education. Thus, it is the right time to rewrite the medical curriculum keeping in mind the need of the new age students to foster a better understanding of the numerous aspects of health care AI, both positive and negative. Therefore, AI systems should be incorporated into undergraduate medical education, postgraduate residency training, and continuing medical education programs to promote awareness of their appropriate use.

Developing curriculum proposals specifically designed to train future doctors on AI would be a valuable contribution in that regard. To do this effectively, educators and healthcare professionals must be equipped with right skills to integrate AI into curriculum design, teaching methods, and assessment practices.

Artificial intelligence is no longer just a topic for computer science, it is now relevant to every field, and medicine is no exception. Today's learners are growing up in a digital world where social connections and interactive learning are deeply valued. As AI becomes increasingly prevalent, all areas of education, including medical training, must adapt accordingly. In this highly connected era, medical education must evolve to keep pace with changes in healthcare, digital advancements, and expectations of new generation of students.

Medical students of the future will need to embrace a new model of education, one that keeps up with the fast-paced growth of technologies, such as AI and machine learning. Leave apart medical education, AI is now entering primary education space as well, wherein the storybooks are narrated by AI voice, children's drawings are corrected by algorithms, and writing prompts are generated automatically.

Today's professors are working with a generation of students who have instant access to answers at their fingertips, often missing out on the deeper understanding that develops through critical thinking, thoughtful reflection, and tackling complex problems. AI is no longer just assisting with assignments, it is generating essays, clinical scenarios by simulation, cost effectiveness, solving cases just on basis of symptomatology, differential diagnosis, giving accurate diagnosis, and even line of treatment plans in a structured and systemic manner. In response, educators must discover and implement appropriate teaching strategies that engage students and sustain the learners' attention and engagement.

On the other hand, overreliance on AI could lead to a decline in essential human interaction, which is important for building empathy, communication skills, and bedside manners. The overuse of AI also poses a significant risk of diminishing students' critical and innovative thinking. Therefore, it is essential to strike a balance between traditional teaching methods and AI-driven approaches. Addressing this issue, NMC has mandated the inclusion of Attitude, Ethics, and Communication Module (AETCOM) in medical curriculum.

Also important is to address challenges like educating the educators themselves through continuous training, infrastructure upgradation, pooling finances, technical issues, and plagiarism as well. At the same time, through the lens of the Hippocratic Oath, there is an ethical responsibility for medical educators, students, and practitioners to embrace AI where it proves effective, be it in promoting analytical thinking, improving diagnostic precision, or ensuring patient safety. When applied responsibly, AI can uphold the fundamental principle of medicine: "to help and do no harm".

CHAPTER 36

Teaching and Learning by Simulation

Shivaprakash Sosale C, Sagar V, Shilpa KL

Learning Objectives

- Define simulation-based medical education (SBME) and its role in pediatrics.
- Describe components, infrastructure, and technologies of a pediatric simulation center.
- Explain curriculum design principles and learning frameworks in pediatric SBME.
- Discuss uses, benefits, and clinical significance of simulation in pediatrics.
- Identify challenges, limitations, and future directions of pediatric SBME.

INTRODUCTION

Simulation-based medical education (SBME) is a type of experiential learning that utilizes simulation to replicate realistic clinical scenarios within a controlled setting. This approach allows trainees to develop both technical and nontechnical skills by engaging with their peers. It also provides them the opportunity to make mistakes in a safe environment and receive corrective feedback either from the simulator or a mentor. Simulation offers a safe environment where both confidence and competence can be continuously developed, with the ultimate goal of achieving excellence in patient care. Simulation has not only become an essential tool for comprehensive medical education, especially in pediatrics but also integrated into pediatric residency and fellowship training programs. Additionally, SBME can serve as a means to enhance the skills of more experienced professionals, such as neonatologists, or improve provider performance through real-time consultations with seasoned clinicians during simulated resuscitation scenarios via telemedicine. However, highly interactive, in-person SBME sessions are needed for procedural skills and teamwork behaviours.[1]

As clinicians and researchers, we are experiencing a significant expansion of diagnostic and prognostic tools, driven by the introduction of cutting-edge technologies, which are becoming increasingly accessible, even for studying rare and complex pediatric diseases. Additionally, as educators, it is now imperative to foster a technology-enhanced environment in simulation-based learning. With this goal in mind, we present key recommendations for reshaping SBME, aiming to usher in a new era for this crucial aspect of pediatric education.

WHAT IS SIMULATION?

It is essential to establish a shared mental model of what simulation entails. David Gaba defines it as "a technique, not a technology, used to replace or enhance real experiences with guided experiences that evoke or replicate significant aspects of the real world in a fully interactive manner."

The term "simulation" can refer to the use of simulated patients, whether through manikins or actors, as well as simulated scenarios. These scenarios can take place in a controlled simulated environment, such as a simulation center, or within an actual clinical setting, known as in-situ simulation.

The recognition of simulation's significance in clinical education stems from its impact on other high-reliability industries, such as aviation, the military, and the oil sector. As our understanding of systems thinking has grown, along with the need to ensure consistently high-quality care across various healthcare settings, simulation has been increasingly utilized for multiple purposes, including the optimization of new healthcare delivery systems.[2]

INTERDISCIPLINARY TEAMWORK AND SKILLS

The healthcare team consists of professionals from various disciplines, including doctors, nurses, physiotherapists, radiologists, radiographers, pharmacists, medical students, and other personnel. The composition of these teams depends on their specific objectives, such as stroke management, trauma care, or acute coronary syndrome intervention. Each team member undergoes training based on their respective discipline; however, integrating them into a cohesive unit is essential for managing patients with complex conditions. No single discipline holds greater importance than another—each member plays a vital role. Simulated team exercises help participants understand their complementary roles, ensuring smooth collaboration and avoiding conflicts. Flexibility in decision-making and interventions is also crucial. Additionally, teamwork and effective communication skills are key components of such training.

Senior staff, who have a broad understanding of team-based approaches, typically serve as simulation trainers. Their role involves objectively assessing team dynamics, providing real-time feedback, and maintaining checklists of key actions and human factors. Video recordings of role-playing exercises can be reviewed to highlight strengths and areas for improvement. Trainers offer constructive feedback, addressing both positive and negative behaviors.

Scenario writers design customized cases for interdisciplinary team training, focusing on specific roles and interactions. These scenarios should be realistic, structured, and comprehensive, incorporating event triggers, environmental distractions, and supporting events. They should be systematically developed with proficiency-based assessments that evaluate both technical and teamwork performance. Furthermore, all training actions should be supported by data and evidence to ensure validity.[3]

HOW TO SET UP A SIMULATION CENTER?

A simulation center represents a long-term investment in medical education, serving various training needs. It can support undergraduate education by facilitating the study of anatomy, physiological functions, and medical examination techniques. Additionally, it is valuable for residency training, helping trainees refine procedural skills, prepare for practical examinations, and complete refresher courses or recertification tests. The center can also be utilized for continuing medical or nursing education, providing hands-on training, or for competency assessments before recruitment.

Establishing a simulation center requires careful planning, starting with a conveniently located site, typically within a hospital or university campus. The architectural design and infrastructure should be developed in collaboration with trainers and end-users to ensure adequate training spaces, rooms with one-way mirrors, and sufficient space for equipment. Video recording capabilities should also be incorporated. Staffing includes full-time technicians and a manager, while trainers are usually part-time medical professionals. The selection of mannequins and equipment should follow thorough demonstrations and trials, ensuring all stakeholders are satisfied. Additionally, securing long-term technical support from vendors is essential.

Different medical simulation technologies that can be integrated into the center include:

- *Human patient simulators*: These full-sized mannequins mimic human physiological functions such as blinking, breathing, and heartbeats. Advanced models interact with learners using computer-guided teaching programs and can display vital signs on monitors, enabling realistic training in scenarios ranging from basic physical examinations to complex trauma management. Some simulators even recognize medication injections via laser bar-code readers and adjust vital signs accordingly.
- *Simulated clinical environments*: Training areas can replicate real-life settings like intensive care units, emergency cubicles, or operating rooms, equipped with necessary medical tools and crash carts. This setup allows trainees to familiarize themselves with realistic environments.
- *Virtual procedure stations*: These stations provide hands-on practice for various procedures, such as bronchoscopy, colonoscopy, and intubation. They can simulate diverse clinical scenarios and pathologies, allowing trainees to practice repeatedly until they master the required techniques.
- *Electronic medical records (EMRs)*: As healthcare institutions increasingly use EMRs to manage patient data, simulation centers can integrate a station for trainees to interact with fictitious patient records. These systems can include medical histories, notes, laboratories results, and even links to radiology reports, offering a comprehensive training experience.

CURRICULUM DEVELOPMENT

Simulation-based medical education has become an essential component of pediatric training programs, serving not only as a training tool but also as a means for both formative and summative assessments. Various studies have explored curriculum development methodologies and simulation delivery, highlighting key principles necessary for optimizing learning outcomes.

Debriefing is widely regarded as a fundamental aspect of simulation training and serves as an example of using simulation for formative assessment. While the timing and structure of debriefing may vary, it should always emphasize reflection, constructive feedback, and a learner-centered plan for improving future performance. A review of best practices in simulation identified debriefing as the most frequently cited factor contributing to successful learning.

Other established frameworks for developing pediatric simulation curriculum include deliberate practice, mastery learning, and rapid cycle deliberate practice, all of which function as summative assessment tools by comparing learner performance to a set benchmark or minimum competency level.[4]

Deliberate practice provides learners with immediate feedback and coaching, allowing them to make necessary adjustments while developing a skill. A key aspect of this approach is repetitive practice, which offers multiple opportunities for skill refinement. This strategy has been applied in pediatrics to enhance CPR performance and improve success rates in lumbar punctures among pediatric residents.

Mastery learning builds upon deliberate practice by requiring learners to continue practicing a skill until they achieve a mastery level, meaning they can perform it competently without coaching. This process may involve rapid or extended repetition. Studies in pediatric resuscitation SBME have shown that, although learning to mastery leads to significant skill acquisition, skills may deteriorate within 6 months, emphasizing the need for ongoing practice. Courses such as Pediatric Advanced Life Support and Trauma Resuscitation in Kids, a Canadian pediatric trauma course, require learners to meet a minimum competency level, with simulation playing a key role in both skill development and assessment. Additionally, the resuscitation training board game has been shown to enhance neonatal resuscitation knowledge retention and has been suggested for summative assessments as an example of serious gaming in pediatric SBME.

A recent advancement in SBME is rapid cycle deliberate practice, which integrates the aforementioned learning principles into a single instructional design. This method involves frequent interruptions or "pauses" in a scenario, allowing the learner to receive corrective feedback before continuing or restarting with improved performance. Pediatric residents have demonstrated improved skill acquisition in resuscitation and septic shock management through this approach, though long-term retention has not shown significant improvement compared to other modalities.

Several expert-reviewed simulation curricula have been published in pediatric fields, particularly in pediatric emergency medicine and pediatric critical care. These curricula include longitudinal programs for pediatric fellows, residents, and emergency medicine trainees. Early pediatric simulation curricula primarily focused on procedural skills, cardiopulmonary resuscitation, trauma, and disaster management. However, more recent innovations in PEM simulation have incorporated objectives related to patient- and family-centered care, breaking bad news, and medical error disclosure. Future pediatric simulation curricula are expected to integrate EMRs, expand into system-wide applications, and extend programs to rural and community-based settings.[4]

WHAT CAN SIMULATION BE USED FOR IN PEDIATRIC TRAINING?

Simulation in pediatric training can be used for:

- Enhancing clinical skills in a controlled environment
- Practicing emergency and resuscitation procedures
- Improving decision-making and critical thinking
- Building confidence in managing pediatric patients
- Providing exposure to rare or complex cases
- Reducing anxiety about making mistakes in real patient interactions
- Enhancing teamwork and communication among healthcare professionals
- Allowing repeated practice without risk to patients

BOX 1: Benefits of simulation.

- *Immersive and experiential learning:* Engages learners through hands-on, realistic scenarios
- *Reflective learning:* Encourages self-assessment and improvement through feedback and debriefing
- *Multifaceted learning:* Develops knowledge, skills, and attitudes simultaneously
- *On-demand learning:* Provides increased exposure to both common and rare medical conditions
- *Safe, risk-free environment:* Enables learning without compromising patient safety
- *Repetitive practice:* Allows learners to refine skills through repeated practice
- *Evaluation of new methods:* Facilitates testing of new equipment, interventions, treatment protocols, and procedures
- *Multidisciplinary team training:* Enhances collaboration and communication among healthcare professionals
- *Standardized assessment:* Enables objective evaluation of learners using consistent clinical scenarios

BENEFITS OF SIMULATION IN PEDIATRICS

For junior trainees, simulation serves as a valuable tool for building confidence in taking patient histories and examining young patients, while for more experienced trainees, it offers exposure to less common scenarios such as pediatric resuscitations, breaking bad news, and safeguarding. By breaking down critical events into manageable learning components, simulation allows for the development and refinement of essential competencies like leadership, prioritization, and communication.

These learning opportunities can be integrated into a comprehensive educational framework using a "digital toolbox" that includes instant messaging and 24/7 access to learning resources such as Webex sessions, podcasts, and vodcasts. Additionally, simulation is increasingly incorporated into blended learning approaches to enhance skill retention and mitigate skill deterioration over time.[5]

Box 1 summarizes the benefits of simulation in pediatrics.

CLINICAL SIGNIFICANCE OF SIMULATION IN PEDIATRICS

The utilization, demand, and necessity of pediatric SBME have significantly increased over the past two decades. A key driving factor is the growing emphasis on patient safety in medicine. This shift has had a direct impact on trainee experiences, leading to greater faculty supervision and a stronger focus on demonstrating competence. Additionally, the commitment to patient safety aligns with the push for practicing evidence-based medicine.

A notable trend in modern healthcare is the effort to minimize unnecessary interventions and reduce iatrogenic complications. In pediatrics, this includes decreasing lumbar puncture rates for neonatal fever, prioritizing bag-mask ventilation over intubation, and reducing appendectomies for uncomplicated appendicitis. While these changes improve patient care, they also contribute to educational gaps by limiting exposure to certain procedures.

Beyond the reduced necessity for certain procedures, medical students and residents face increasing work-hour restrictions. The evolving medical education landscape places a stronger emphasis on work-life balance and trainee mental health, which may further reduce opportunities for hands-on learning. Pediatrics, in particular, already has fewer high-acuity resuscitation cases compared to adult medicine. Given these constraints, high-yield simulation training has become essential for exposing trainees to rare cases and procedures

BOX 2: Designing a simulation.

- *Identify the learning need*—determine the specific knowledge, skills, or competencies to be addressed
- *Logistics of the activity*—outline participant roles, required equipment, and other logistical considerations
- *Define learning outcomes and educational theory*—establish clear learning objectives and the theoretical framework supporting the session
- *Setting and background*—provide context for the simulation, including relevant clinical or situational details
- *Briefing for participants*—prepare the narrator, participants, and any simulated patients with necessary instructions
- *Immersion in the simulation*—ensure engagement, maintain appropriate levels of control, and prioritize a safe learning environment
- *Expected observations*—identify key actions, responses, or interventions anticipated during the session
- *Session conclusion*—wrap up the simulation effectively, reinforcing key learning points
- *Debriefing and feedback approach*—use structured debriefing to facilitate reflection, discussion, and improvement strategies

without extending the duration of medical education.

DESIGNING SIMULATION

Every simulation-based learning activity should be structured around four interconnected components:

1. *Briefing*—preparing learners by setting expectations and objectives.
2. *Immersion*—engaging in the simulation-based experience.
3. *Debrief*—reflecting on performance with guided discussion and feedback.
4. *Action plan*—implementing strategies to improve future performance.

To ensure effectiveness, each simulation session should be designed using a standardized template. This allows for the development of a structured series of simulation-based learning activities, ensuring constructive alignment between the intended learning outcomes (ILOs), the immersive experience, the debriefing process, and the feedback provided.

Box 2 illustrates an example of design of simulation.

CHALLENGES IN IMPLEMENTATION OF SIMULATION

Despite the growing enthusiasm for SBME, several barriers continue to hinder its widespread adoption. The most frequently cited challenges include resource constraints related to time, financial investment, and limited access to simulation centers or equipment.

Establishing a simulation center and training facility requires significant resources, including the cost of purchasing equipment, securing physical space, and allocating faculty and staff time for simulation sessions. However, data on the financial aspects of simulation-based learning are scarce. A systematic review found that only 6% of studies reported simulation costs, with a mere 1.6% comparing these costs to other educational interventions. This lack of data makes it difficult to convince healthcare budget decision-makers to invest in the initial expenses, though demonstrating a strong return on investment may be a more persuasive approach.

In pediatrics, the potential financial benefits of simulation-based training include preventing deaths, reducing significant safety events, avoiding intensive care admissions, and shortening hospital stays. Additional cost savings may come from mitigating legal expenses, reducing ongoing medical care costs for harmed patients, and improving workforce productivity by ensuring better long-term health outcomes for surviving patients. Even beyond catastrophic savings, efficiency improvements—such as streamlining processes, eliminating redundant work, and enhancing medication practices—can further justify the investment.

However, if the primary driver for simulation-based training is patient safety, then financial benefits may not be the ultimate objective. Instead, the ethical responsibility of preventing harm, saving lives, and upholding the principle of "first, do no harm" should be the foremost priority.

LIMITATIONS OF USING SIMULATION

Identifying both opportunities and challenges is the first step in successfully implementing SBME. Addressing these barriers can lead to significant benefits. It is well known that establishing and maintaining a dedicated simulation center requires substantial financial investment, time, and manpower. Additionally, setting up a simulation session is resource intensive. One of the primary limitations of SBME is its learner-dependent nature, requiring active participation and engagement for effective learning.

A major challenge lies in integrating simulation-based training into the existing medical curriculum. Further research is needed to determine the optimal amount of simulation exposure and to develop standardized guidelines that ensure its educational effectiveness. Additionally, trained faculty with expertise in debriefing techniques and assessment tools—such as checklists and global rating scales—are essential for maximizing learning outcomes. Ongoing studies continue to assess the transferability of skills acquired in simulation to real clinical settings.[6]

FUTURE OF SIMULATION IN PEDIATRICS

Further research is needed to explore the use of simulation for assessment purposes. Many hospitals and medical schools have integrated high-fidelity simulation into their educational curricula. Studies utilizing simulation-based assessment tools have shown that these assessments are valid and reliable indicators of clinical performance and resident competency.

However, the clinical significance of performance measured in a simulated environment remains uncertain. More evidence is required to determine whether simulation training directly enhances physicians' ability to manage real-life critical events. Additionally, a key area for future research is evaluating whether simulation-based training leads to measurable improvements in patient safety and clinical outcomes. Although there is growing enthusiasm for simulation as a means of enhancing medical training and patient safety, definitive evidence demonstrating its direct impact on patient outcomes is still lacking. Addressing this gap will require significantly more research.[7]

Simulation-based medical education is a rapidly evolving field, driven by the need for more efficient training methods. Various medical disciplines, including clinicians and nurses, are increasingly prioritizing high-quality simulation to maximize the effectiveness of educational interventions.

The implementation of a medical simulation curriculum can involve multiple trainees, particularly in fostering teamwork among nurses, clinicians, and pharmacists. Effective communication is a critical skill for leadership and collaboration in medical settings. Simulation has been successfully utilized to improve team communication in pediatric healthcare, leading to better patient outcomes.

CONCLUSION

In conclusion, simulation-based training is increasingly being adopted as an instructional methodology worldwide. Many pediatric and neonatal units are incorporating SBME into their educational programs. While it cannot replace direct clinical exposure, simulation offers the advantage of repetitive practice in a low-risk environment. Its immersive and hands-on approach addresses some of the limitations of traditional training models. By improving human performance, enhancing professional confidence, and minimizing patient risks, SBME is transforming medical education in the Western world. It is now time to explore and embrace this innovative teaching approach in the Indian subcontinent.

KEY POINTS

- Simulation-based education originated in the aviation and space industries. Over the past two to three decades, SBME has become increasingly vital in pediatrics.
- Effective use of simulation technology for specific learning objectives requires careful planning.
- Best practices in SBME include debriefing with feedback, deliberate practice, and mastery learning.
- Deliberate practice involves immediate feedback or coaching to ensure proper execution of skills.
- Simulation is particularly effective for teaching pediatric cardiopulmonary resuscitation, procedural skills, trauma care, and disaster management.
- More innovative applications in pediatrics include training in delivering bad news, medical error disclosure, family-centered care, and system integration.
- Early and frequent integration of SBME in pediatric medical and residency education can help bridge learning gaps, such as differences in pathophysiology and training for rare procedures and clinical scenarios.
- Pediatric procedures can be taught to a minimum competency level using validated checklists and Global Rating Scales to assess learner performance.
- Simulation also plays a crucial role in evaluating and enhancing communication skills.
- The growing demand for simulation education is driven by factors such as work hour restrictions, heightened safety measures, and reduced exposure to high-acuity patient cases.

REFERENCES

1. Spadea M, Ciantelli M, Fossati N, et al. Enhancing the future of simulation-based education in pediatrics. Ital J Pediatr. 2021;47:36.
2. Clerihew L, Rowney D, Ker J. Simulation in paediatric training. Arch Dis Child Educ Pract Ed. 2016;101(1):8-14.
3. Lateef F. Simulation-based learning: Just like the real thing. J Emerg Trauma Shock. 2010;3(4):348-52.
4. Davila U, Price A. Past Present and Future of Simulation in Pediatrics. Treasure Island (FL): StatPearls Publishing; 2025. [online] Available from https://www.ncbi.nlm.nih.gov/books/NBK559082 [Last accessed January, 2026].
5. Cheng A, Duff J, Grant E, et al. Simulation in paediatrics: An educational revolution. Paediatr Child Health. 2007;12(6):465-8.
6. Kalaniti K, Campbell DM. Simulation-based medical education: time for a pedagogical shift. Indian Pediatr. 2015;52(1):41-5.
7. Ojha R, Liu A, Rai D, et al. Review of Simulation in Pediatrics: The Evolution of a Revolution. Front Pediatr. 2015;3:106.

CHAPTER 37

Evidence-based Medicine and Teaching

Sarthak Das, Archana Malik, Saroj Kumar Tripathy

INTRODUCTION

Evidence-based medicine (EBM) represents a significant paradigm shift in healthcare, merging clinical expertise with the most current and relevant research evidence and integrating patient preferences into clinical decision-making. First formally defined by Sackett et al. in 1996, EBM has become the cornerstone of modern clinical practice and medical education.[1] In today's dynamic healthcare environment, the practice of EBM is essential for improving patient outcomes, optimizing healthcare delivery, and fostering lifelong learning among medical professionals.

Teaching EBM to medical students and healthcare professionals not only enables them to become competent clinicians but also promotes critical thinking, analytical skills, and a culture of inquiry. As the volume of medical literature expands exponentially, future practitioners must be trained to sift through data efficiently and make evidence-informed decisions. With the advent of competency-based medical education (CBME) in India and globally, the integration of EBM into the curriculum has gained renewed importance. This chapter aims to explore the principles of EBM, the pedagogical methods for teaching it, challenges in its implementation, and strategies for its integration into the current educational landscape.

WHAT IS EVIDENCE-BASED MEDICINE?

Evidence-based medicine is defined as "the conscientious, explicit, and judicious use of current best evidence in making decisions about the care of individual patients".[1] It involves a structured approach to clinical problem-solving by integrating the best available research evidence with clinical expertise and patient values. The process of EBM includes five steps: (1) Formulating a clinical question, (2) Searching for the best evidence, (3) Appraising the evidence, (4) Applying the evidence in clinical practice, and (5) Evaluating the performance.[2]

This approach ensures that healthcare is both up-to-date and individualized. It also fosters a culture where clinical decisions are not based solely on tradition, opinion, or outdated practices but are instead rooted in current scientific knowledge and contextual realities.

RELEVANCE OF EVIDENCE-BASED MEDICINE IN MEDICAL EDUCATION

The rapid expansion of medical information, growing healthcare complexities, and the demand for quality, cost-effective care have made EBM more relevant than ever. Medical education must prepare students to be not just consumers of knowledge but also discerning appraisers of scientific evidence. Incorporating EBM in the curriculum instills critical skills such as literature searching, biostatistical reasoning, critical appraisal, and the application of research findings to clinical practice.[3]

In competency-based curricula, such as the Indian Medical Graduate (IMG) framework under CBME, EBM is crucial for fostering self-directed learning, reflective practice, and professional development.[4] Teaching EBM aligns with core competencies like patient care, medical knowledge, communication skills, professionalism, and systems-based practice.

TEACHING STRATEGIES FOR EVIDENCE-BASED MEDICINE

- *Didactic lectures and seminars*: Traditional lectures are useful for introducing the principles of EBM, including the hierarchy of evidence, study designs, and basic statistical concepts. Seminars and journal clubs can promote interactive learning.
- *Flipped classroom*: In this model, students review EBM resources, video lectures, or readings before class and engage in problem-solving or critical appraisal during class time. This method encourages active learning and better retention.[5]
- *Team-based learning (TBL)*: TBL fosters collaborative learning and improves critical thinking. Students work in teams to solve clinical scenarios using EBM principles.
- *Problem-based learning (PBL)*: EBM can be integrated into clinical case discussions, where students are encouraged to identify learning needs, formulate clinical questions, and seek evidence.
- *Point-of-care learning*: Embedding EBM teaching in clinical rounds or bedside teaching helps students connect theory with real-world practice.
- *Critical appraisal workshops*: Hands-on workshops where students learn to interpret different study types, understand biostatistics, and evaluate study quality are effective.
- *Use of digital tools*: Online databases (PubMed and Cochrane Library), mobile apps (UpToDate and BMJ Best Practice), and evidence synthesis tools (GRADEpro) are essential for practical EBM teaching.
- *Simulation-based learning*: Simulated clinical scenarios incorporating EBM decisions help in reinforcing skills in a safe and controlled environment.
- *Mentorship and role modeling*: Faculty members practicing and emphasizing EBM in their clinical decisions serve as powerful role models for students.

INTEGRATION OF EVIDENCE-BASED MEDICINE IN UNDERGRADUATE AND POSTGRADUATE CURRICULUM

The Medical Council of India (now National Medical Commission) has advocated for the integration of EBM into the CBME curriculum. Undergraduate students can be introduced to EBM concepts during foundation courses and clinical postings. At the postgraduate level, EBM should be embedded in thesis writing, clinical audits, and multidisciplinary team discussions.[6]

For effective integration, the following framework can be adopted:

- Early introduction to EBM in foundation and preclinical years.
- Gradual increase in complexity with clinical exposure.
- Practical assignments such as critically appraised topics (CATs).

- Assessments through objective structured clinical examination (OSCE), multiple-choice questions (MCQs), and reflective writing.
- Use of portfolios to track progress in EBM competencies.

CHALLENGES IN TEACHING EVIDENCE-BASED MEDICINE

- *Lack of trained faculty*: Not all faculty members are familiar with the principles or practice of EBM.
- *Limited resources*: Access to journals, databases, and EBM tools may be restricted, especially in resource-limited settings.
- *Time constraints*: Integrating EBM in an already packed curriculum can be challenging.
- *Student engagement*: Not all students may appreciate the value of EBM or possess the skills to navigate complex literature.
- *Assessment difficulties*: Measuring EBM competencies objectively can be difficult.

OVERCOMING CHALLENGES

- *Faculty development programs (FDPs)*: Training and sensitizing faculty in EBM principles and pedagogy.
- *Institutional support*: Ensuring access to resources, journals, and databases.
- *Curriculum alignment*: Embedding EBM within existing clinical modules.
- *Use of technology*: Leveraging mobile apps, online platforms, and digital libraries.
- *Student-centered approaches*: Encouraging peer-led sessions, small group discussions, and reflective practice.

ROLE OF EVIDENCE-BASED PRACTICE IN CLINICAL DECISION-MAKING

Evidence-based medicine empowers clinicians to make informed decisions that improve patient outcomes. It reduces unwarranted practice variation, encourages the use of effective interventions, and helps phase out outdated or harmful practices. The EBM approach facilitates shared decision-making, where clinicians and patients work together, considering both the scientific evidence and patient preferences.[7]

Moreover, EBM supports clinical guidelines development and health policy decisions, ensuring consistency and accountability in healthcare delivery.

IMPACT OF EVIDENCE-BASED MEDICINE ON LEARNER DEVELOPMENT[8]

Training in EBM improves:

- Critical thinking and problem-solving skills
- Self-directed learning habits
- Communication skills through evidence-informed patient counseling
- Ethical reasoning by aligning clinical decisions with the best evidence and patient values
- Preparedness for lifelong learning

RECENT ADVANCES AND GLOBAL TRENDS IN EVIDENCE-BASED MEDICINE EDUCATION[8,9]

Globally, institutions are adopting innovative methods to teach EBM:

- *Massive open online courses (MOOCs)*: Platforms like Coursera and FutureLearn offer free EBM courses.
- *Integration with artificial intelligence (AI)*: AI tools are being used to curate and synthesize evidence.
- *EBM competency frameworks*: Developed by organizations like CanMEDS and AAMC.
- *Inclusion in licensing examinations*: Many countries have incorporated EBM in national board examinations.

India is also witnessing a growing emphasis on EBM, with several medical colleges offering workshops and certificate courses in research methodology and critical appraisal. The Indian Council of Medical Research (ICMR) and NMC encourage EBM through faculty development and curriculum reforms.

EVIDENCE-BASED MEDICINE AND TEACHING: RELEVANCE TO INDIAN COMPETENCY-BASED MEDICAL EDUCATION CURRICULUM

With the implementation of the CBME curriculum by the National Medical Commission (NMC) in India in 2019, the paradigm of medical teaching and learning has undergone a transformative shift. At the heart of CBME lies the emphasis on developing not just knowledge but also the skills and attitudes necessary for holistic and evidence-informed clinical practice. Within this framework, EBM becomes not just a tool but a core professional competency for undergraduate medical students in India.[1]

In the CBME model, IMGs are expected to become lifelong learners who are competent to apply the best available evidence in real-time clinical settings. This aligns with the global understanding of EBM as defined by Sackett et al., as "the conscientious, explicit, and judicious use of current best evidence in making decisions about the care of individual patients".[1] Indian CBME envisions early introduction of EBM principles in the foundation course itself, followed by vertical integration across preclinical, paraclinical, and clinical years.[10]

The Attitude, Ethics, and Communication (AETCOM) module—which is a critical pillar of CBME—also encourages the practice of EBM by fostering critical thinking, shared decision-making, and ethical reasoning based on scientific evidence. For instance, students are now taught to search for literature on PubMed, appraise journal articles, understand levels of evidence, and apply findings during clinical discussions, case presentations, and journal clubs.[11]

Practical implementation of EBM in India, however, is not without challenges. Heterogeneity in faculty training, limited access to high-quality resources, language barriers, and variable digital infrastructure in rural and semiurban institutions remain areas of concern. Therefore, capacity building of faculty through medical education units (MEUs), FDPs, and the use of simplified, context-specific teaching tools is necessary.[10,11]

Nationally, there is a growing repository of Indian medical research databases such as the ICMR, MedIND, and IndMed that should be integrated into EBM teaching, especially for region-specific diseases and treatment protocols. Moreover, Indian students must be trained not only to appraise global evidence but also to recognize the gaps in Indian data and contribute to contextually relevant research during their undergraduate research projects [ICMR Short Term Studentship (STS), or student research programs].[12]

Another important CBME mandate is reflective practice, which can be seamlessly linked with EBM by encouraging students to reflect on how evidence informed their clinical reasoning, decisions, and patient interactions. Portfolios, logbooks, and case-based discussions (CBDs) can be utilized to assess students' integration of EBM into practice.[1,10-12]

In summary, the CBME curriculum provides a fertile ground for EBM to thrive in India. The synergy of early exposure, structured modules like AETCOM, assessment innovations, and faculty development have the potential to transform today's Indian medical student into a competent and evidence-informed doctor of tomorrow.

CONCLUSION

Evidence-based medicine is a critical skill for healthcare professionals in the 21st century. Its integration into medical education ensures that future doctors are not only skilled in diagnosis and treatment but are also equipped to appraise, apply, and generate evidence. Teaching EBM requires innovative, student-centered approaches and institutional support. As the healthcare landscape continues to evolve, the role of EBM in enhancing clinical decision-making, improving patient care, and fostering professionalism will only grow. By embedding EBM into the fabric of medical education, we prepare learners for a future defined by scientific rigor, ethical responsibility, and patient-centered care.

REFERENCES

1. Sackett DL, Rosenberg WM, Gray JA, et al. Evidence based medicine: what it is and what it isn't. BMJ. 1996;312(7023):71-2.
2. Straus SE, Glasziou P, Richardson WS, et al. (Eds). Evidence-Based Medicine: How to Practice and Teach EBM, 5th edition. Elsevier; 2018.
3. Green ML. Graduate medical education training in clinical epidemiology, critical appraisal, and evidence-based medicine: a critical review of curricula. Acad Med. 1999;74(6):686-94.
4. Medical Council of India. Competency-Based Undergraduate Curriculum for the Indian Medical Graduate, Volume I-III. New Delhi: MCI; 2018.
5. Chen HC, Priest KC, Batten JN, et al. Student perceptions of flipped classroom in graduate medical education. Med Educ. 2017;51(6):649-59.
6. Ilic D, Maloney S. Methods of teaching medical trainees evidence-based medicine: a systematic review. Med Educ. 2014;48(2):124-35.
7. Montori VM, Guyatt GH. Progress in evidence-based medicine. JAMA. 2008;300(15):1814-6.
8. Young T, Rohwer A, Volmink J, et al. What are the effects of teaching evidence-based health care (EBHC)? Overview of systematic reviews. PLoS One. 2014;9(1):e86706.
9. Prasad V, Vandross A, Toomey C, et al. A decade of reversal: an analysis of 146 contradicted medical practices. Mayo Clin Proc. 2013;88(8):790-8.
10. National Medical Commission. (2019). Competency Based Undergraduate Curriculum for the Indian Medical Graduate. [online] Available from https://www.nmc.org.in/information-desk/for-colleges/ug-curriculum/ [Last accessed January, 2026].
11. Medical Council of India. (2019). AETCOM Booklet. [online] Available from https://www.nmc.org.in/wp-content/uploads/2020/08/AETCOM_book.pdf [Last accessed January, 2026].
12. ICMR Short Term Studentship (STS) Program. [online] Available from https://sts.icmr.org.in/ [Last accessed January, 2026].

CHAPTER

38 Using Artificial Intelligence in Medical Education

Ghanshyam Das, Harish K Pemde

Learning Objectives

By the end of this chapter, the learner should be able to:

- Define artificial intelligence and describe major AI subtypes.
- Describe key applications of AI in medical education.
- Explain how AI can support personalized learning, clinical reasoning, feedback, and preparation for AI-enabled healthcare practice.
- Discuss major challenges and risks of AI use in medical education.
- Outline ethical and regulatory considerations when using student and patient data with AI tools in educational settings.

INTRODUCTION

Medical education has undergone profound evolution over the past century, driven largely by advances in science, technology, and pedagogy. Over the past few decades, artificial intelligence (AI) and its applications have grown rapidly in a changing digital ecosystem where expectations are rising and are fueled by social media and medical practitioners.[1] Today, *AI* represents the next major transformative force. As health systems face increasing patient complexity, exploding biomedical knowledge, and demands for efficiency, AI offers unprecedented opportunities to support learners, educators, and clinicians. In this context, medical education must prepare future doctors not only to use AI tools but also to understand, evaluate, and collaborate.

Yet, despite enthusiasm and clear potential, the incorporation of AI in medical education raises questions. How should AI be incorporated into curricula? What skills must learners develop to use AI? How do we ensure that AI tools do not introduce bias or reduce critical thinking? And how can educators preserve the patient-centered focus of medical training along with AI?

This chapter explores the applications, benefits, risks, and future objectives of AI in medical education, and provides a resource for educators and learners navigating this field.

Artificial intelligence in medical education spans algorithms that interpret imaging, systems that convert large volumes of clinical data into meaningful insights, and generative language models capable of tutoring, producing patient case scenarios. These tools help—not replace—the human elements of empathy, reasoning, and ethics that are important to medical professionalism.

Several factors drive the incorporation of AI in AI-enabled clinical tools now increasingly being to teaching and learning. First, the medical knowledge pool changes rapidly, far outpacing human capacity for memorization. Second, the emphasis on competency-based education aligns well with AI systems that can personalize instruction and track learner progress over time. Third, AI-enabled clinical tools are now increasingly being used and demand that future doctors be able to critically understand and interpret algorithmic outputs in a given clinical context.

This chapter has been enhanced using AI.

APPLICATIONS OF ARTIFICIAL INTELLIGENCE IN MEDICAL EDUCATION

Intelligent Tutoring Systems

Artificial intelligence-driven tutoring platforms can analyze learners' strengths and weaknesses, providing instructions accordingly. These systems deliver customized quizzes, explanations, and remediation exercises in real time. For example, chatbot-style tutors powered by large language models (LLMs) can simulate a personal tutor, offering explanations of physiology or pharmacology topics. Unlike static e-learning modules, they adapt based on user performance patterns.

Virtual Patients and Clinical Simulations

Virtual patient simulations along with natural language processing allow learners to practice interviewing, diagnosing, and counseling patients in a safe virtual environment. Immersive patient simulators (IPSs) enable a representation of a virtual counterpart in a three-dimensional "game-like" virtual environment where students can freely interact in real time with virtual patients.[2] These systems can respond dynamically to student questions, adjusting patient symptoms, or history based on clinical reasoning. This improves decision-making skills and offers standardized exposure to rare or complicated cases that may not be common.

Radiology and Pathology Training

Machine-learning algorithms trained on medical images can help learners in pattern recognition. For example, an AI tool may highlight suspicious areas on an X-ray or histopathology slide, prompting learners to reflect on their differential diagnoses. These systems can also prepare thousands of examples, helping students to gain knowledge beyond clinical experience.

Assessment and Competency Tracking

Automated scoring tools can evaluate written assignments, OSCE/DOAP, or clinical documentation. Speech-recognition systems can analyze communication skills, providing reflection/feedback on clarity, empathy, and structure in selected settings and with appropriate validation. Furthermore, AI can track competency progression, identifying weak areas requiring reinforcement and predicting performance.

Administrative and Workflow Support

Beyond direct teaching, AI helps educational administration. Systems can generate schedules, analyze examination data, and prepare tasks such as generating individualized learning plans. This reduces workload on faculty, allowing them to dedicate more time to mentorship and personalized instruction **(Table 1)**.

TABLE 1: Domains of learning and AI application.

Domain	*AI applications*	*Examples*
Teaching and learning	Personalized learning	Adaptive learning platforms
Assessment	Automated grading and feedback/reflection	MCQ scoring and OSCE scoring
Simulation	Virtual patients and simulators	AI-driven mannequins and VR surgery sims
Curriculum support	Content generation	Case creation, quizzes, and summaries
Administrative	Timetable and student analytics	Predicting at risk students

BENEFITS AND OPPORTUNITIES

Personalized Learning

The most important advantage of AI is its ability to tailor education to each learner's pace, style, and needs. Students who struggle with specific concepts receive targeted content, while advanced learners can progress more rapidly. This individualized approach supports *proper* learning and reduces disparities. Machine learning-related content can be embedded within a larger curricula focused on competence in using information technology to improve patient care.[3]

Enhanced Clinical Reasoning Training

Through large datasets and predictive modeling, AI can expose to diverse clinical scenarios, enhancing diagnostic accuracy, and decision-making skills. By comparing student reasoning with expert pathways, AI can identify gaps and cognitive biases.

Improved Access and Equity

Artificial intelligence-powered learning tools can reach students in remote areas, reducing reliance on local faculty availability. Simulations and virtual patients can substitute for limited clinical exposure. AI can democratize high-quality medical education globally.

Real-time Feedback and Reflection

Immediate feedback is crucial for skill development, yet is often limited by faculty availability. AI can provide instantaneous, consistent assessments, especially in domains like communication skills, documentation, and pattern recognition. Students can reflect more frequently, supporting continuous improvement. To address the challenges and fully harness AI's potential, educational strategies must be grounded in structured frameworks. Kern's Six-Step Approach to curriculum development emphasizes on assessment, goal setting, instructional design, implementation, evaluation, and feedback.[7]

Preparing the Future Workforce

Modern health systems integrate AI into diagnostics, treatment, and patient monitoring. Training medical students to understand algorithmic principles, evaluate accuracy, and recognize limitations ensures that they become competent new-age doctors. Early exposure to AI tools helps doctors to work effectively with such systems **(Figs. 1 and 2)**.

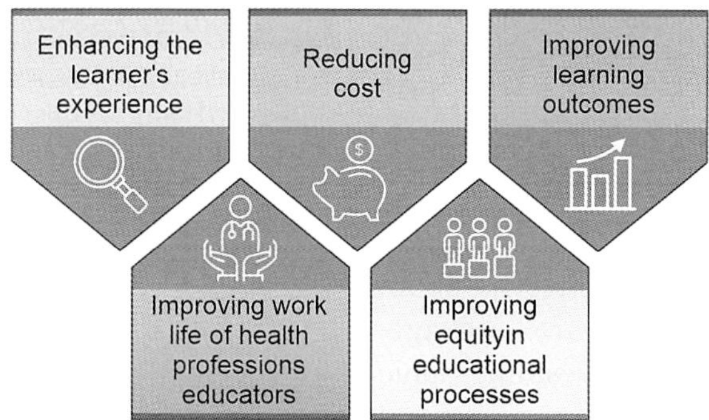

Fig. 1: Benefits of AI.

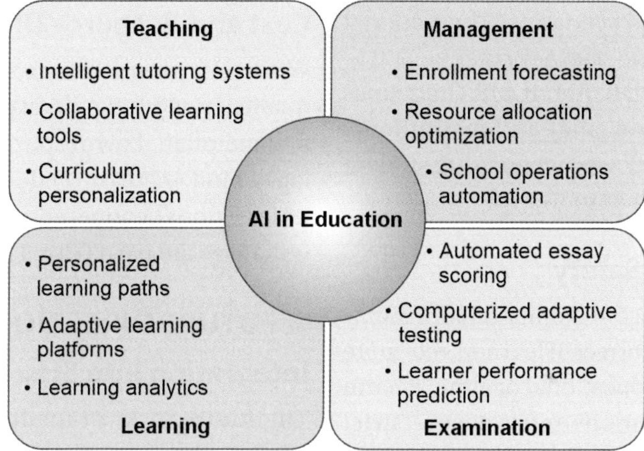

Fig. 2: Benefits of AI in education.

CHALLENGES, RISKS, AND ETHICS

Overreliance and Depletion of Critical Thinking

One danger is that students may accept AI-generated insights uncritically, decreasing their clinical acumen. Cognitive autonomy refers to the clinician's ability to make independent judgments, analyze data, and formulate decisions based on reasoning rather than external cues.[4] Educational programs must emphasize that AI is a *tool*, not an oracle. Learners must be trained to question, verify, and criticize algorithmic output.

Bias and Fairness Issues

Artificial intelligence systems trained on biased or incomplete data may perpetuate inequities. One of the biggest challenges with LLMs like ChatGPT is the occurrence of inaccurate information or so-called hallucinations. These inaccuracies arise from how LLMs generate text by predicting likely word sequences from their training data, without a built-in mechanism to verify factual accuracy. To prevent hallucinations, educators have proposed various methods, like training models on more diverse data, using adversarial training methods, and human-in-the-loop approaches.[5] Educators must ensure transparency in data sources and include bias-awareness training also into curricula.

Privacy and Data Protection

Training AI systems often requires student and patient data, raising concerns about confidentiality, and secure storage. Institutions must balance educational value with strict compliance to privacy laws and ethical guidelines. De-identified or synthetic data can help avoid risks but are not always ideal for real-world scenarios. The national regulations [e.g., Data-Privacy Data-Protection Act (DPDP) Act; ICMR Guidelines on use of AI in medicine] and institutional policies must be followed when using student or patient data with AI tools.

Reliability and Safety

Artificial intelligence recommendations may occasionally be incorrect. If learners rely more on such systems, educational or clinical harm may result. Institutions must ensure strict validation of AI tools before implementation and maintain oversight by trained educators. For high-stakes use, AI tools should undergo external validation and ongoing monitoring of performance. It should be ensured that an appropriate human expert verifies the AI conclusions and AI-generated reports and data, etc. before using the same. This concept of human in the loop (HiTL) should always be ensured.

Faculty Readiness and Cultural Resistance

Adoption of AI requires faculty training, technological literacy, and institutional investment. Some educators fear that AI will replace traditional teaching or decrease professional identity. Effective implementation requires faculty acceptance, clear communication of AI's role, and continued professional development.

BOX 1: Challenges and risks.

- Overreliance and depletion of critical thinking
- Bias and fairness issues
- Privacy and data protection
- Reliability and safety
- Faculty readiness and cultural resistance
- Cost and resource disparities

Cost and Resource Disparities

While AI promises greater equity, high-quality systems can be expensive to develop and maintain. Low-resource institutions may lag behind, increasing educational disparities unless global cooperation and open-source initiatives are used **(Box 1)**.

FUTURE DIRECTIONS

Integration into Standard Curricula

The future of AI in medical education lies not in standalone tools but in incorporation across the curriculum. Early foundational courses may cover algorithmic principles, data literacy, and ethical AI usage. Current implementations demonstrate that LLMs' applications span across medical education, clinical decision support, diagnostics, and patient care, while highlighting critical challenges in privacy, ethics, and factual accuracy that require resolution for integration into healthcare and medical education.[6] Assessments will evaluate a learner's ability to critically evaluate AI outputs. However, in undergraduate education, their use should be carefully supervised and aligned with learning outcomes rather than used primarily for assignment generation.

Human–Artificial Intelligence Collaboration Models

Education will effectively train students to work alongside AI. This includes understanding when to trust an algorithm, when to override it, and how to communicate AI-informed decisions to patients with clarity and empathy. Such collaboration will emphasize on real clinical practice, where AI augments clinician judgment rather than replacing it.

Artificial Intelligence-assisted Research Training

Artificial intelligence tools can support students to explore datasets, generate ideas for study design, and assist in literature searches, but must not replace critical appraisal and scientific integrity. This may increase student-led research and broaden participation in academics. Ethical and methodological training are essential to ensure strict scholarship.

Global Harmonization and Standards

As AI tools are increasingly used, medical colleges will need to establish evidence-based guidelines for their development, validation, deployment, and evaluation. Collaborative international standards can ensure quality, reduce redundancy, and address safety and bias.

Evolving Role of the Medical Educator

Rather than diminishing the educator's role, AI enhances it. Faculty can focus more on mentorship, professional identity formation, and complex clinical reasoning. Educators will help students to navigate AI-generated insights, maintain ethics, and cultivate compassion.

CONCLUSION

Artificial intelligence shows promise in improving medical education through personalization, enhanced simulation, and exposure to diverse clinical scenarios. It prepares learners for a future in which AI is used in healthcare. Yet, its implementation demands critical thinking, ethical vigilance, and continuous evaluation. As medical education integrates AI, its success will depend not only on technological sophistication but on preserving the humanity of profession. By embracing AI thoughtfully, mentors can shape a future in which doctors are better equipped, more reflective, and more capable of delivering high-quality patient care.

KEY POINTS

- Artificial intelligence in medical education includes tools for adaptive learning, intelligent tutoring, virtual and augmented simulations, automated assessment, curriculum support, and administrative analytics, all intended to augment rather than replace teachers and clinicians.
- Properly designed AI systems can personalize learning, expose students to diverse and rare clinical scenarios, provide frequent formative feedback, and help prepare graduates for AI-enabled clinical environments.
- Overreliance on generative AI and other tools risks erosion of critical thinking, cognitive autonomy, and clinical reasoning; students must be trained to question and verify AI outputs rather than accept them uncritically.
- AI systems can perpetuate or amplify existing biases and inequities when

trained on unrepresentative data; educators should address bias, fairness, and transparency explicitly in teaching and in tool selection.

- Use of AI in education raises important privacy and data-protection issues; student and patient data should be de-identified when possible and handled according to legal and institutional frameworks.
- Safe and effective AI integration requires faculty development, institutional support, and continuous evaluation of AI tools' educational impact and safety, particularly when tools influence clinical decisions or assessments.
- Future curricula will likely embed AI concepts longitudinally, emphasizing human–AI collaboration, ethical and professional use, and the educator's role as mentor, critical guide, and guardian of patient-centered care.

REFERENCES

1. Chan KS, Zary N. Application of artificial intelligence in medical education: Current status and future directions. JMIR Med Educ. 2019;5(1):e13028.
2. Kleinert R, Heiermann N, Plum PS, et al. Web-Based Immersive Virtual Patient Simulators: Positive Effect on Clinical Reasoning in Medical Education. J Med Internet Res. 2015;17(11):e263.
3. Kolachalama VB, Garg PS. Machine learning and medical education. NPJ Digit Med. 2018;1:54.
4. Izquierdo-Condoy JS, Arias-Intriago M, Tello-De-la-Torre A, et al. Generative Artificial Intelligence in Medical Education: Enhancing Critical Thinking or Undermining Cognitive Autonomy? J Med Internet Res. 2025;27:e76340.
5. Ji Z, Lee N, Frieske R, Yu T, Su D, Xu Y, Ishii E, Bang YJ, Madotto A, Fung P. Survey of hallucination in natural language generation. ACM computing surveys. 2023 Mar 3;55(12):1-38.
6. Maity S, Saikia MJ. Large Language Models in Healthcare and Medical Applications: A Review. Bioengineering (Basel). 2025;12(6): 631.
7. Ahsan Z. Integrating artificial intelligence into medical education: a narrative systematic review of current applications, challenges, and future directions. BMC Med Educ. 2025;25:1187.

Index

Page numbers followed by *f* refer to figure, *fc* refer to flowchart and *t* refer to table.

A

B

C

D

E

M

T

U

V

W

Y

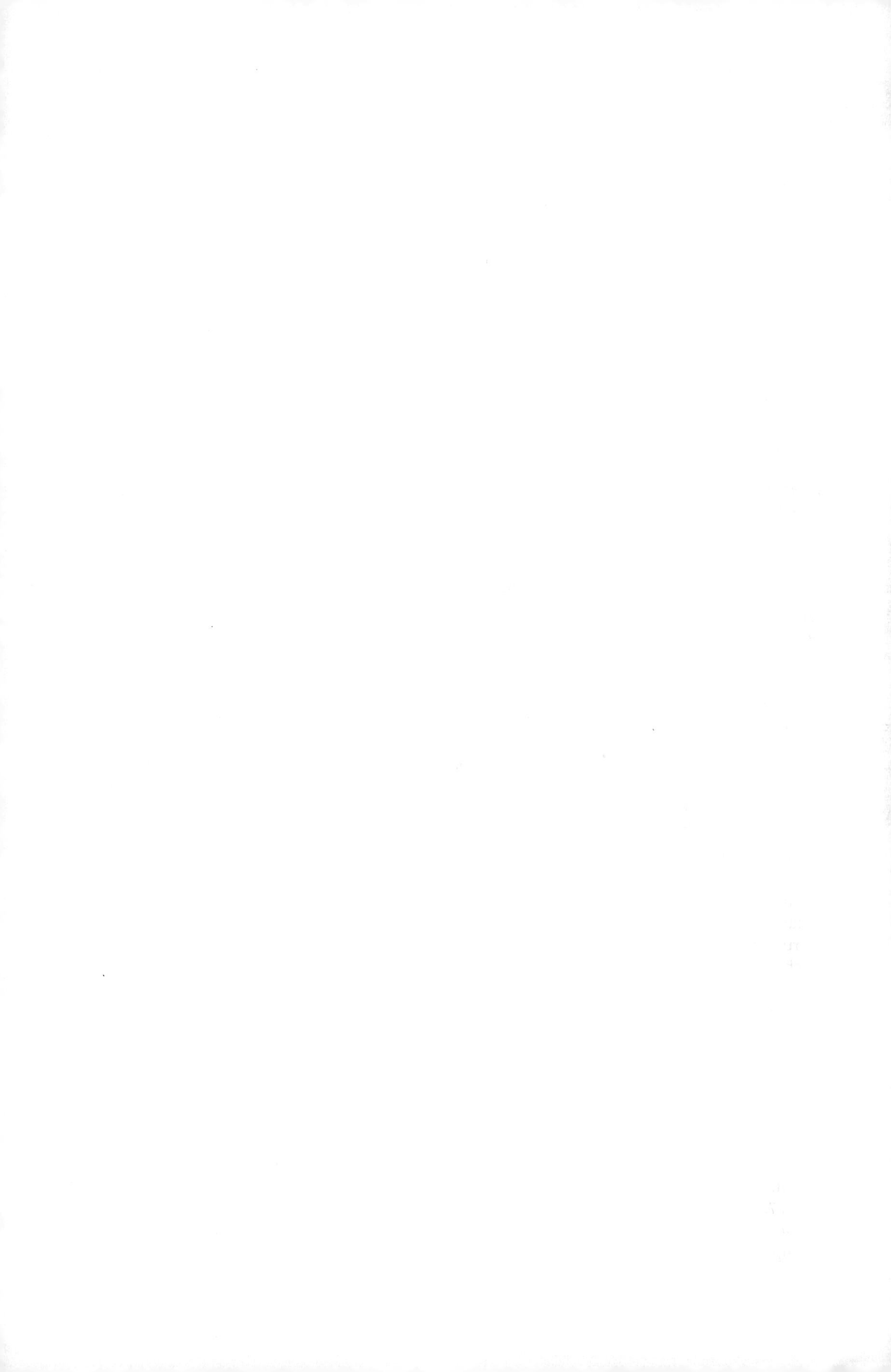